D1325830

ATTACHMENT THEORY AND RESEARCH

Also Available

Adult Attachment:
Theory, Research, and Clinical Implications
Edited by W. Steven Rholes and Jeffry A. Simpson

The Evolution of Mind:
Fundamental Questions and Controversies
Edited by Steven W. Gangestad and Jeffry A. Simpson

Attachment Theory and Research

New Directions and Emerging Themes

edited by
Jeffry A. Simpson
W. Steven Rholes

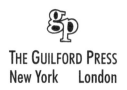

THE GUILFORD PRESS
New York   London

© 2015 The Guilford Press
A Division of Guilford Publications, Inc.
370 Seventh Avenue, Suite 1200, New York, NY 10001
www.guilford.com

Printed in the United States of America

This book is printed on acid-free paper.

Last digit is print number: 9 8 7 6 5 4 3 2 1

Library of Congress Cataloging-in-Publication Data

Attachment theory and research : new directions and emerging themes / edited by
Jeffry A. Simpson, W. Steven Rholes.
    pages cm
  Includes bibliographical references and index.
  ISBN 978-1-4625-1217-1 (hardback)
  1. Attachment behavior. I. Simpson, Jeffry A. II. Rholes, W. Steven (William
Steven)
  BF575.A86A8195 2015
  155.9′2—dc23

2014044248

About the Editors

Jeffry A. Simpson, PhD, is Professor of Psychology and Director of the Doctoral Minor in Interpersonal Relationships (IREL) at the University of Minnesota. His research focuses on adult attachment processes, human mating, idealization in relationships, empathic accuracy in relationships, social influence in relationships, and how interpersonal experiences earlier in life affect adult health and relationship outcomes. He has previously served as editor of the journal *Personal Relationships* and as associate editor and editor for the *Journal of Personality and Social Psychology: Interpersonal Relations and Group Processes*. In addition, he has served on grant panels at the National Science Foundation (NSF), and the National Institute of Mental Health (NIMH), and as chair of the Social, Personality, and Interpersonal Relations grant panel at NIMH. Dr. Simpson is a recipient of the Berscheid–Hatfield Award for Midcareer Achievement in the Study of Relationships from the International Association for Relationships Research and of the Carol and Ed Diener Award for Midcareer Achievement in Social Psychology from the Society for Personality and Social Psychology. He is also the president of the International Association for Relationship Research. His programs of research have been funded by grants from the NSF, NIMH, the National Institute on Aging, and the Marsden Foundation in New Zealand.

W. Steven Rholes, PhD, is Professor in the Department of Psychology at Texas A&M University. He has conducted research in social cognition, children's social development, and adult attachment. In 1992, Dr. Rholes, with Jeffry A. Simpson, published one of the first studies to confirm predictions about avoidant attachment style, using behavioral observations as evidence. For more than 20 years, the impact of attachment styles on emotional support sought and provided by members of romantic couples has been the central focus of his research, with more recent research focusing on couples during the transition to parenthood. Dr. Rholes has served as both department head and associate dean during this period.

Contributors

Gurit E. Birnbaum, PhD, School of Psychology, Interdisciplinary Center (IDC) Herzliya, Herzliya, Israel

Jude Cassidy, PhD, Department of Psychology, University of Maryland, College Park, College Park, Maryland

Tracy L. Dalgleish, PhD, CPsych, Greenbelt Family Health Team, Ottawa, Ontario, Canada

Cassandra C. DeVito, MS, Department of Psychological and Brain Sciences, University of Massachusetts, Amherst, Amherst, Massachusetts

Lisa M. Diamond, PhD, Department of Psychology, University of Utah, Salt Lake City, Utah

Guy Doron, PhD, School of Psychology, Interdisciplinary Center (IDC) Herzliya, Herzliya, Israel

Mary Dozier, PhD, Department of Psychological and Brain Sciences, University of Delaware, Newark, Delaware

Tsachi Ein-Dor, PhD, School of Psychology, Interdisciplinary Center (IDC) Herzliya, Herzliya, Israel

Brooke C. Feeney, PhD, Department of Psychology, Carnegie Mellon University, Pittsburgh, Pennsylvania

R. Chris Fraley, PhD, Department of Psychology, University of Illinois at Urbana–Champaign, Champaign, Illinois

Fiona Ge, MS, Department of Psychological and Brain Sciences, University of Massachusetts, Amherst, Amherst, Massachusetts

Omri Gillath, PhD, Department of Psychology, University of Kansas, Lawrence, Kansas

Cindy Hazan, PhD, Department of Human Development, Cornell University, Ithaca, New York

Brittany K. Jakubiak, MS, Department of Psychology, Carnegie Mellon University, Pittsburgh, Pennsylvania

Susan M. Johnson, EdD, CPsych, Emeritus, Department of Psychology, University of Ottawa, and International Center for Excellence in Emotionally Focused Therapy, Ottawa, Ontario, Canada; Marital and Family Therapy Program, Alliant University, San Diego, California

Jason D. Jones, MS, Department of Psychology, University of Maryland, College Park, College Park, Maryland

Gery C. Karantzas, PhD, School of Psychology, Deakin University, Burwood, Victoria, Australia

Marie-France Lafontaine, PhD, School of Psychology, University of Ottawa, Ottawa, Ontario, Canada

Edward P. Lemay, Jr., PhD, Department of Psychology, University of Maryland, College Park, College Park, Maryland

Jana Lembke, BA, Department of Psychological and Brain Sciences, University of Massachusetts, Amherst, Amherst, Massachusetts

Sarah Merrill, PhD, Department of Human Development, Cornell University, Ithaca, New York

Mario Mikulincer, PhD, School of Psychology, Interdisciplinary Center (IDC) Herzliya, Herzliya, Israel

Nickola C. Overall, PhD, School of Psychology, University of Auckland, Auckland, New Zealand

Ramona L. Paetzold, DBA, Department of Management, Texas A&M University, College Station, Texas

Paula R. Pietromonaco, PhD, Department of Psychological and Brain Sciences, University of Massachusetts, Amherst, Amherst, Massachusetts

W. Steven Rholes, PhD, Department of Psychology, Texas A&M University, College Station, Texas

Caroline K. P. Roben, PhD, Department of Psychological and Brain Sciences, University of Delaware, Newark, Delaware

Glenn I. Roisman, PhD, Institute of Child Development, University of Minnesota, Minneapolis, Minnesota

Phillip R. Shaver, PhD, Department of Psychology, University of California, Davis, Davis, California

Jeffry A. Simpson, PhD, Department of Psychology, University of Minnesota, Minneapolis, Minneapolis, Minnesota

Meredith Van Vleet, PhD, Department of Psychology, Carnegie Mellon University, Pittsburgh, Pennsylvania

Vivian Zayas, PhD, Department of Psychology, Cornell University, Ithaca, New York

Contents

Introduction

New Directions and Emerging Themes in Attachment Theory and Research

W. Steven Rholes
Jeffry A. Simpson

Few theories and areas of research have been more prolific during the past decade than the attachment field. John Bowlby's (1969/1982, 1973, 1980, 1988) comprehensive theory explaining the conditions under which parents and children, romantic partners, and close friends form, build, maintain, and sometimes dissolve attachment bonds "from the cradle to the grave" (Bowlby, 1979, p. 129), and the ensuing flood of research that now supports major principles of attachment theory, rank among the most important intellectual achievements in the psychological sciences today. This volume showcases the latest theoretical and empirical work from some of the field's top scholars, who are tackling a wide variety of important questions and issues from an attachment theory perspective. As you will see, the chapters in this book span a breathtaking panorama of different models, processes, topics, and outcomes, all of which are grounded in key principles, hypotheses, and/or findings associated with Bowlby's highly generative theory or recent conceptual extensions of it.

When authors were asked to contribute chapters to this book, we requested that each chapter be organized to address three sets of issues. First, we wanted each chapter to highlight the most important principles, ideas, and/or findings within the realm of the topic or issue that the chapter was intended to address. Second, we asked authors to identify the most important and novel emerging themes relevant to their specific topic or

1

issue. Third, we requested that authors propose new, promising directions toward which future research should be directed. As editors, we viewed this third theme as particularly important, because we wanted this volume to serve as a roadmap for future theory and research within each domain canvassed in this book. The final outcome of this enterprise—the comprehensiveness, novelty, and sheer quality of the chapters that this cast of authors produced—more than met our high expectations. We believe that you will agree once you read the groundbreaking chapters in this book.

Two Core Themes

Though the issues and topics covered by the chapters in this volume are diverse, they cluster around two core themes: (1) classic, long-standing themes and issues that have defined attachment theory and research since Bowlby, Ainsworth, Main, Hazan, Shaver, and others opened the theoretical floodgate that has produced the rich empirical terrain of the current attachment field; and (2) novel extensions of attachment theory and its basic principles to new domains and outcomes of inquiry. We now discuss where and how each chapter fits within these two core themes.

Classic Themes

One long-standing theme in the attachment field is whether and how early experiences with caregivers affect social development into adulthood, especially romantic relationships. In Chapter 1, Fraley and Roisman explore how early attachment experiences shape differences in the way in which people feel, think, and behave in romantic relationships in early adulthood. They focus on two developmental pathways that may connect early attachment experiences with romantic relationship functioning in early adulthood: (1) the development of social competence and (2) the formation of intimate friendships. They also discuss several emerging themes in developmental research, such as identifying the developmental factors that link early social experiences with later developmental outcomes, distinguishing different mediation pathways between early experiences and later outcomes, and using multiple-wave studies to test whether and how associations between early experiences and later outcomes either decay or stabilize over time.

Another perennial theme is how attachment processes are implicated in the development of sexual pair bonding in adult romantic relationships. In Chapter 3, Zayas, Merrill, and Hazan note that romantic partners often act as both attachment figures and sexual partners, yet research on sex and adult attachment have advanced independently. As a consequence, not much is known about whether and how the sexual mating system interfaces with the development of attachment-based pair bonds in romantic relationships. Zayas and her colleagues suggest that the neural and physiological systems operative during sexual intercourse overlap with those underlying attachment bonds, which partially explains why sexual interactions produce physiological and endocrinological states that evoke attachment security. They suggest that if sex occurs repeatedly across time with the same partner, these systems become "conditioned," thereby explaining the formation of pair bonds.

A third mainstay theme is whether and how attachment and dependence operate (either independently or jointly) to affect romantic relationship functioning and outcomes. In Chapter 8, Feeney, Van Vleet, and Jakubiak propose that virtually all partners in close relationships must deal with dependence issues, regardless of whether they are conscious versus unconscious, deliberate versus accidental, or explicit versus implicit. They then address several critical questions: Is dependence good or bad for partners and relationships? Is there an optimal level of dependence that one should strive for in close relationships? And if so, what affects the attainment of optimal dependence? Feeney and her colleagues answer these questions from an attachment perspective and then highlight some promising avenues for future research on optimal dependence in close relationships.

Another classic theme is whether and how different forms of stress influence the development and expression of basic attachment processes and outcomes. Diamond opens Chapter 4 by noting that the attachment system purportedly evolved to regulate responses to danger and threat in the service of facilitating infant survival. She then reviews evidence concerning how early caregiving may shape "enduring profiles" of stress reactivity in the autonomic system and the hypothalamic–pituitary–adrenocortical (HPA) axis of the endocrine system. Following this, she examines whether the quality of infant–caregiver attachment affects the development of these systems independently of other contextual influences, such as infant adversity, poverty, maltreatment, and neglect. She then explores connections between attachment theory and adaptive calibration principles, which propose that children who display stronger physiological stress reactivity (in response to early life adversity) should show certain beneficial outcomes if they experience more nurturance or support later in life. Diamond concludes by discussing this model's implications for understanding stress-related plasticity and adaptation in attachment insecurity across the life course.

A fifth key theme in the attachment literature is whether and how attachment security can be instilled in people. In Chapter 5, Mikulincer and Shaver suggest that feeling secure is a "resilience resource" and a building block of good mental health and social adjustment. They first review what is known about contextually boosting a person's sense of security in laboratory experiments and field studies; they then describe their model of attachment system activation and functioning in adulthood. Following this, Mikulincer and Shaver review research revealing that experimentally induced security has positive effects on emotion regulation, self- and other-appraisals, mental health, and prosocial behavior. They conclude by discussing studies showing that real-life interpersonal contexts that strengthen a person's sense of attachment security can produce beneficial changes in psychological functioning.

Novel and Emerging Themes

One emerging theme in the attachment field is the integration of neuroscience methods and theories with the traditional approaches to the study of close relationships and the body of knowledge that has grown from such traditional methods. Chapter 2 addresses this theme: Gillath argues that incorporating natural science methods into social science has facilitated an interdisciplinary transformative approach to understanding the functioning of close relationships. In his chapter, he reviews principles of neuroscience that are relevant to attachment, as well as the tools and methods used in neuroscience. He also discusses the growing efforts to synthesize traditional research on close relationships with neuroscience research. He then discuses several theoretical advances and emerging themes and models in the field of attachment neuroscience, and proposes new and promising directions for future research.

A second group of emerging themes concerns how people regulate their romantic relationships, express their sexuality, and parent their children. In Chapter 6, Overall and Lemay explore multiple ways in which dyadic regulation processes may operate within romantic relationships. They first discuss regulation processes that focus on threat (e.g., inducing guilt to obtain reassurance), along with those that focus on being highly attentive to the needs and fears of insecurely attached persons. Overall and Lemay conclude that both types of processes can generate beneficial outcomes or can produce costs in romantic relationships. They end their chapter by highlighting the various benefits and costs of dyadic regulation processes, and illustrating how damaging effects can occur.

In Chapter 7, Birnbaum addresses how the sexual and attachment systems interface within romantic relationships. She begins by reviewing literature that has examined the reciprocal link between the attachment system and the sexual system. Following this, she describes how relationship quality may be affected by sexuality and the quality of sex. Birnbaum concludes her chapter with a discussion of the dual role of sex—as a factor that holds relationships together, and as a force that encourages people to contemplate and sometimes pursue alternative partners in a world of rapidly changing societal trends.

Jones, Cassidy, and Shaver address the important topic of parenting from an attachment perspective in Chapter 9. They begin by discussing attachment theory, especially connections between the attachment and caregiving behavioral systems. They then summarize the theoretical and empirical links between parents' self-reported attachment styles and parenting variables, focusing on three features of parenting: parental behaviors, emotions, and cognitions. This is followed by a detailed description some of their own recent research on attachment and parenting. They conclude the chapter by proposing several promising directions for future research.

Another major new theme is how attachment principles can be used to understand what happens in organizational and work settings. In Chapter 10, Paetzold surveys approximately 20 years of attachment research in organizational settings. Her review shows that attachment anxiety and avoidance are associated with a number of workplace difficulties, including negative health outcomes, problematic team and leader–follower interactions, and increased turnover intentions. The chapter also considers measurement issues and unresolved conceptual issues for better understanding the impact of attachment processes on organizations.

Still another growing area of research centers on relations between attachment and health. In Chapter 11, Pietromonaco, DeVito, Ge, and Lembke propose a framework in which attachment-based regulatory strategies and relationship behaviors produce health-related reactions ranging from the physiological level to the behavioral level, which in turn affect the probability of disease. The authors then review relevant literature that has evaluated the tenability of the predictions generated by their framework. With respect to suggestions for future research, Pietromonaco and colleagues emphasize the need to test additional behavioral and physiological moderators of disease effects.

Remaining within the health sphere, Karantzas and Simpson discuss applications of attachment theory to the emerging field of aged care. In Chapter 12, they explain key concepts from attachment theory and then discuss their application to the aged-care context. The primary concepts discussed include felt security, proximity seeking, and the stress–diathesis model. They also review the relatively small literature on attachment and aged care. The authors discuss in detail the issue of measuring attachment orientations among the elderly. They conclude their chapter with an extended discussion of the new directions for attachment research with elderly populations.

The final novel theme addressed in this volume is how attachment principles might be used to understand psychotherapy, improve therapy, and develop more effective interventions. Ein-Dor and Doron point out in Chapter 13 that while attachment anxiety and avoidance are associated with vulnerability to a wide range of mental disorders, attachment theory has had relatively little to say about how insecure attachment orientations result in such a wide variety of different disorders (multifinality). The theory also has trouble explaining why a person with one attachment profile develops one disorder, whereas another person with the same profile develops another disorder or no disorder at all (divergent trajectories). Ein-Dor and Doron develop and present a transdiagnostic model to address these issues. Within the context of this model, they discuss contexts and mediating processes that may explain multifinality and divergent trajectories.

Two chapters address psychotherapy issues. In Chapter 15, Johnson, Lafontaine, and Dalgleish describe how and why attachment theory serves as the basis for emotionally focused therapy (EFT). The authors then review then empirical studies that provide support for some of EFT's core principles. Among other things, they explore changes in attachment responses and styles, and examine how strengthening the attachment bond can affect other important aspects of the relationship. The authors also describe ways in which therapists can use attachment theory to guide their understanding of their clients' communications during therapy sessions. A brief case study is included to illustrate the change processes that can be produced by EFT.

In Chapter 14, Dozier and Roben discuss attachment-based interventions with at-risk infants and young children. The authors then cover three major issues regarding interventions. The first centers on foundational issues needed to create successful attachment-based interventions. The second involves a description of several current attachment-based intervention programs; this section shows a remarkable variety of programs all based to a greater or lesser degree on attachment theory. The third addresses dissemination of successful programs from the laboratory to field settings, and explains the great difficulties in crossing this boundary.

Conclusion

As the chapters in this book confirm, one of the most dramatic changes in the past decade has been the rapid extension of attachment principles, ideas, processes, and findings to myriad topics in areas outside developmental and social/personality psychology (where attachment theory and research originally flourished). Core attachment principles, hypotheses, and ideas—those stemming from both the normative and the individual-difference components of attachment theory—have infiltrated areas within the neurosciences, family social science, the health sciences, the clinical sciences (including therapy and intervention work), the scientific study of sex and sexuality, and even the organizational sciences. Attachment theory and its empirical findings, in other words, are now being more broadly applied to address significant questions, issues, and problems in a wide variety of areas within the purview of the psychological sciences. This is an important new direction, because many of these areas can benefit from a comprehensive lifespan theory that explains not only how normative principles and processes, but also how individual variations *around* normative principles and processes, can help us to better understand why people think, feel, and behave as they do in different situations and at different stages of life. The next decade is likely to reveal how well attachment theory and its core principles are able to clarify, resolve, and answer some of these long-standing questions, and where other theories, models, or principles are needed to more fully explain certain phenomena or outcomes more fully. If Bowlby were alive today, we suspect that he would be pleased to see his grand theory being incorporated into so many different fields that are attempting to solve so many diverse and important problems and issues.

In conclusion, when we started planning this book, our aspiration was that the authors of each invited chapter would provide broad and comprehensive coverage of the most important theories, models, principles, and research findings relevant to the topic focused on by each chapter. In addition, we hoped that the authors would offer useful "roadmaps" that future researchers interested in each topic could navigate. As editors, we are delighted with what this outstanding set of authors has delivered. We sincerely hope that you—the reader of this novel and cutting-edge volume— will concur.

References

Bowlby, J. (1969/1982). *Attachment and loss: Vol. 1. Attachment.* New York: Basic Books.

Bowlby, J. (1973). *Attachment and loss: Vol. 2. Separation.* New York: Basic Books.

Bowlby, J. (1979). *The making and breaking of affectional bonds.* New York: Methuen.

Bowlby, J. (1980). *Attachment and loss: Vol. 3. Loss.* New York: Basic Books.

Bowlby, J. (1988). *A secure base.* New York: Basic Books.

1

Early Attachment Experiences and Romantic Functioning

Developmental Pathways, Emerging Issues, and Future Directions

R. Chris Fraley
Glenn I. Roisman

Some adults are involved in well-functioning romantic relationships. They are able to provide support for their partners, resolve conflict effectively, and generally find their relationships satisfying and rewarding. In contrast, other people's romantic relationships are characterized by conflict, dissatisfaction, and regret. Why is it that some relationships flourish, whereas others fail to do so?

In this chapter, we examine the ways in which early attachment experiences help to organize individual differences in the way people feel, think, and behave in romantic relationships. First, we draw briefly upon Bowlby's attachment theory to review what is known about the developmental antecedents of romantic relationship functioning. In the next part of the chapter, we discuss two of the major developmental pathways that connect attachment experiences early in life with romantic relationship functioning in adulthood: the development of social competence and the formation of intimate friendships. We review research on how early attachment experiences help support the development of these interpersonal resources. In addition, we review research that shows how these resources, in turn, support the development of romantic functioning in adulthood.

In the final portion of the chapter, we discuss ongoing issues and debates in research on early experience and development. Specifically, we explain some of the inferential ambiguities that can arise when researchers investigate the legacy of early experiences per se. We also outline some potential problems that can emerge when investigators are trying to translate theoretical ideas about developmental processes into testable statistical models. Throughout our discussion, we highlight not only what we consider the important challenges in this area of work, but what we consider promising directions for future research. We begin by reviewing some of the foundational ideas in attachment theory, focusing on some of the basic ideas that framed Bowlby's understanding of how early experiences become entrenched in human development.

Early Attachment Experiences and the Canalization of Developmental Pathways

Bowlby was interested in understanding the nature of the bond that develops between infants and their caregivers, and the implications of that bond for social and personality development across the lifespan. He and his colleagues (Bowlby, Robertson, & Rosenbluth, 1952) noticed that children who had been separated from their primary caregivers frequently expressed intense anxiety and despair, often vigorously trying to regain their missing caregivers by crying, clinging, and searching. To explain these behaviors, Bowlby (1969/1982) drew extensively from ethological theory, arguing that such "protest" reactions function to restore and maintain proximity to a primary attachment figure—a strategy that would be adaptive for infants born without the capacity to defend or care for themselves.

The Attachment Behavioral System

Bowlby (1969/1982) posited that such reactions are regulated by an innate motivational system—the attachment behavioral system—organized by natural selection to promote the safety and survival of infants. According to Bowlby (1969/1982), the internal dynamics of the attachment system are similar to those of a homeostatic control system, in which a set goal is maintained by the constant monitoring of signals with continuous behavioral adjustment. In the case of the attachment system, the set goal is *physical or psychological proximity*. When a child perceives the attachment figure to be nearby and responsive, he or she is generally playful, uninhibited, and sociable. However, when he or she perceives a threat to the relationship or his or her well-being, the child seeks the attention and comfort of the primary caregiver. From an evolutionary perspective, these dynamics facilitate proximity between child and caregiver, which helps to ensure the child's safety and protection, and ultimately his or her reproductive fitness (also see Zayas, Merrill, & Hazan, Chapter 3, this volume).

During the early months of life, the degree of security an infant experiences is believed to depend largely on exogenous signals, such as the proximate availability and responsiveness of primary caregivers. Over repeated interactions, however, children develop a set of knowledge structures, or *internal working models*, that represent those interactions and contribute to the endogenous regulation of the system (Bretherton & Munholland, 1999). These representations enable a child to simulate a variety of response options to determine which course of action might best facilitate certain goals (e.g., regaining the attention of the caregiver).

Importantly, these cognitive structures also reflect what the child has learned about the responsiveness and availability of caregivers over the course of repeated interactions. If caregivers are generally warm, responsive, and consistently available, the child learns that others can be counted on when needed. Consequently, he or she is likely to explore the world confidently, initiate warm and sociable interactions with others, and find security in the knowledge that a caregiver is available if needed. In short, the child has developed a secure working model of attachment. If attachment figures are cold, rejecting, unpredictable, frightening, or insensitive, however, the child learns that others cannot be counted on for support and comfort, and this knowledge is embodied in insecure working models of attachment. The child is likely to regulate his or her behavior accordingly— either by excessively demanding attention and care, or by withdrawing from others and/or attempting to achieve a high degree of self-sufficiency (DeWolff & van IJzendoorn, 1997).

The Canalization of Developmental Trajectories

Importantly, Bowlby believed that the transactions between children and their social environments have a reinforcing effect on the working models that children construct. Drawing on Waddington's (1957) ideas about cell development (see Fraley & Brumbaugh, 2004, for a review), Bowlby argued that an individual's developmental pathway becomes increasingly *canalized* or buffered over time, such that minor disturbances only temporarily nudge an individual off his or her developmental course; the individual gradually reverts to the trajectory that was previously established.

Bowlby found the concept of canalization useful in his theorizing about personality development. He often wrote of *degrees of canalization* as a way to reconcile the ideas that natural selection may favor developmental processes that unfold in a relatively deterministic way on the basis of predictable features of the environment, but that ultimately organisms need to be flexible enough to adapt to varying ecologies by calibrating themselves against early environmental inputs. In the context of personality development, Bowlby believed that several processes function to canalize developmental pathways to varying degrees. He separated these into two classes. The first were concerned with the *caregiving environment* itself. Specifically, Bowlby argued that if the individual's caregiving environment is relatively stable, it is unlikely that the child's developing models of the world will be disconfirmed. The powerful nature of these constraints was emphasized by Bowlby's (1973) observation that a child is typically born into a family in which he or she has the same parents, the same neighborhood, and the same ecology for long periods of time. In fact, empirical research demonstrates that the quality of the caregiving environment is relatively stable across time (Fraley, Roisman, & Haltigan, 2013). Bowlby believed that in the absence of significant transitions (e.g., parental divorce, moving to a new town, loss of an attachment figure), the caregiving environment itself will be sufficiently stable to support the canalization of specific developmental pathways.

The second kind of canalization process involves *social-cognitive* mechanisms. One reason Bowlby believed that developmental pathways become increasingly canalized over time is that the basic cognitive processes underlying relational cognition are self-confirming. If a child has learned over the course of his or her interactions with primary caregivers that other people are generally responsive and well intentioned, the child, when presented with a potentially ambiguous social interaction, is likely to interpret this interaction in a way that is consistent with the working models he or she already holds. Moreover, as those expectations and norms become reinforced over time, they become increasingly resistant to change. In other words, the developing child functions much like a Bayesian: As he or she accumulates evidence in favor of specific assumptions, some assumptions are weighted more and others are weighted less. As a result, it takes increasingly strong and persistent feedback to undermine those assumptions, and the child's developmental pathway becomes more entrenched over time.

Two Major Pathways between Early Attachment Experiences and Romantic Functioning

One of the central ideas in attachment theory is that early attachment experiences set the stage for the way people think, feel, and behave in their romantic relationships in adulthood. Indeed, emerging evidence from longitudinal studies suggests that the way people function in their romantic relationships may have its roots in early attachment experiences. For example, Roisman, Collins, Sroufe, and Egeland (2005) studied a sample of young adults from the Minnesota Longitudinal Study of Risk and Adaptation (MLSRA) who had participated in the Strange Situation with their primary caregivers as infants. They found that young adults who had secure attachment histories were more likely to produce coherent discourse regarding their romantic relationship in the Current Relationship Interview (CRI; Crowell & Owens, 1996) and had higher-quality romantic functioning as observed in standard conflict and collaboration tasks. Using data from the same sample, Simpson, Collins, Tran, and Haydon (2007) found that early attachment experiences, as indexed by Strange Situation classifications at 12 months of age, predicted the extent to which people experienced negative emotions in their romantic relationships at ages 20–21. Similarly, Salvatore, Kuo, Steele, Simpson, and Collins (2011) found that individuals who had been securely attached at 12–18 months of age were able to recover from conflict more effectively than those with insecure attachment histories. (See also Salo, Jokela, Lehtimäki, & Keltikangas-Järvinen, 2011, and Zayas, Michel, Shoda, & Aber, 2011, for additional research on early parental experiences and romantic functioning.)

Although there are various perspectives on how early experiences are transformed into patterns of adaptive and less adaptive functioning in romantic relationships, one theme is that early attachment experiences have their effects via at least two major pathways by facilitating (1) the development of social competence, and/or (2) the development of close friendships. In the next sections, we review research on each of these pathways. Specifically, we review research suggesting that early attachment experiences are associated with the development of both social competence and close friendships. In addition, we review research indicating that these two pathways, in turn, are associated with relationship functioning in adulthood.

Early Attachment Experiences and Social Competence

Broadly defined, *social competence* refers to the set of social, emotional, and cognitive skills needed for adaptation to a broad array of developmental contexts and challenges (Waters & Sroufe, 1983). A guiding theme in attachment theory is that the development of social competence is fundamental for navigating romantic relationships effectively. For one person to serve as an attachment figure for another person—or to use him or her as an attachment figure—one must be able to take the other person's perspective, have empathy, and be able to resolve conflict in effective ways.

Bowlby believed that supportive and responsive interactions between parents and their children are crucial for children's development of these broad skills. For example, he believed that a child's sense of self (i.e., whether the child perceives him- or herself as lovable) is rooted in the history of transactions between parents and children. In addition, the child's ability to regulate emotions in an appropriate way is rooted in early relational experiences. In the following sections, we review research that has addressed the pathways between (1) early experience and social competence, and (2) social competence and romantic functioning.

Pathways between Early Attachment and Social Competence

An important line of work in attachment research concerns the relations among early attachment histories and emotional understanding and perspective-taking skills. Laible and Thompson (1998), for example, had young children watch three puppets enact a variety of vignettes; at the end of each story, each child was queried about the protagonist puppet's feelings. They found that children with secure attachment histories exhibited greater emotional understanding than children without secure attachment histories. This suggests that the ways in which children had internalized their histories of attachment experiences may have influenced their ability to understand another's point of view of others and their own emotional view of the world.

Research has also found that children with secure attachment histories are more empathic than others. Kestenbaum, Farber, and Sroufe (1989), for example, studied children's free-play interactions and coded cases in which a child was visibly distressed and how he or she behaved. They found that children with secure attachment histories were more likely than those with avoidant histories to behave in empathic ways in the presence of distressed children.

Children with histories of insecure attachment have been found to behave with more anger, greater aggression and hostility, and less empathy in both structured and more naturalistic situations. For example, Troy and Sroufe (1987) found that children with avoidant attachment histories were more likely to victimize their peers. McElwain, Cox, Burchinal, and Macfie (2003) found that children with insecure attachment histories were more likely to exhibit instrumental aggression when interacting with peers at 36 months of age.

In summary, these findings are consistent with the notion that early attachment experiences provide a framework for the development of social competence. Children who have secure attachment histories are more likely than those who do not to exhibit the kinds of competencies that might enable them to successfully negotiate a variety of interpersonal tasks. Compared to children with insecure attachment histories, children with secure histories exhibit greater emotional understanding, are better able to take the perspective of other individuals, are more empathic, and express less anger and hostility.

Pathways between Social Competence and Romantic Functioning

In social-psychological research, the association between social competence and relationship functioning has primarily been investigated by using concurrent assessments. Bartholomew and Horowitz (1991), for example, found that individuals who had higher self-confidence and who expressed greater interpersonal warmth were more likely to hold secure working models of close relationships in adulthood. Research has also found that individuals who are more empathically accurate in their relationships (Simpson et al., 2011) or who are better able to seek and provide support during stressful and challenging situations (Collins & Feeney, 2000) are more likely to have securely functioning romantic relationships.

There is also longitudinal research linking social competence to relationship functioning. Simpson and his colleagues (2007), for example, examined peer competence and romantic functioning, using data from the MLSRA. Peer competence was assessed at grades 1, 2, and 3 by using teacher ratings of how well target children resembled a prototypical child who "was well liked and respected by peers, had mutual friendships, demonstrated understanding of other children's perspectives and ideas, and constructively engaged peers in activities" (p. 359). Romantic functioning was assessed in a number of ways at ages 20–23, including the emotional tone of the relationship (i.e., the relative balance of positive to negative affect) and behavioral observations of couple behavior. They found that individuals who had higher peer competence ratings in childhood had higher romantic relationship process scores, less negative affect, and a higher ratio of positive to negative emotional experiences.

Using longitudinal data from the National Institute of Child Health and Human Development (NICHD) Study of Early Child Care and Youth Development (SECCYD), we (Fraley, Roisman, & Haltigan, 2013) examined trajectories of social competence from early childhood (54 months) through age 15 years. We found that individuals who exhibited greater social competence in early childhood (rated by parents and teachers) were more likely to be secure at age 18 on measures of self-reported attachment styles, compared to those who exhibited less social competence in early childhood. In addition, children who became more socially competent across time were more likely to be secure at age 18. Taken together, these studies indicate that social competence, assessed in a variety of ways in early childhood and adolescence, is associated with romantic functioning in adulthood.

Early Attachment Experiences and Close Friendship Relationships

The individual projects his/her representation of relationships onto future
social contacts, leading to a repetition and confirmation of expected cycles
of behavior. All in all, this process leads to the carry-over of basic relationship
styles into future relationships.
                              —SHULMAN, ELICKER, AND SROUFE (1994, p. 343)

A key idea in Bowlby's theory is that early attachment experiences set the stage for the way in which the child navigates interpersonal contexts. This includes not only the child's interactions with primary attachment figures, but other contexts in which issues concerning trust and intimacy emerge, including relations with teachers and mentors (Ainsworth, 1989), siblings (Teti & Ablard, 1989), and, importantly, close friends.

Close friendships serve a number of important developmental functions. For example, friendships can provide a context in which one explores new skills and interests, builds alliances, bolsters self-esteem, and reinforces emerging identities (Shulman et al., 1994). The process of forming and maintaining a close friendship, however, is not a trivial matter. One must be capable of managing conflict, offering support, adopting the other's perspective, and engaging in appropriate levels of self-disclosure and reciprocity. Indeed, research indicates that these kinds of social competencies play a role in facilitating the development of well-functioning friendships (e.g., Boling, Barry, Kotchick, & Lowry, 2011; Simpson et al., 2007).

Close friendships are also of special interest from an attachment perspective because they are some of the first extrafamilial contexts in which issues concerning intimacy, trust, and support are explored. According to some theorists, close friendships are often testing grounds for transferring attachment-related features and functions away from parents (Zeifman & Hazan, 2008). As such, the experiences that take place in the context of friendship relationships may constitute a key "transfer station" in shaping the development of expectations for trust, intimacy, and support in romantic relationships.

According to attachment theorists, repeated experiences of supportive, responsive care in early attachment relationships may support the development of the skills necessary for developing and maintaining high-quality friendships. In the sections below, we review research on the pathways between early attachment experiences and the quality of friendship relationships in childhood and adolescence. In addition, we examine research on how friendship experiences and perceptions are related to views of romantic relationships and relationship functioning.

Pathways between Early Attachment Experiences and Friendship

Research suggests that early attachment experiences may play an important role in shaping the quality of peer interactions and close friendships. Children classified as secure in the Strange Situation are more likely to have stable play partners, demonstrate greater reciprocity, and exhibit empathy toward peers during the preschool years (Kestenbaum et al., 1989). Research has also found that secure infant–parent attachment is related to lower levels of child–friend aggression at age 3 (McElwain et al., 2003) and fewer negative interactions with close friends at age 5 (Youngblade & Belsky, 1992).

There are many potential pathways through which early attachment experiences may shape the functioning of friendship relationships. One pathway that has been investigated extensively by McElwain and her colleagues concerns mental state talk. To be effective in their friendships, children need to take into consideration their friends' beliefs, desires, and feelings. One way in which children can acquire these competencies is through supportive exchanges with caregivers—that is, exchanges in which they communicate about psychological states in a supportive, uncritical manner. McElwain, Booth-LaForce, and Wu (2011) examined the association between early attachment experiences and the nature of mind talk in parent–child interactions at 24 months of age. They found that children with secure attachment histories were more likely to have mothers who engaged in cognitive talk (i.e., they were more likely to reference feelings, desires, and plans appropriately). In turn, children whose mothers engaged in more cognitive talk at 24 months of age were more likely to have high-functioning friendships at 54 months, as indexed by more positive friendship interactions across time.

Nonetheless, questions remain about whether early attachment security is uniquely associated with the quality of friend relationships or with social competence more generally. On the one hand, Schneider, Atkinson, and Tardif (2001) conducted a meta-analysis of research on the association between child–parent attachment and children's peer relations; they found that the small to moderate associations they observed were larger for children's close friendships than for their relations with other peers. On the other hand, a more recent meta-analysis by Groh et al. (2014) observed that while early attachment significantly contributed to children's social competence with friends and nonfriends, the magnitude of the effect was larger for *nonfriends* than friends. In short, the assumption that close friendship functioning, in particular, is more strongly linked to children's attachment histories than the way they relate to and are viewed by their peers more generally is not supported by the most recent meta-analytic evidence.

Pathways between Friendship Functioning and Romantic Functioning

Research also indicates that the functioning of relationships with friends may shape the way in which romantic relationships function. According to Furman, Simon, Shaffer, and Bouchey (2002), adolescents develop expectations for and assumptions about romantic relationships based, in part, on their experiences in close friendships. Consistent with this assumption, adolescents who hold relatively secure views of their parents are also likely to hold secure views of close friendships and romantic relationships (Furman et al., 2002). Importantly, however, individual differences in the views people hold of their friendships are associated with views of romantic relationships even when variations in parental representations are taken into account. Thus, although it is possible that early attachment experiences help set the stage for the functioning of friendship relationships, the unique experiences that adolescents have in those friendships also play a role in shaping expectations and attitudes toward emerging romantic relationships. Indeed, Furman et al. (2002) conclude that "views of friendships may mediate the links between views of relationships with parents and those of romantic relationships" (p. 250).

Prospective data that bear on this issue come again from the study by Simpson et al. (2007). Simpson and his colleagues assessed the quality of friend relationships in adolescence in the MLSRA through an interview in which participants discussed their close friendships, how much they trusted and disclosed to their friends, and the extent to which they felt that their friends were authentic. They found that the quality of those friendships was positively correlated with various indices of romantic relationship functioning in early adulthood.

In addition, an analysis of data from the SECCYD (Fraley, Roisman, Booth-LaForce, Owen, & Holland, 2013) examined children's perceptions of friendship quality with their self-identified best friend. The Friendship Quality Questionnaire (FQQ; Parker & Asher, 1993) was administered at grades 3, 4, 5, and 6 and at age 15 years. The FQQ assesses various aspects of friendship quality, including validation and caring, conflict resolution, help and guidance, and intimate exchange. Using growth curve modeling, we found that individuals who had high-quality friendships early in life were more likely to report security in their romantic relationships at age 18 years. In addition, individuals whose friendship relationships increased in quality over time were more likely to report security in their romantic relationships at age 18.

Emerging Themes, Conceptual Challenges, and Directions for Future Research

As we have seen, attachment theory suggests that two important paths bridge early attachment experiences and adaptive functioning in close relationships: the development of social competence and the development of close friendships. Although this particular portrayal of developmental processes is useful, it is obviously incomplete for the purposes of explaining the full range of factors that lead to variation in romantic functioning. We now discuss some of the ambiguities involved in understanding the relations among these central theoretical constructs. In addition, we discuss some broader issues and debates involved in the study of developmental pathways. Part of our goal is to highlight what we consider to be some of the emerging issues in this area. However, we also hope to call attention to what we consider to be some interesting directions for future research.

Ambiguities Concerning the Causal Structure of Developmental Pathways

One of the challenges in uncovering the antecedents of romantic functioning is that it is not clear what kinds of developmental models are necessary for modeling the relations among the variables of interest. Our review is implicitly guided by the first panel of Figure 1.1. This model assumes that

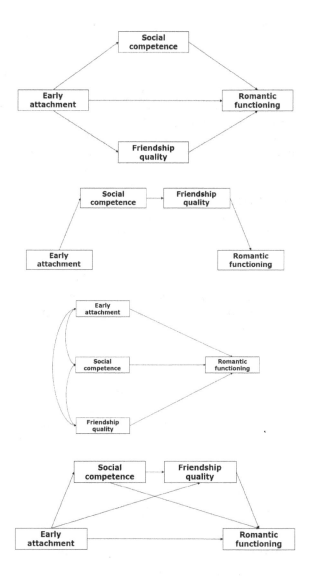

FIGURE 1.1. Alternative ways of organizing the pathways among early caregiving experiences, social competence, friendship quality, and romantic functioning.

early attachment experiences help shape romantic functioning via two key processes: the development of social competence and the development of close friendships. But there are alternative ways to arrange the pieces of this map, and, conceptually, these are equally compelling. For example, the second panel of Figure 1.1 illustrates a model articulated by Simpson et al. (2007). This model is similar to the first, with one exception. Namely, it holds that the development of social competence also shapes the development of close friendships. Simpson and his colleagues (2007) refer to this as a "double mediation model," because it assumes two mediational steps in the link between early experiences and romantic relationship functioning. A different way to organize these variables is to assume that each one has the potential to influence romantic functioning, but without specifying any explicit causal relations among them. The third panel of Figure 1.1 illustrates a basic model assuming that all three factors may contribute to variation in romantic functioning, and that the three predictors may be related to one another for unspecified reasons. A fourth way to frame these relations is to assume that they are all causally related to one another within the constraints provided by the temporal ordering of the variables. The fourth panel of Figure 1.1 illustrates a case in which each temporally prior variable influences all the variables that follow it in time. Romantic functioning is affected by social competence both directly and indirectly through its influence on friendship quality.

Which of these models is the most appropriate way to conceptualize the pathways that lead from early attachment experiences to romantic functioning? We are not sure that this question can be answered adequately on the basis of existing research. Simpson and his colleagues have advocated for the double mediation model illustrated in the second panel of Figure 1.1. They also examined some alternative models, including the one illustrated in the third panel. From their analyses, they concluded that the double mediation model best fits the data. Drawing upon data from the same sample, Englund, Kuo, Puig, and Collins (2011) examined a direct path between early attachment and friendship functioning, but did not find statistically significant paths between early attachment and social competence or between social competence and friendship quality in the context of the other constructs in the model. We and our colleagues (Fraley, Roisman, Booth-LaForce, et al., 2013) have adopted the third model because we feel that it makes the fewest assumptions. However, we did not find an association between early caregiving experiences and friendship relationships. That said, we found that increases in the quality of caregiving over time were associated prospectively with increases in the quality of friendships.

In summary, the jury is still out regarding the optimal way to model the relations among these various factors. We believe that resolving these issues is a valuable direction for future research. Having said that, we wish to emphasize two caveats. First, the specific models under discussion do not take time into account explicitly. Children's attachment experiences are not constrained to the first few years of life, and if their attachment-related experiences with parents have an impact on their subsequent relationships, it is the cumulative history of those experiences rather than the early history alone that may be relevant (Sroufe, Egeland, Carlson, & Collins, 2005). The models we have illustrated depict variables that reflect a "snapshot in time," without regard for how they continue to evolve and interact with one another. The second point is that these models do not take into consideration a host of other factors that are likely to be relevant for understanding the ways in which early attachment experiences translate into romantic functioning. A useful direction for future research involves articulating what kinds of factors have been omitted and uncovering their contributions to the developmental processes of interest.

Alternative Mediational Structures and Their Implications for Understanding Developmental Pathways

A second major issue concerns the conceptualization of the junctures in these developmental pathways. One way to conceptualize resources (e.g., the development of social competence) is that they provide scaffolding or support for the developmental pathway on which an individual is traveling. In other words, they can serve as agents of canalization. A child with a secure attachment history, a high degree of social competence, and intimate friendships, for example, may be more likely to exhibit well-functioning romantic relationships than someone who lacks this developmental history.

But these kinds of processes are also discussed as transition points in the developmental literature. They represent junctures at which people can potentially deviate from pathways they have already established. Although a person with a secure attachment history is more likely than someone with an insecure attachment history to develop high levels of social competence, this process is probabilistic, not deterministic (Sroufe, 1997). Thus some children with secure attachment histories will not develop adequate social skills; conversely, some children with insecure attachment histories will develop appropriate social competence. These developmental junctures can either reinforce a specific developmental trajectory or alter it. What are the implications for that distinction for testing theories and building statistical models of developmental processes?

Let us consider a simplified version of the problem. Let us assume that romantic functioning (y) is a function of early attachment experiences (x) and various residual factors, with a regression weight of $b = .30$. If we assume that the variances of each variable are 1.00, the expected correlation between x and y is equal to b or .30. Now let us make the model slightly more complex. Let us assume that x has its influence on y, in part, due to z_1 (e.g., social competence). And for the sake of simplicity, let us assume that the value of the paths (b) are equivalent and are equal to .30. Using covariance algebra, we find in this simple three-variable model that the expected association between x and y is now .30 × .30 = .09. If we hold everything constant, adding a single juncture or mediator *reduces* the expected correlation between x and y. If we add a second mediator (e.g., a double mediation model) such that $x \rightarrow z_1 \rightarrow z_2 \rightarrow y$, the expected correlation grows even smaller (i.e., .30 × .30 × .30 = .027). These dynamics are illustrated in the upper portion of Figure 1.2.

In short, if we attempt to flesh out the developmental pathway between early attachment experiences and romantic functioning in adulthood by *adding mediators along a common developmental pathway*, the expected association between early experiences and later outcomes necessarily decreases. In fact, if we assume that we do not adjust the value of the paths, the expected correlation between x and y approaches zero as the number of mediators increases. We refer to such mediational chains as *horizontally*

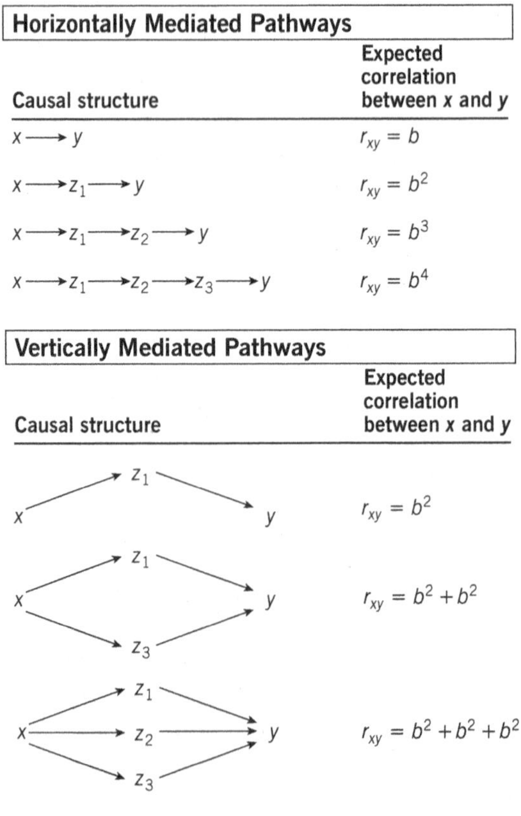

FIGURE 1.2. Horizontally mediated and vertically mediated pathways.

mediated pathways from this point forward. This result implies that a model positing various junctures along a common pathway is more likely to create discontinuities in development than to create sustained effects of early experiences. Horizontally mediated pathways are incompatible with the theoretical assumption that these various mechanisms sustain the effects of early experiences across time.

There is an alternative way to specify mediators, however. Consider the lower portion of Figure 1.2. These diagrams illustrate models in which the mediators are added vertically. As such, we refer to such chains as *vertically mediated pathways*. Notice that as we add mediators vertically, the expected association between early attachment experiences and romantic functioning *increases*. For example, if we assume that all the paths are equal to .30 in the four-variable model, the expected correlation between early experience and adult functioning is .09 + .09 = .18. If we make the same assumptions for the five-variable model, the expected correlation rises to .09 + .09 + .09 = .27. Why do vertically mediated pathways make the expected correlation between x and y more robust? In this kind of model, early experiences play an *organizing role* across multiple life domains, including social competence, peer relations, and a variety of other factors. If those domains also influence the outcome of interest, then those mechanisms buffer the relationship between x and y.

In summary, there are alternative ways to formalize developmental pathways. When one adds horizontally mediated pathways to a model, one is implicitly claiming that such factors function to reduce the expected association between early experiences and romantic functioning. When one adds vertically mediated pathways, in contrast, one is implicitly claiming that such factors serve to buttress or support the association between early experiences and romantic functioning. Statistically, these additions provide multiple pathways through which the indirect effects of early experience can accumulate and shape later outcomes. By calling attention to this issue, we hope not only to make researchers aware of the difference, but to alert researchers to the possibility of alternative developmental models that can be examined.

Developmental Cascades

Developmental cascades "refer to the cumulative consequences for development of the many interactions and transactions occurring in developmental systems that result in spreading effects across levels, among domains at the same level, and across different systems or generations" (Masten & Cicchetti, 2010, p. 491). Developmental cascades represent one process by which the effects of one variable may become manifest in various outcomes downstream. The middle panel of Figure 1.3 represents an example of potential cascade effects that could exist among the kinds of variables

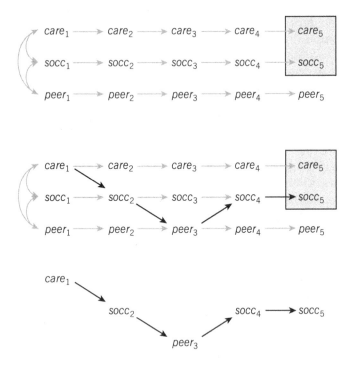

FIGURE 1.3. Developmental cascades and their effects on promoting the associations between developmental outcomes. Abbreviations: *care*, caregiving environment; *socc*, social competence; *peer*, quality of peer friendships. The various subscripts refer to different time points.

discussed in this chapter. According to this model, early caregiving experiences have their effects on social competence downstream via multiple routes. For example, there is a direct effect of early caregiving on social competence. In addition, that particular effect passes on to friendship quality, which feeds back into social competence at a later point in time. The net result of this cascade is that the association between caregiving and social competence at later points in time is stronger than it would be in the absence of such cascades; such pathways potentially enable the effects of certain experiences to accumulate.

For the sake of discussion, we focus on the way in which the association between caregiving and social competence evolves over time. Let us assume that each of the three variables of interest (i.e., caregiving, social competence, and friendship quality) is relatively stable over time, such that the autoregressive paths between each variable and itself (e.g., $care_1$ → $care_2$) is equal to .60. Moreover, let us assume that the three variables are correlated with one another at the initial assessment (r = .30). In the absence of any cascading effects, the expected correlations among the three variables are .30 at the first time wave, .11 at the second, .04 at the third, .01 at the fourth, and .01 at the fifth (see the top panel of Figure 1.3).

Now assume that the quality of the caregiving environment at the first wave predicts social competence at the second wave, such that the regression coefficient is .30. In addition, using the same magnitude of coefficient, let us assume that social competence, in turn, influences friendship functioning, and eventually trickles back to social competence downstream. Now the correlation between caregiving and social competence in the first wave is .30, .29 in the second, .10 in the third, .05 in the fourth, and .02 in the fifth. In other words, compared to a situation in which there are no cascading effects, the presence of developmental cascades helps to boost the association between the two variables of interest.

One reason why the concept of developmental cascades is important is that cascade effects, if specified correctly, function as vertically mediated pathways. If early experiences are modeled such that they organize multiple potential constructs (e.g., social competence and friendship quality), those factors will help sustain certain effects for a longer period of time than they would subsist in the absence of such effects. However, cascade effects alone, when specified in this fashion, cannot sustain coordinated effects indefinitely. As the predicted associations reveal, the shared associations among caregiving and social competence gradually decrease and will continue to do so unless there are ongoing and persistent transactional pathways among the constructs. Moreover, in such a model, the effects of early experiences will eventually wash out. This kind of model, while building in vertically mediated pathways, also includes horizontally mediated pathways and their respective consequences compete with one another (see below).

There is a lot to be learned about developmental pathways by studying cascade effects across time. Moreover, although the concept of developmental cascades has been discussed most extensively in the developmental literature (e.g., Masten et al., 2005), there is potentially a lot of value in studying cascades in intensive longitudinal studies in the social-psychological literature. Adopting such models, for example, would allow researchers to investigate the ways in which conflicts in romantic relationships exert downstream effects indirectly via their influence on other resources (e.g., time spent apart, verbal communication).

The Legacy of Early Experiences

One of the challenges of understanding the way in which early attachment experiences translate into subsequent adaptation has to do with issues of developmental timing. Specifically, when most scholars speak of the potential impact of early attachment experiences on subsequent outcomes, they implicitly (and sometimes explicitly) are suggesting that experiences that take place early in life are more influential in shaping personality development than comparable experiences that take place later in time.

Nonetheless, it is not as straightforward as it might seem to test the hypothesis that early experiences per se play a unique role in development. There are two obstacles to studying these issues. First, many longitudinal analyses do not take into consideration the idea that multiple assessment waves are needed to separate alternative models of how early experiences influence subsequent outcomes. Second, many studies do not distinguish timing from time.

Do Early Experiences Have Enduring or Transient Effects on Developmental Outcomes?

The traditional methodological approach to studying development is, paradoxically, incapable of answering this basic question. A typical prospective, longitudinal study measures experiences at some point during childhood and assesses the consequences of those experiences at a later point in time. If childhood experiences are related to later outcomes, researchers conclude that those experiences played a role in organizing development. If they are only weakly related or unrelated to later outcomes, researchers assume that those experiences were largely inconsequential (see Fraley, Roisman, & Haltigan, 2013).

Some of our theoretical work, however, indicates that the size of a single association is not informative with respect to the potential effects of early experiences. It is possible for early experiences to relate to an outcome later in time because they matter early in life and the outcome itself is stable. If this is the case, the association between measures of early experience and measures of subsequent adaptation will get increasingly small across time, approaching zero in the limit (see panel A of Figure 1.4). Alternatively, if early experiences continue to play an ongoing role in adaptation due to a canalization-like process, the association between early experiences and subsequent outcomes may decay at first, but should stabilize at a nonzero value (see panel B of Figure 1.4).

Notice that the difference between alternative developmental models lies in their asymptotic predictions about the patterning of effects across time. A single effect size can be accommodated by both predictions. For example, the association of .22 between early experiences and adaptation at age 7 illustrated in panels A and B of Figure 1.4 neatly falls on both trajectories. As such, the only way to test alternative developmental models concerning the legacy of early experiences is to examine the associations between early experiences and subsequent outcomes across multiple occasions across time.

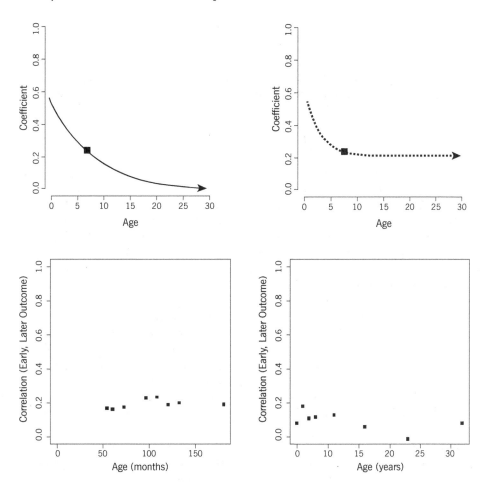

FIGURE 1.4. Alternative ways of conceptualizing the legacy of early experiences in interpersonal functioning. Panel A (top left) illustrates a situation in which the effects of early experiences on an outcome of interest decay across time, approaching zero in the limit. Panel B (top right) illustrates a situation in which the effects of early experiences on an outcome of interest are sustained across time, approaching a nonzero value across increasing intervals. Panel C (bottom left) represents the empirical correlations between early sensitivity and mothers' reports of social competence across various ages, based on data from the NICHD SECCYD as reported in the Fraley, Roisman, and Haltigan (2013) study. Panel D (bottom right) illustrates the empirical correlations between early caregiving and social competence across various ages, based on data from the MLSRA as reported in the Raby, Roisman, Fraley, and Simpson (in press) study.

We have explored these ideas with data from the NICHD SECCYD. For example, we (Fraley, Roisman, & Haltigan, 2013) examined whether the long-term effects of early maternal sensitivity on social competence and academic ability were more likely to fade gradually over time (suggesting that early caregiving supports development early in life, but does not have canalizing effects) or to stabilize at a nonzero value as children aged (suggesting canalization effects). We found that variation in early parental sensitivity predicted social competence in a relatively stable way across time (see panel C of Figure 1.4).

Although the Fraley, Roisman, and Haltigan (2013) analyses illustrate the potential value in examining the implications of alternative models of developmental pathways, the research was not able to examine the association between early experiences and attachment functioning in adulthood per se. In a project better suited for that purpose, we (Raby, Roisman, Fraley, & Simpson, in press) used data from the MLSRA to determine whether early caregiving experiences were prospectively related to measures of social competence—including romantic functioning in adulthood—across multiple assessment occasions. Parental sensitivity was assessed as a composite of sensitive parenting coded from parent–child interactions across several occasions when children were between the ages of 3 and 42 months. Social competence was assessed by using teachers' rankings of target children's social competence on multiple occasions between kindergarten and age 16. Importantly, measures of romantic functioning at ages 23 and 32 years were used as indicators of social competence in adulthood. This is based on the developmental view that part of what early attachment experiences help to organize is optimal functioning for age-appropriate developmental tasks. In young and middle adulthood, that includes functioning in romantic relationships. These analyses revealed that early caregiving experiences predicted social competence in an enduring manner over time. Specifically, children who had supportive caregiving experiences early in life were more likely than those who did not to have well-functioning romantic relationships in adulthood. And, importantly, those effects were more consistent with a developmental model assuming that the effects of early experiences become canalized than with a model not making that assumption.

Separating Timing from Time

A second way to explore the potential role of early experiences in particular is by attempting to separate *timing* from *time*. To clarify this distinction, let us consider the timing of parental divorce. Parental divorce is a prototypical example of the disruption of family and attachment relationships—one that has the potential to have complex and negative consequences for child development. Does the timing of parental divorce matter in shaping the development of interpersonal functioning? Namely, are the downstream consequences of parental divorce greater if the divorce takes place early in a child's life as opposed to later? A traditional way of addressing this question is to study a sample of children of a common age (e.g., 14–16 years old) and split children from divorced families into two groups: those whose parents divorced when a child was under the age of 5, and those whose parents divorced when a child was 5 or older. The key limitation of this approach is that the two groups differ not only in the age at which their parents divorced (i.e., the *timing* of parental divorce), but in the *amount of time* that has transpired since the divorce. The first group, for example, has had more time for the potential negative consequences of divorce to manifest and accumulate. Although the accumulation of negative consequences is a legitimate pathway through which early parental divorce could have its effects on developmental outcomes, one might expect such effects to exist regardless of whether the divorce took place early or later in the child's life. The evidence for canalization effects per se would be stronger if the timing of the event (age of parental divorce) could be separated from the effects of time per se (i.e., the amount of time that has transpired since the event).

One way to untangle these distinct effects is by studying people who vary in the age at which their parents divorced (i.e., developmental timing) and the length of time that has transpired since the divorce took place (i.e., time). Fraley and Heffernan (2013) examined this issue by assessing the attachment security of adults with the Experiences in Close Relationships— Relationship Structures (ECR-RS)—a self-report measure of attachment styles that can be used to assess security in a variety of relational domains (e.g., parental, romantic). They found that that people who reported that their parents had divorced when they were younger were more insecure in their relationships with their parents now than people whose parents had divorced when they were older. Importantly, this association was observed even after Fraley and Heffernan statistically controlled for the amount of time that had passed since the divorce. The *timing* of parental divorce mattered. These findings are consistent with the view that attachment disruptions that take place early in life can be uniquely influential in shaping developmental outcomes.

Fraley and Heffernan (2013) did not find that the timing of parental divorce per se had an impact on people's security in their romantic relationships. People whose parents had divorced, however, were slightly more likely to be insecure in their romantic attachment styles. Our point is not to dwell on these findings in particular, but to highlight the import of the methodological strategy itself. Specifically, one potentially valuable way to address the question of whether early experiences in particular leave a relatively enduring residue on interpersonal functioning is by identifying specific events of interest and examining their timing while taking into consideration the amount of time that has transpired since the event in question. Without taking the amount of time that has transpired into account, one cannot separate the potential effects of early experience per se from the amount of time that has elapsed since the event took place.

Separating the Unpredictability and Valance of Early Caregiving Environments as a Way of Understanding Relationship Functioning

According to life history theory (e.g., Stearns, 1992), organisms of most species have to allocate effort to potentially competing life tasks, such as growth and reproduction. Importantly, some of these tasks exist in competition with one another due to limited resources. For example, an organism cannot easily invest its energy in reproduction while simultaneously investing its energy in somatic growth. As such, organisms often make tradeoffs with respect to their development.

Historically, life history theory was often used to understand differences between species with respect to reproductive behavior. In recent years, however, a number of evolutionary biologists and psychologists have begun to use the theory as a way of understanding the way in which individual organisms within a species may make these tradeoffs as a function of their developmental ecology (Kaplan & Gangestad, 2004). People's life history strategies are believed to fall along a dimension that can be characterized as running from slow to fast. Individuals who adopt slower strategies are more likely to invest in stable sexual relationships, to have fewer children, and to invest more time and resources in each child. In contrast, individuals who follow faster life history strategies are more likely to have multiple sexual partners, to have greater numbers of children, and to invest less time and energy in each child.

According to life history theory, one factor that shapes the development of slow versus fast strategies is the predictability of the early caregiving environment. Specifically, it is assumed that developing organisms take cues from their early caregiving environment about whether the environment is predictable, sustainable, and safe. When the environment is relatively difficult, natural selection may favor organisms that reproduce sooner and which invest fewer resources in individual offspring. When the environment is less difficult, natural selection may favor organisms that have fewer children and invest more heavily in the ones that they do.

According to Ellis, Figueredo, Brumbach, and Schlomer (2009), difficult environments can be characterized with respect to two distinct dimensions. The first, *harshness*, refers to the overall quality of the caregiving environment, which can be indexed by socioeconomic status (SES). The second, *unpredictability*, refers to the instability of the early environment. An unpredictable or unstable environment, for example, may be characterized by frequent changes in parental employment, residential mobility, and parental divorce and remarriage.

Simpson, Griskevicius, Kuo, Sung, and Collins (2012) recently presented analyses that highlight the importance of this distinction, using longitudinal data from the MLSRA. They operationalized harshness as SES, as coded across three time points early in a child's life. Unpredictability was operationalized by different measures, including changes in the mother's employment status, changes in residence, and changes in cohabitation status. A variety of outcome variables were examined, including the number of sexual partners that individuals reported when they were 23 years old, aggressive behavior at age 23, criminal activities and behavior at age 23, and age of first intercourse. They found that one of the strongest predictors of sexual and risky behavior at age 23 was having an unpredictable environment between the ages of 0 and 5 years. Specifically, people who had less predictable and rapidly changing environments early in life exhibited a faster life history strategy at age 23 by having more sexual partners, as well as engaging in more aggressive and delinquent behaviors.

We believe that the distinction between valence and predictability is a potentially valuable one for future research. Moreover, it provides a useful way to bridge variation in early experiences with individual differences in romantic functioning. We hope future researchers can explore these distinctions in more depth.

Genetic Influences and Gene × Environment Interactions on Relationship Functioning

There is a growing body of research on how individual differences in basic personality traits, such as neuroticism, are related to romantic functioning. For example, individuals who score higher on neuroticism are more likely than others to report dissatisfaction in their marriages (Karney & Bradbury, 1997) and to report negativity (Caughlin, Huston, & Houts, 2000). These findings have led some scholars to question whether the kinds of developmental processes we have discussed might be better understood as potentially heritable dispositional effects instead of developmental ones. Thus another valuable direction for future research involves untangling the relative contributions of heritable and experiential factors in shaping interpersonal development. Because this research area is likely to evolve in interesting directions as researchers move from classic twin designs to designs involving specific genetic variants, we now outline some current trends, highlight some future directions, and emphasize some caveats.

Heritability and the Quality of Parent–Child Relationships

Empirical research based on twin designs suggests that there is not strong evidence for the heritability of the quality of infant–caregiver relationships. Some of our research has addressed this issue by analyzing the twin subsample of the Early Childhood Longitudinal Study—a nationally representative and longitudinal study of children. In one study (Roisman & Fraley, 2006), for example, we used standard behavior genetic models to partition the variance in the observed quality of infant–caregiver relationships when children were 9 months of age. We found that the estimated contribution of additive genetic effects to the quality of infant–caregiver relationships was close to zero. In contrast, the estimated contribution of shared environment effects was close to 40%, and the estimate of the nonshared environmental effects was 59%.

In follow-up analyses from this sample, we (Roisman & Fraley, 2008) found that infant attachment security observed at 24 months was largely a function of shared and nonshared environmental influences; the estimated additive genetic variance in security was close to zero. In addition, the estimated additive genetic variance in parenting quality rated at 24 months was also close to zero. This study further decomposed the covariation between parenting quality and attachment security, and found that the association between these two variables was largely due to shared and nonshared environmental influences (Roisman & Fraley, 2008; see also Fearon et al., 2006).

In summary, although it is premature to rule out the hypothesis that heritable factors might explain some of the variation in early attachment experiences, the findings to date suggest that this hypothesis does not offer a viable account for variation in the quality of early parent–child relationships or in the security of a child's attachment pattern. Moreover, analyses do not support the assumption that additive genetic factors account for the covariation between parenting quality and attachment security. Although heritable factors might explain some portion of individual differences in romantic functioning later in life (e.g., Donnellan, Burt, Levendowsky, & Klump. 2008), they do not appear to *confound* the inference that parent–child experiences also contribute to interpersonal development.

Molecular Genetic and Gene × Environment Research

One of the exciting developments in the last decade has been the study of specific genetic variants (e.g., single-nucleotide polymorphisms [SNPs] and variable number tandem repeats) and their relation to various phenotypes, either as genetic effects or in interaction with environmental effects (e.g., gene × environment [G × E] interactions). Some of this research suggests that there may be specific genetic variants underlying some of the variation in romantic functioning. For example, Gillath, Shaver, Baek, and Chun (2008) found that anxious attachment in adulthood was associated with a polymorphism of the *HTR2A* serotonin receptor gene.

Although we find much of this research fascinating, we offer several caveats. One of the most important issues to consider is that there are many intervening processes between genes and interpersonal behavior. For example, genes code for the production of mRNA, which plays a role in the development of proteins, which play a role in the organization of the nervous system, and so on (Slavich & Cole, 2013). Effects at any of these junctures can be modulated by various factors that influence transcription and methylation. The existence of so many links (i.e., horizontally mediated links) makes it unlikely a priori that the association between any one genetic variant and a specific, multiply determined outcome will be very large. Indeed, there is a growing consensus in the study of molecular genetics that the association between specific polymorphisms and phenotypic outcomes is extremely small—smaller, in some cases, than a Pearson correlation of .02 (see Gibson, 2012). Thus the only way to reliably detect such findings in the context of null hypothesis significance testing is to use extremely large sample sizes—sample sizes that far exceed what is routine in social, developmental, and personality research. To detect an effect of .02 with 80% power, for example, one would need at least 15,455 participants. (And that estimate does not account for the alpha adjustments that one might wish to use for testing multiple genetic variants instead of a single variant.) Moreover, with small sample sizes, it is easy to falsely detect an association that does not exist (e.g., Simmons, Nelson, & Simonsohn, 2011; Roisman, Booth-LaForce, Belsky, Burt, & Groh, 2013). Thus, even if bivariate genetic effects are really small, it should not be surprising if there are a few sizable ones reported in the literature. Nonetheless, the point is that nonreplicated findings of genetic associations are not particularly informative. If research-ers are to pursue the way in which specific genetic variants shape romantic functioning, we strongly recommend the use of large sample sizes.

Another exciting direction is the examination of G × E interactions. One reason why G × E research has the potential to be valuable for studying the ways in which early experiences might shape interpersonal functioning later in life is that such models treat both genetic and environmental factors as legitimate contributors to phenotypic variation. In contrast, biometric models based on twin designs often pit genetic and environmental factors against one another, such that higher variance estimates of one component necessitate lower variance estimates for other components.

One emerging area of investigation in G × E research involves the examination of alternative interaction models. The classic model, often referred to as a *dual-risk* or a *diathesis–stress* model, assumes that some individuals possess vulnerabilities that may make them more susceptible to negative environmental experiences (e.g., neglectful caregiving) than other individuals. In the context of G × E research, these vulnerabilities are often construed as genetic risk factors, but historically they have often been stud-ied as cognitive risk factors (e.g., Abramson et al., 2002). Another model that has been gaining attention in recent years is *differential susceptibility* theory (e.g., Belsky & Pleuss, 2009) or the theory of *biological sensitiv-ity to context* (e.g., Boyce & Ellis, 2005). According to these frameworks, many of the factors that investigators have identified as potential risk factors are not risk factors per se, but are better construed as plasticity factors. In other words, although some individuals might be at greater risk for developing poor interpersonal skills in difficult caregiving environments, those same people are more likely than others to thrive in supportive caregiving environments. They are differentially susceptible to environmental influences, for better and for worse.

Salo et al. (2011) found an interaction between variation in *HTR2A* and maternal nurturance, such that individuals who carried two T alleles of the *HTR2A* rs6313 SNP exhibited a stronger inverse association between maternal nurturance at age 10 and avoidant attachment measured 21–27 years later. These individuals were more likely both to benefit from early maternal nurturance and to be harmed by the relative lack of nurturance. We (Fraley, Roisman, Booth-LaForce, et al., 2013) found a similar effect— that increases in maternal sensitivity over childhood and adolescence predicted lower levels of avoidance at age 18 among individuals who carried two T alleles of *HTR2A* than among C allele carriers. However, we found that even C carriers exhibited a negative association between increases in maternal sensitivity and avoidance, suggesting that the basic effect held for people with both genetic variants.

We believe that this kind of work has the potential to be of great interest in the near future, but again we offer some caveats. As in the molecular genetic work discussed previously, there is a lot of room for "discovering" things that are not replicable. Specifically, the number of genetic variants that can be studied is large, and the set of G × E interactions that can be tested is even larger. Because this work is relatively new, it is difficult to articulate and defend strong predictions a priori. This makes it particularly important that researchers think carefully about sample sizes and attempt to replicate any findings that they uncover before weaving those findings into the knowledge base of psychology.

References

Abramson, L. Y., Alloy, L. B., Hankin, B. L., Haeffel, G. J., MacCoon, D. G., & Gibb, B. E. (2002). Cognitive vulnerability–stress models of depression in a self-regulatory and psychobiological context. In I. H. Gotlib & C. L. Hammen (Eds.), *Handbook of depression* (pp. 268–294). New York: Guilford Press.

Ainsworth, M. S. (1989). Attachments beyond infancy. *American Psychologist, 44*, 709–716.

Bartholomew, K., & Horowitz, L. (1991). Attachment styles among young adults: A test of the four-category model. *Journal of Personality and Social Psychology, 61*, 226–245.

Belsky, J., & Pluess, M. (2009). Beyond diathesis stress: Differential susceptibility to environmental influences. *Psychological Bulletin, 135*, 885–908.

Boling, M. W., Barry, C. M., Kotchick, B. A., & Lowry, J. (2011). Relations among early adolescents' parent–adolescent attachment, perceived social competence, and friendship quality. *Psychological Reports, 109*, 819–841.

Bowlby, J. (1969/1982). *Attachment and loss: Vol. 1. Attachment.* New York: Basic Books.

Bowlby, J. (1973). *Attachment and loss: Vol. 2. Separation: Anxiety and anger.* New York: Basic Books.

Bowlby, J., Robertson, J., & Rosenbluth, D. (1952). A two-year-old goes to the hospital. In R. S. Eisler, A. Freud, H. Hartmann, & E. Kris (Eds.), *Psychoanalytic study of the child* (Vol. 7, pp. 82–94). New York: International Universities Press.

Boyce, W. T., & Ellis, B. J. (2005). Biological sensitivity to context: A. An evolutionary–developmental theory of the origins and functions of stress reactivity. *Development and Psychopathology, 17*, 271–301.

Bretherton, I., & Munholland, K. A. (1999). Internal working models in attachment relationships: A construct revisited. In J. Cassidy & P. R. Shaver (Eds.), *Handbook of attachment: Theory, research, and clinical applications* (pp. 89–111). New York: Guilford Press.

Caughlin, J. P., Huston, T. L., & Houts, R. M. (2000). How does personality matter in marriage?: An examination of trait anxiety, interpersonal negativity, and marital satisfaction. *Journal of Personality and Social Psychology, 78*, 326–336.

Collins, N. L., & Feeney, B. C. (2000). A safe haven: An attachment theory perspective on support seeking and caregiving in intimate relationships. *Journal of Personality and Social Psychology, 78*, 1053–1073.

Crowell, J., & Owens, G. (1996). *Current Relationship Interview.* Unpublished manuscript, State University of New York at Stony Brook.

DeWolff, M., & van IJzendoorn, M. (1997). Sensitivity and attachment: A meta-analysis on parental antecedents of infant attachment. *Child Development, 68*, 571–591.

Donnellan, M. B., Burt, S. A., Levendosky, A., & Klump, K. (2008). Genes, personality, and attachment in adults: A multivariate behavioral genetic analysis. *Personality and Social Psychology Bulletin, 34*, 3–16.

Ellis, B. J., Figueredo, A. J., Brumbach, B. H., & Schlomer, G. L. (2009). Fundamental dimensions of environmental risk. *Human Nature, 20*, 204–268.

Englund, M. M., Kuo, S. I., Puig, J., & Collins, W. A. (2011). Early roots of adult competence: The significance of close relationships from infancy to early adulthood. *International Journal of Behavioral Development, 35*, 490–496.

Fearon, R. M. P., van IJzendoorn, M. H., Fonagy, P., Bakermans-Kranenburg, M. J., Schuengel, C., & Bokhorst, C. L. (2006). In search of shared and non-shared environmental factors in security of attachment: A behavior-genetic study of the association between sensitivity and attachment security. *Developmental Psychology, 42*, 1026–1040.

Fraley, R. C., & Brumbaugh, C. C. (2004). A dynamical systems approach to understanding stability and change in attachment security. In W. S. Rholes & J. A. Simpson (Eds.), *Adult attachment: Theory, research, and clinical implications* (pp. 86–132). New York: Guilford Press.

Fraley, R. C., & Heffernan, M. E. (2013). Attachment and parental divorce: A test of the diffusion and sensitive period hypotheses. *Personality and Social Psychology Bulletin, 39*, 1199–1213.

Fraley, R. C., Roisman, G. I., Booth-LaForce, C., Owen, M. T., & Holland, A. S. (2013). Interpersonal and genetic origins of adult attachment styles: A longitudinal study from infancy to early adulthood. *Journal of Personality and Social Psychology, 104*, 817–838.

Fraley, R. C., Roisman, G. I., & Haltigan, J. D. (2013). The legacy of early experiences in development: Formalizing alternative models of how early experiences are carried forward over time. *Developmental Psychology, 49*, 109–126.

Furman, W., Simon, V. A., Shaffer, L., & Bouchey, H. A. (2002). Adolescents' working models and styles with parents, friends, and romantic partners. *Child Development, 73*, 241–255.

Gibson, G. (2012). Rare and common variants: Twenty arguments. *Nature Reviews Genetics, 13*(2), 135–145.

Gillath, O., Shaver, P. R., Baek, J. M., & Chun, S. D. (2008). Genetic correlates of adult attachment style. *Personality and Social Psychology Bulletin, 34*, 1396–1405.

Groh, A. M., Fearon, R. P., Bakermans-Kranenburg, M. J., van IJzendoorn, M. H., Steele, R. D., & Roisman, G. I. (2014). The significance of attachment security for children's social competence with peers: A meta-analytic study. *Attachment and Human Development, 16*(2), 103–136.

Kaplan, H. S., & Gangestad, S. W. (2005). Life history theory and evolutionary psychology. In D. M. Buss (Ed.), *The handbook of evolutionary psychology* (pp. 68–95). Hoboken, NJ: Wiley.

Karney, B. R., & Bradbury, T. N. (1997). Neuroticism, marital interaction, and the trajectory of marital satisfaction. *Journal of Personality and Social Psychology, 72*, 1075–1092.

Kestenbaum, R., Farber, E., & Sroufe, L. A. (1989). Individual differences in empathy among preschoolers' concurrent and predictive validity. In N. Eisenberg (Ed.), *New Directions for Child Development: No. 44. Empathy and related emotional responses* (pp. 51–56). San Francisco: Jossey-Bass.

Laible, D., & Thompson, R. (1998). Attachment and emotional understanding in preschool children. *Developmental Psychology, 34*, 1038–1045.

Masten, A. S., & Cicchetti, D. (Eds.). (2010). Developmental cascades [Special issue]. *Development and Psychopathology, 22*(3), 491–715 (Part 1); 22(4), 717–983 (Part 2).

Masten, A. S., Roisman, G. I., Long, J. D., Burt, K. B., Obradović, J., Riley, J. R., et al. (2005). Developmental cascades: Linking academic achievement and externalizing and internalizing symptoms over 20 years. *Developmental Psychology, 41*, 733–746.

McElwain, N. L., Booth-LaForce, C., & Wu, X. (2011). Infant–mother attachment and children's friendship quality: Maternal mental-state talk as an intervening mechanism. *Developmental Psychology, 47*, 1295–1311.

McElwain, N. L., Cox, M. J., Burchinal, M. R., & Macfie, J. (2003). Differentiating among insecure mother–infant attachment classifications: A focus on child–friend interaction and exploration during solitary play at 36 months. *Attachment and Human Development, 5*, 136–164.

Parker, J. G., & Asher, S. R. (1993). Friendship and friendship quality in middle childhood: Links with peer group acceptance and feelings of loneliness and social dissatisfaction. *Developmental Psychology, 29,* 611–621.

Raby, K. L., Roisman, G. I., Fraley, R. C., & Simpson, J. A. (in press). The enduring predictive significance of early sensitivity: Social and academic competence through age 32 years. *Child Development.*

Roisman, G. I., Booth-LaForce, C., Belsky, J., Burt, K. B., & Groh, A. M. (2013). Molecular-genetic correlates of infant attachment: A cautionary tale. *Attachment and Human Development, 15,* 384–406.

Roisman, G. I., Collins, W. A., Sroufe, L. A., & Egeland, B. (2005). Predictors of young adults' representations of and behavior in their current romantic relationship: Prospective tests of the prototype hypothesis. *Attachment and Human Development, 7,* 105–121.

Roisman, G. I., & Fraley, R. C. (2006). The limits of genetic influence: A behavior-genetic analysis of infant–caregiver relationship quality and temperament. *Child Development, 77,* 1656–1667.

Roisman, G. I., & Fraley, R. C. (2008). A behavior-genetic study of parenting quality, infant attachment security, and their covariation in a nationally representative sample. *Developmental Psychology, 44,* 831–839.

Salo, J., Jokela, M., Lehtimäki, T., & Keltikangas-Järvinen, L. (2011) Serotonin receptor 2A gene moderates the effect of childhood maternal nurturance on adulthood social attachment. *Genes, Brain and Behavior, 10,* 702–709.

Salvatore, J. E., Kuo, S. I., Steele, R. D., Simpson, J. A., & Collins, W. A. (2011). Recovering from conflict in romantic relationships: A developmental perspective. *Psychological Science, 22,* 376–383.

Schneider, B. H., Atkinson, L., & Tardif, C. (2001). Child–parent attachment and children's peer relations: A quantitative review. *Developmental Psychology, 37,* 86–100.

Shulman, S., Elicker, J., & Sroufe, L. A. (1994). Stages of friendship growth in preadolescence as related to attachment history. *Journal of Social and Personal Relationships, 11,* 341–361.

Simmons, J., Nelson, L., & Simonsohn, U. (2011). False-positive psychology: Undisclosed flexibility in data collection and analysis allow presenting anything as significant. *Psychological Science, 22,* 1359–1366.

Simpson, J. A., Collins, W. A., Tran, S., & Haydon, K. C. (2007). Attachment and the experience and expression of emotions in romantic relationships: A developmental perspective. *Journal of Personality and Social Psychology, 92,* 355–367.

Simpson, J. A., Griskevicius, V., Kuo, S. I., Sung, S., & Collins, W. A. (2012). Evolution, stress, and sensitive periods: The influence of unpredictability in early versus late childhood on sex and risky behavior. *Developmental Psychology, 48,* 674–686.

Simpson, J. A., Kim, J. S., Fillo, J., Ickes, W., Rholes, W. S., Oriña, M. M., et al. (2011). Attachment and the management of empathic accuracy in relationship-threatening situations. *Personality and Social Psychology Bulletin, 37,* 242–254.

Slavich, G. M., & Cole, S. W. (2013). The emerging field of human social genomics. *Clinical Psychological Science, 1,* 331–348.

Sroufe, L. A. (1997). Psychopathology as an outcome of development. *Development and Psychopathology, 9,* 251–268.

Sroufe, L. A., Egeland, B., Carlson, E. A., & Collins, W. A. (2005). *The development of the person: The Minnesota Study of Risk and Adaptation from Birth to Adulthood.* New York: Guilford Press.

Stearns, S. C. (1992). *The evolution of life histories.* New York: Oxford University Press.

Teti, D. M., & Ablard, K. E. (1989). Security of attachment and infant–sibling relationships: A laboratory study. *Child Development, 60,* 1519–1528.

Troy, M., & Sroufe, L. A. (1987). Victimization among preschoolers: The role of attachment relationship history. *Journal of the American Academy of Child and Adolescent Psychiatry, 26,* 166–172.

Waddington, C. H. (1957). *The strategy of the genes.* London: George Allen & Unwin.

Waters, E., & Sroufe, L. A. (1983). Social competence as a developmental construct. *Developmental Review, 3,* 79–97.

Youngblade, L. M., & Belsky, J. (1992). Parent–child antecedents of 5-year-olds' close friendships: A longitudinal analysis. *Developmental Psychology, 28,* 700–713.

Zayas, V., Mischel, W., Shoda, Y., & Aber, J. L. (2011). Roots of adult attachment: Maternal caregiving at 18 months predicts adult attachment to peers and partners. *Social Psychological and Personality Science, 2,* 289–297.

Zeifman, D., & Hazan, C. (2008). Pair bonds as attachments: Reevaluating the evidence. In J. Cassidy & P. R. Shaver (Eds.), *Handbook of attachment: Theory, research, and clinical applications* (2nd ed., pp. 436–455). New York: Guilford Press.

2

The Neuroscience of Attachment

*Using New Methods to Answer Old
(and New) Questions*

Omri Gillath

What can electrical activity along the scalp, blood flow to specific brain areas, levels of chemicals in a synapse or the bloodstream, and the structure of one's double helix tell us about abstract concepts such as love, security, and attachment? If we consider the recent upsurge in research focusing on the micro-level analysis of attachment, the answer is—a lot. Building on the knowledge base and methods developed within cognitive psychology, neuroscience, psychophysiology, genetics, endocrinology, and immunology, scholars have started to provide a new and exciting set of answers to fundamental questions related to attachment theory and research. Issues such as "How do attachment bonds develop?", "Why do people have a specific attachment style?", "What is attachment security?", and "Is attachment an emotion or a motivation?" have gained renewed interest while being considered from new angles. Research can now begin to answer questions such as these by examining the systems and processes underlying attachment.

Neuroscience is an interdisciplinary area, which builds on and exchanges ideas with such fields as psychology, computer science, psycho-neuroimmunology, neuroendocrinology, and genetics. In the current chapter, I start with a brief summary of the leading principles and ideas relevant to attachment and its investigation via neuroscientific tools. I follow this summary with a literature review that highlights different techniques (such as brain imaging and genetic mapping) and different sources of information (such as animal models and computer simulations used to study attachment processes). These examples represent current endeavors to fill important gaps in attachment theory and research. I then discuss some of the theoretical advancements and emerging themes and models in this area of investigation, and finish the chapter by proposing some new and promising directions for future research.

Leading Principles and Ideas

Attachment theory (e.g., Ainsworth, Blehar, Waters, & Wall, 1978; Bowlby, 1969/1982) and the extensive literature it has spawned (for reviews, see Cassidy & Shaver, 2008; Mikulincer & Shaver, 2007a) grew out of Bowlby's psychoanalytic training and practice. It involves an innovative integration of psychoanalytic object relations theories with cognitive and developmental psychology, cybernetic systems theory, and primate ethology (Bowlby, 1969/1982). From its conception, Bowlby (1969/1982) described attachment by using biological and neural terms, such as the *behavioral system*. A behavioral system is a biologically based, evolved inborn program in an individual's central nervous system that governs the selection, activation, and termination of behavioral sequences. These behavioral sequences produce a predictable and generally functional change in the person–environment relationship that results in a set goal being met (e.g., getting access to resources, avoiding harm).

The main function of the *attachment behavioral system* is to promote survival by motivating proximity-seeking behaviors, especially when an individual faces threats or stressors (Bowlby, 1969/1982). The system's set goal is a state of safety and security. Threats or stressors can interfere with the set goal, which in turn activate the attachment system. Once activated, the system motivates people to regain safety and security. The primary strategy to do that is via seeking proximity to a stronger, wiser other—usually a primary caregiver or a relationship partner—whom Bowlby termed an *attachment figure*. When proximity is obtained and safety regained, people tend to feel relieved and secure. Repeatedly experiencing this scenario typically results in the development of secure mental representations or *internal working models* (IWMs) of oneself (as being worthy of love and care) and others (as caring and likely to help in times of need). These mental representations, once solidified and relatively stable, play a role in multiple domains such as emotion regulation, close relationship functioning, and the operation of other behavioral systems (e.g., exploration and caregiving). Thus attachment security broadens people's perspectives or skills, which in turn foster better mental health and self-actualization (see Mikulincer & Shaver, Chapter 5, this volume).

Not all interactions with attachment figures are positive and result in a sense of greater attachment security. According to Ainsworth et al. (1978), there are significant individual differences in attachment system dynamics and functioning, based on the repeated interactions people experience with their attachment figures. When attachment figures are sensitive, available, and responsive in times of need, people feel they can confidently rely on them. This, in turn, facilitates the development of a sense of connectedness and security. In contrast, when attachment figures are not reliably available and supportive, people are likely to feel a sense of attachment insecurity. Being chronically insecure, in turn, is associated with pursuing *secondary attachment strategies*—those that deactivate or hyperactivate the attachment system—instead of the primary strategy of proximity seeking.

Ainsworth et al. (1978) identified two types of insecurity. When caregivers tend to be cold and rejecting in times of need, people who seek proximity and support from them are likely to develop an *avoidant attachment style* characterized by distrust of relationship partners, strong striving for independence, and emotional distancing. People high on attachment avoidance tend to downplay the importance of emotions and relationship-related issues and to use deactivating strategies. These strategies involve dismissal of threat and attachment-related cues and suppression of attachment-related thoughts, emotions, and memories.

When caregivers tend to be intrusive and to provide inconsistent and insensitive support, people are likely to develop an *anxious attachment style* characterized by chronic worries related to relationship partners not being available in times of need. People high on attachment anxiety tend to perceive themselves as worthless and helpless, are hypervigilant to relationship-related cues, and use hyperactivating secondary strategies. These strategies include high sensitivity to signs of rejection, intense appeals to attachment figures, and obsessive reliance on them as a source of safety and support.

Attachment styles, which are often conceptualized in terms of a two-dimensional space with attachment anxiety and avoidance as its axes, can be assessed with reliable and valid self-report scales such as the Experiences in Close Relationships (ECR; Brennan, Clark, & Shaver, 1998). In studies using such measures, attachment styles have been associated in theoretically predictable ways with relationship variables such as quality and length, affect regulation strategies, and many other outcomes (for reviews, see Cassidy & Shaver, 2008; Mikulincer & Shaver, 2007a). People who score low on both attachment dimensions tend to be secure or have a *secure* attachment style. Attachment security is associated with greater self-confidence, better personal adjustment, more effective emotion regulation, good communication with relationship partners, generous and helpful behavior, and more satisfying relationships. When I refer to people as *anxious, avoidant,* or *secure* throughout this chapter, I mean that they score relatively high on attachment anxiety or avoidance, or they score low on both (secure).

Though individual differences are important, and numerous studies have examined the correlates of attachment styles, a full understanding of attachment requires an understanding of its normative processes (Bowlby, 1969/1982; Zayas & Hazan, 2015). This aspect of attachment includes processes such as activation of the attachment system, the formation and maintenance of attachment bonds, and the functioning of attachment security. To study these processes, researchers have used experimental manipulations to activate particular attachment IWMs (e.g., Baldwin, Keelan, Fehr, Enns, & Koh Rangarajoo, 1996). Using this approach, it was found that subtle experimental manipulations can increase or decrease a person's sense of attachment security and insecurity, which in turn affects cognitions, physiology, and behavior (for reviews, see Gillath, Selcuk, & Shaver, 2008; Mikulincer & Shaver, 2007b).

For example, researchers have found that words such as *love*, *hug*, and *affection*; memories of social and emotional support from loving relationship partners; the names of a person's security-providing attachment figures; or drawings/photographs depicting a parent's love for a child all tend to increase people's short-term sense of security and decrease their short-term anxiety and avoidance (e.g., Gillath, Hart, Noftle, & Stockdale, 2009). These changes affect other behavioral systems as well. For example, enhancement of attachment security results in increases in authenticity, prosocial tendencies, and exploration (e.g., Elliot & Reis, 2003; Gillath, Sesko, Shaver, & Chun, 2010). Furthermore, the effects of security primes remain statistically significant even when researchers control for dispositional neuroticism, positive affect, and self-esteem (e.g., Mikulincer, Hirschberger, Nachmias, & Gillath, 2001). Although these findings focus on temporary changes in attachment, there is evidence to suggest that similar processes can have long-lasting effects (for a review, see Gillath et al., 2008).

The majority of research on attachment has dealt with its macro-level processes (Levinger, 1994). Research and analysis at the macro level have focused on the associations that environment, context, and experience (e.g., dyad, family, society, culture) have with, or their effects on, attachment processes and outcomes. For example, how does growing up in a poor, dangerous neighborhood affect one's attachment style (Del Giudice, 2009)? Conversely, research and analysis at the micro level have focused on the associations that neurons, hormones, genetics, and so on have with, or their effects on, attachment processes and outcomes. For example, how does hippocampus size or blood flow correlate with people's attachment style scores? To fully understand attachment, one must look beyond (or below) the macro-level processes and into the micro-level processes (Levinger, 1994), which is now being done in research on the neuroscience of attachment.

Investigating the Neuroscience of Attachment

To study attachment at the micro level, researchers have used the methods and knowledge base developed within cognitive psychology (attention, memory, control, inhibition, etc.), psychophysiology (including animal models), and social/affective neuroscience. Researchers engaged in such investigations seek answers to questions such as "Do people have an innate tendency to develop a specific attachment style?", "How and when do attachment bonds and styles develop?", "Is attachment based on a unique neural or cognitive system, or are people using existing systems (such as thought control or emotion regulation) and applying general skills and tendencies to the specific domain of attachment?", and "What is attachment security and how does it work?" To answer these questions, researchers use a diverse set of methods and techniques ranging from brain activation to levels of oxytocin in the blood or saliva. Below I briefly review some answers that research using micro-level strategies or methods has provided.

Tools, Methods, and Techniques

There are different ways to study brain functioning, including functional magnetic resonance imaging (fMRI), electroencephalography (EEG), near infrared spectroscopy (NIRS), positron emission tomography (PET) or computed tomography (CT) scans, and transcranial magnetic stimulation (TMS). To date, researchers have mainly used fMRI and EEG to study the underlying mechanisms of attachment (e.g., Canterberry & Gillath, 2012; Zhang, Li, & Zhou, 2008). Neuroimaging can help researchers achieve a better understanding of issues that cannot be clarified by using non-neuroscientific methods, and it tests models and hypotheses about attachment that are otherwise difficult to test. For that to happen, an extensive mapping of the brain regions and processes involved in attachment needs to occur, and the contribution of each region or neural system/process must be identified. With such mapping, researchers can understand how general processes take place and their contribution to attachment. For example, how do people form new social ties and based on that how they form attachment bonds. In turn researchers can examine ways to change or improve attachment-related processes such as bonding or emotion regulation. Likewise, knowing which brain regions or processes are involved in certain attachment-related behaviors allows for comparisons between people who have different attachment styles and helps us better understand the sources of the differences between them, as demonstrated below. Next I provide a few examples of research focused on central topics in the attachment literature that have used neuroscientific methods.

Brain Imaging: fMRI, EEG, and Volumetry

As mentioned above, the IWM is a central construct in attachment theory. According to Bowlby (1969/1982), who created the construct to capture people's different attachment-related mental representations, IWMs allow people to understand the past and plan/prepare for the future (e.g., Brumbaugh & Fraley, 2006). This conceptualization suggests that attachment includes a top-down regulation process that modulates people's emotions, thoughts, and behavior. Despite ample work on IWMs (e.g., Bretherton & Munholland, 2008), our understanding of them has changed very little beyond Bowlby's original conceptualization. For example, it is still unclear what mechanisms allow the formation of IWMs and their updating over time, how IWMs differ from other cognitive structures and processes such as schemas, and how their top-down cognitive process differs from general top-down processes. Using neuroimaging can help provide answers to some of these questions that have not been answered by more traditional methods.

For example, in one of the first studies to examine the neural correlates of attachment style, we (Gillath, Bunge, Shaver, Wendelken, & Mikulincer, 2005) found that regulation of attachment-related thoughts was associated with activation in the prefrontal cortex (PFC)—an area involved in various cognitive processes that are not necessarily related to attachment (e.g., Miller & Cohen, 2001). Thus, when people were trying to stop thinking about rejection and separation from a romantic partner, we found activation in brain areas associated with attention, conflict monitoring, and working memory (e.g., the dorsolateral PFC, the medial PFC, and the anterior cingulate cortex [ACC]; see also Anderson et al., 2004). These patterns of activation are similar to the ones identified when people suppress non-attachment-related thoughts, suggesting that IWMs and their associated top-down regulatory mechanisms are manifestations of general regulatory processes used to cope with attachment-related material (for a fuller discussion, see Gillath, Giesbrecht, & Shaver, 2009).

Neuroimaging studies not only shed light on the processes associated with the attachment system; they also allow the comparison of these processes among people who have different attachment styles. For example, in the same study (Gillath et al., 2005) we found that while most participants exhibited activation in the medial PFC and ACC when suppressing attachment-related thoughts (which is similar to the activation pattern viewed when suppressing other general thoughts, such as "white bears"), avoidantly attached people showed a different pattern of activation. Specifically, whereas less avoidant people deactivated various brain regions such as the subgenual cingulate cortex (SCC; known to be associated with the regulation of emotion; Anderson et al., 2004; Drevets, 2000), when suppressing attachment-related thoughts, avoidantly attached people did not.

We interpreted this lack of deactivation as related to the constant suppression that highly avoidant people engage in—suppression of emotions and relationship-related thoughts.

Neuroimaging methods have also provided insight into another central component of attachment theory: the formation of attachment bonds and identification of attachment figures. Specifically, two brain areas appear to be involved in these processes—the amygdala and hippocampus. The attachment system, as mentioned above, is activated when people feel threatened. When the system is active, people look for help and for someone who can provide safety and security, such as an attachment figure. To do that, people need to quickly process information, identify the risk and a potential solution, and learn to associate a specific person with this solution—that is, with the provision of help or soothing.

The amygdala underlies all these processes. Activation in the amygdala is associated with processing of emotional or salient material, paying attention to novel stimuli, and consolidation of new memories through tagging (i.e., labeling something as important or meaningful; see Phelps & LeDoux, 2005). For example, when a child experiences stress and then receives help, these events are associated with heightened activation in the amygdala. The amygdala is thought to tag such events as meaningful and the people who provided help as important, making recall of these people more likely in the future (Lemche et al., 2006). Lemche and colleagues (2006) demonstrated that when people were exposed to cues of insecurity, the amygdala was indeed active—presumably as people processed the risk and retrieved images to help them cope. Other studies have found neighboring brain regions, such as the anterior temporal pole—known to be associated with emotion perception and response—to be activated when people are exposed to attachment-insecurity-related cues (e.g., Gillath et al., 2005; Vrticka & Vuilleumier, 2012).

Retrieval of images or scenarios is thought to take place in the hippocampus, which is also involved in creating associations between internal states (e.g., feeling secure or distressed) and cues in the environment (e.g., having a caregiver around; Kennedy & Shapiro, 2004), and with the consolidation of memories. Together, the amygdala and hippocampus allow the formation of an association between close others and meaningful events and experiences, which contributes to the perception of these others as attachment figures (e.g., Buchheim et al., 2006; Lemche et al., 2006; Vrticka, Andersson, Grandjean, Sander, & Vuilleumier, 2008).

The attachment system recruits these general abilities to generate lifelong associations regarding the roles of others in one's life (e.g., caregiver, stranger) and to tag specific people as more significant than others—as attachment figures. By better understanding the mechanisms involved in the conditioning and processing of emotional information in the amygdala, the temporal pole, and the hippocampus, we might be able to help people form better attachment bonds and help those who have problems with creating such bonds (e.g., Romanian orphans; Chisholm, 1998).

A third example of the value of neuroscience to the understanding of attachment involves emotion regulation. People who have different attachment styles cope differently and exhibit different emotion regulation strategies (e.g., suppression, enhancement). For example, anxiously attached people tend to be highly emotional and overwhelmed by their emotions, whereas securely attached people have a weaker emotional reaction to distressing information (Nash, Prentice, Hirsh, McGregor, & Inzlicht, 2014). A number of explanations have been suggested for these behaviors, but it remains unclear why anxiously attached people manifest emotions so intensely—is it due to higher sensitivity? Lower ability to control? Or both? Using neuroimaging, we (Gillath et al., 2005) have found that when people are asked to suppress their negative thoughts and emotions during an emotion regulation task, anxiously attached people exhibit lower activation in the orbitofrontal cortex (OFC). The OFC is associated with emotion regulation skills, the lower activation found in anxiously attached people could hence be interpreted as lesser engagement of this area in the process among anxiously attached people. This, in turn, suggests that the extreme emotional reactions of anxiously attached people are due to their lack of ability to regulate emotions (Gillath et al., 2005; Warren et al., 2010).

A final example involves our understanding of security priming. Whereas most of the research on attachment in general, and attachment neuroscience more specifically, has focused on attachment styles (anxiety and avoidance), less is known about the enhancement of attachment security and especially its underlying neural mechanisms. To address this gap, we (Canterberry & Gillath, 2012) recently examined people's brain activation as we exposed them to attachment-security-related primes. Behavioral studies have provided ample evidence to suggest that the enhancement of attachment security has a host of beneficial outcomes for personal and relational well-being (for reviews, see Gillath et al., 2008; Mikulincer & Shaver, 2007b). In our study we suggested and tested the proposal that the benefits associated with security are the outcome of three processes—cognitive, affective, and behavioral. Indeed, we found that security priming led to distributed, co-occurring activation in brain areas reflective of these cognitive, affective, and behavioral processes (e.g., the PFC, parahippocampus, and temporal and parietal gyri). These patterns of activation related to security were moderated by attachment styles. For example, attachment avoidance was associated with activation in areas related to encoding and retrieval (parahippocampal gyrus), suggesting that avoidantly attached people were making increased memory retrieval attempts during the exposure to the prime, perhaps reflecting a lack of easily accessible secure models.

These findings, while consistent with the existing attachment literature, go beyond behavioral findings to demonstrate that all three components (cognitive, affective, and behavioral) operate simultaneously. Thus security seems to act as a mental resource derived from multiple sources that facilitates pro-relational and prosocial tendencies. Furthermore, the findings provide support for the idea that security priming is not merely a shift in the cognitive accessibility of security-related concepts. Rather, it seems to activate a system of emotions, cognitions, and motives all contributing to growth and well-being (see also Eisenberger et al., 2011; Karremans, Heslenfeld, van Dillen, & Van Lange, 2011).

These are only a few examples of the rapidly growing literature on brain regions and mechanisms involved in bonding and attachment processes (see also Coan, 2008). There are additional regions involved in attachment processes, such as the nucleus accumbens (e.g., Aron et al., 2005), the ACC (dorsal ACC; e.g., DeWall et al., 2012; Warren et al., 2010, and rostral ACC; Eisenberger & Lieberman, 2004), the dorsolateral PFC (e.g., Gillath et al., 2005; Warren et al., 2010), and the insula (e.g., DeWall et al., 2012). These areas are thought to be involved in emotions related to attachment and bonding, such as love and desire (reward) or rejection and fear (punishment), and their regulation. Knowing which brain regions are involved in each of these processes and how they work together can improve the design of attachment-related interventions. For example, one reason why anxiously attached people show lower activation in the OFC when trying to suppress thoughts may have to do with specific neurotransmitters and receptors in the OFC. If this is the case, neurotransmitters could be modulated with chemical or pharmaceutical interventions. This, in turn, could potentially assist anxiously attached people to cope better with their emotions and feel less insecure.

A different approach for using neuroscience to better understand the attachment system and attachment styles is to focus on brain laterality and brain structure or volume. For example, using EEG, Dawson and colleagues (2001) found that insecurely attached infants, as compared with secure ones, exhibited reduced left frontal brain activity. Reduced activity in the left frontal brain is associated with negative emotions and depression (Hellige, 1993). Dawson et al. suggested that the reduced activation they found among insecure infants represents a greater tendency to use withdrawal-type emotion regulation strategies (turning away from the external environment) and a failure to use appropriate approach regulation strategies (e.g., approaching an attachment figure when needed).

Cohen and Shaver (2004) using a divided visual field task found similar differences in brain laterality among adults. Specifically they found that avoidantly attached adults as compared with nonavoidant adults made more errors when judging positive attachment-related words presented to the right hemisphere (which is often associated with negative emotions; e.g., Ahern & Schwartz, 1985). These findings suggest that attachment history and style may affect the way people process attachment-related

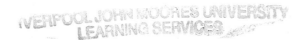

information in the brain. Cohen and Shaver suggest that because avoidantly attached people have less experience with positive attachment-related information, they are more likely to make more errors, especially in the hemisphere that has less to do with processing of positive information.

EEG can also be used to study specific neural reactions to events by investigating event-related potentials (ERPs), such as P3 or N1 (the letter represents positive–negative polarity, and the number represents the latency in hundreds of milliseconds from the event). ERPs are caused by cognitive processes that involve, among others, memory, expectation, attention, and change in mental states. For example, when Zhang et al. (2008) examined people's reactions to facial expressions, they found that attachment styles were related to differences in several components (N1, N2, P2, and N400), suggesting that people who had different attachment styles differed in terms of both early automatic encoding and late elaborative retrieval of emotional content. Thus avoidant participants showed a less negative N1 and N400 compared to anxious and secure participants. N1 is thought to represent level of attention (Hillyard, Teder-Sälejärvi, & Münte, 1998). From these results, one might conclude that avoidant individuals devote less attention to emotional stimuli than secure or anxious people do.

In a similar manner, Dan and Raz (2012) found differences on C1 (C for Component; it can be either positive or negative; C1 is the first visual ERP component that peaks between 50–100ms) and P1 mean amplitudes at occipital and posterior-parietal channels in response to angry faces versus neutral faces, but only among people high on avoidance. The processing biases toward angry faces (in the P1 component) and toward neutral faces (in the C1 component) among avoidant people suggest that only avoidant participants have the capacity to identify cues at such early stages of information processing, which allows them to apply their deactivating strategies (also see Niedenthal, Brauer, Robin, & Innes-Ker, 2002). Focusing on anxious individuals, Zayas, Shoda, Mischel, Osterhout, and Takahashi (2009) and Zilber, Goldstein, and Mikulincer (2007) demonstrated attachment anxiety to be associated with later ERP components, such as N400 and the late positive potential (LPP). For example, Zayas et al. (2009) found that when participants were exposed to attachment-related cues, rejection-related words (e.g., *dismissing*) elicited greater N400 amplitudes than acceptance-related words (e.g., *supporting*) among women high on anxiety and low on avoidance. N400 is thought to reflect the amount of semantic processing elicited by a stimulus. People tend to process more when the stimulus is unexpected or have a greater personal significance. Zayas et al. concluded that anxiously attached women perceive rejection cues as more personally significant, posing greater threat to the self.

In addition to looking at brain activation, either per region (fMRI), per hemisphere (in laterality studies), or at a specific time point (ERPs), researchers have also investigated brain structure or volume. For instance, we (Quirin et al., 2010) found that attachment insecurity is associated with a smaller hippocampal cell density. This finding is compatible with a neurotoxic model of stress-induced cell reduction in the hippocampus. According to this model, unresponsive and insensitive caregiving promotes insecure attachment and simultaneously induces high stress for long periods of time. In turn, chronic high stress and high levels of cortisol (stress-related hormone) result in smaller hippocampus size. Benetti and colleagues (2010) found similar results, such that attachment anxiety was associated with a decrease in gray matter in the anterior temporal pole. Activations in this area and the anatomically adjacent hippocampus were found to be associated with greater attachment anxiety (Gillath et al., 2005), providing convergent validity for the relevance of these brain areas for attachment anxiety.

Tharner and colleagues (2011) also examined brain volume. However, they did it by using a different methodology and a longitudinal rather than a cross-sectional design, which currently is extremely rare in attachment neuroscience. Utilizing ultrasound imaging, they assessed infants' brain volumes when they were 6 weeks old, followed them until they were 14 months old, and then used the Strange Situation (see Ainsworth et al., 1978) to assess their attachment pattern (style). They found that infants who had a larger gangliothalamic ovoid, which comprises the basal ganglia (including the caudate, putamen, nucleus accumbens) and the thalamus, were at lower risk of developing attachment disorganization—regardless of their general brain development/maturity. The basal ganglia are thought to connect higher cortical regions, such as the PFC and lower motor areas, and are believed to be involved in voluntary motor action and learning (e.g., Redgrave, Prescott, & Gurney, 1999). To achieve the set goals of the attachment system, specific behaviors such as crawling, reaching out, and crying must take place. The inability to select and execute such goal-directed attachment behavior is a salient characteristic of attachment disorganization (Main & Solomon, 1990). The smaller volume of these brain structures may contribute to this inability and, in turn, to the development of disorganized attachment. Tharner and colleagues suggest that either intrauterine influences (e.g., stress) or genetics (e.g., a dopamine receptor gene, DRD4) may underlie the subcortical volume differences they identified in their study.

Together, the findings described above emphasize the importance of investigating brain volume separately and with other sources of information (e.g., brain functioning and genetics) to achieve a full understanding of how attachment develops over time and functions. The existing findings suggest that attachment styles are associated with differences in brain volume, and that smaller volume in specific areas is related to disorganized (basal ganglia) or anxious attachment (hippocampus). More research is needed to understand how these structural differences come to be. Are they innate? Do they develop in response to environmental cues? As suggested by Tharner et al. (2011), probably both are true. No study to date, however, has examined this.

Although they are not the focus of this chapter, it is important to note that *physiological correlates* (e.g., heart rate, blood pressure, skin conductance, and glucocorticoid levels) can also shed light on the neuroscience of attachment (e.g., Powers, Pietromonaco, Gunlicks, & Sayer, 2006; see Diamond & Fagundes, 2010, for a review). For example, we (Quirin et al., 2010) have made claims, based on our findings of brain volume differences, regarding the association between attachment insecurity and the hypothalamic–pituitary–adrenocortical (HPA) axis system. These claims have received ample support from studies using physiological markers (e.g., heart rate, blood pressure), which have repeatedly found associations between attachment insecurity and stronger physiological reaction (e.g., higher HPA activity), especially following relational stressors (e.g., Powers et al., 2006). These findings, which demonstrate regulation failures or deficits among insecurely attached people, can be explained in terms of the decreased volume or increased activity in specific brain areas. To do that, studies that combine neural and physiological indices should be carried out. Such studies will allow scholars to tie the relatively new and sometimes unclear neural findings with the broad knowledge base on human physiology. As suggested by Tharner et al. (2011), an additional needed step is to connect the neural (and physiological) findings with genetics.

Genes, Neurotransmitters, and Hormones

There are different ways to utilize knowledge about genes, neurotransmitters, and hormones to investigate attachment. First, researchers can use *behavioral genetic* methods to estimate genetic and environmental contributions to attachment anxiety, avoidance, and security. Second, using *molecular genetic* methods, investigators can examine correlations between attachment cognitions and behaviors on the one hand, and *polymorphisms*[1] on genes that regulate the release, reuptake, or degradation of hormones and neurotransmitters or affect the density of receptors of these hormones and neurotransmitters on the other. Third, researchers can correlate the *blood or saliva levels* of neurotransmitters or hormones with people's attachment-related behaviors or styles. Finally, going back to brain structure and functioning discussed above, researchers can use the distribution of receptors for neurotransmitters such as serotonin, dopamine, oxytocin, and vasopressin in the brain to identify brain regions most likely to be associated with attachment processes and outcomes. For example, the

---

[1] Polymorphisms can be homozygous (having identical alleles at corresponding chromosomal loci) or heterozygous (having dissimilar alleles).

nucleus accumbens, which is rich in all of these neurotransmitter receptors, plays a role in various processes associated with attachment and bonding (e.g., Young & Wang, 2004). In what follows, I focus mainly on the first two methods.

Whereas some early studies using behavioral genetics found little evidence for heredity or genetic influence, and more support for shared environment influence on infant attachment (e.g., O'Connor & Croft, 2001), more recently researchers have started to provide evidence to support the influence of genetics on adult attachment styles. For example, Crawford et al. (2007) found that 40% of the variance in adult attachment anxiety was accounted for by genetic influences, and Donnellan, Burt, Levendosky, and Klump (2008) found that additive genetic effects accounted for 45% of the variability in attachment anxiety and 39% of the variability in avoidance. These findings suggest that a person's attachment style is at least partially the outcome of his or her genetics, and that this genetic contribution to attachment manifests itself mainly in adulthood.

To turn to molecular genetics, the three main genetic candidates that scholars have been studying with regard to attachment are dopamine, serotonin, and oxytocin (but see Troisi et al., 2012, for findings on mu-opioid). Dopamine is involved in the motivation–reward system and in goal-related behavior (e.g., Berridge, 2007) as well as in social and relational behaviors (e.g., Schneier et al., 2000). We (Gillath et al., 2008) found that attachment anxiety was associated with polymorphisms of dopamine (*DRD2*), and Lakatos and colleagues (2002) found an association between dopamine (*DRD4*, the 7-repeat allele) and the likelihood of disorganized attachment. Bakermans-Kranenburg and van IJzendoorn (2011) highlight the interactions of dopamine (receptor *DRD2, DRD4*, and transporter *DAT*) with environmental conditions to affect attachment outcomes. For example, children who have less efficient dopamine-related genes do worse in negative environments than those without genetic risk, and they are more likely to be disorganized or insecure with regard to their attachment style. However, children with these genes have also been found to profit more from nurturing environmental conditions.

Serotonin, the second gene candidate, also influences affect (Gross et al., 2002) and social behavior (Raleigh, Brammer, & McGuire, 1983). In line with this research, serotonin was associated with greater attachment avoidance by Gillath and colleagues (2008) and with greater anxiety by Salo, Jokela, Lehtimäki, and Keltikangas-Järvinen (2011) and Fraley, Roisman, Booth-LaForce, Owen, and Holland (2013). Both Salo et al. and Fraley et al. found that this association was moderated by environmental factors (defined as either maternal nurturance or maternal sensitivity). Caspers et al. (2009) found an association between the serotonin short *5HTTLPR* allele and increased risk for disorganized attachment. They interpreted this as being consistent with the role of serotonin in modulating the frontal–amygdalar circuitry (see also Cicchetti, Rogosch, & Toth, 2011).

Oxytocin also plays a central role in social behavior and specifically in attachment. Costa and colleagues (2009) found associations between the GG genotype of *OXTR* single-nucleotide polymorphisms (SNPs; *6930G >A* or *9073G >A*) and scores on the Attachment Style Questionnaire factors, such that it was negatively associated with Confidence (attachment security) and positively associated with Need for Approval (anxiety) and Relationship as Secondary (avoidance). In contrast, Chen and Johnson (2012) found (only among females) that those who had at least one copy of the A allele of *OXTR rs2254298* reported greater attachment anxiety than females who had two copies of the G allele. However, neither we (Gillath et al., 2008) nor Fraley et al. (2013) found an association between attachment and *OXTR* (see also Bakermans-Kranenburg, & van IJzendoorn, 2014).

Together, these findings suggest that despite Bowlby's (1982) conceptualization of attachment style as a blank slate at birth (i.e., the view that people have an equal or similar potential to develop a secure or insecure attachment style, based on their interactions and the environment), some people might be more predisposed than others to develop (in)secure attachment styles. Combining the findings just described with those from the previous section on neuroimaging, I suggest that specific polymorphisms may affect the development and function of specific brain areas, which in turn are associated with certain attachment styles (see Figure 2.1).

A major problem with many of these findings, however, is their reliance on correlational designs. To deal with this issue, researchers have recently started to use experimental methods to study the links between neurotransmitters and attachment variables, mainly focusing on oxytocin. To do so, they have examined the effects of intranasal oxytocin (compared with placebo) on attachment-related behaviors. For example, Bartz et al. (2010) found that oxytocin affected attachment cognitions (e.g., remembering one's mother as being more caring and close), but that these effects were moderated by attachment styles. Thus people low on attachment anxiety remembered their mothers as more close and caring after oxytocin induction (vs. placebo), whereas people high on attachment anxiety remembered their mothers as less caring and close after the same manipulation. Similarly, while oxytocin induction increased the ease of imagining a secure-script scenario (someone else being deeply compassionate to the self), this was moderated by attachment styles, with insecure individuals having less positive experiences after the induction (Rockliff et al., 2011). De Dreu (2012) also found that oxytocin interacted with attachment styles; however, it interacted mainly with avoidance. Specifically, among people who scored higher on avoidance, oxytocin induction reduced betrayal aversion, and increased trust and cooperation compared to the placebo group.

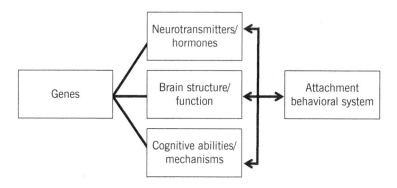

FIGURE 2.1. Attachment as a function of genes and brain structure and function. Genes include dopamine *(DRD2, DRD4, DAT)*, serotonin *(5HT)*, oxytocin *(OXTR)*, and catechol-O-methyltransferase *(COMT)*, among others. Brain structure/function includes volume, connectivity, and mechanisms in areas such as the hippocampus, amygdala, dorsal ACC, SCC, and OFC. Cognitive abilities/mechanisms include attention, emotion regulation, thought control, self-regulation, and IWMs.

Animal Models

There is a very broad literature on animal models of bonding, attachment, and close relationships (e.g., Carter et al., 2005), which I only briefly touch upon. Animal models constitute a powerful method for studying the social brain and the neurobiological mechanisms underlying social relationships, attachment included (e.g., Bales, Maninger, & Hinde, 2012). For instance, oxytocin, which is thought to be a central player in human attachment and bonding, was first examined in animal models (see Carter et al., 2005; Insel & Young, 2001). In studies using animal models, researchers use observational methods to identify bonding (social or pair-bonding) behaviors such as separation distress and soothing, or relationship/attachment styles. Animal models of attachment and pair bonding created by Michael Meaney and others are crucial in our understanding of the roles epigenetics and neural mechanisms play in these systems and behaviors (see Bagot et al., 2009; Bales et al., 2012; Carter et al., 2005; Lim & Young, 2006). Meaney's work demonstrated that parental behavior affects gene expression in the rat pup, which in turn affects the future parenting behavior of the pup when it reaches adulthood. The major advantages of this approach over work based on humans are the abilities to (1) study intergenerational effects in much shorter time frames, (2) use genetic or chemical manipulations that would be hard or impossible to use in humans, (3) inflict lesions, and (4) perform postmortem analysis that would be prohibited, more difficult, or unethical in humans—all of which permit clearer inferences about causality. Thus animal models provide additional angles that permit better and deeper understanding of the structures, mechanisms, and functions involved in attachment processes and outcomes in ways that typically are not possible with human participants.

Theoretical Models

Although the research in the domain of attachment neuroscience is relatively young, important findings have started to accumulate, and researchers have developed preliminary conceptual models to organize these findings. For example, Fonagy, Luyten, and Strathearn (2011) suggest a developmental, biobehavioral *switch model*, not focused specifically on attachment, but rather on its associations with *mentalization* (i.e., the ability to understand the mental state of oneself and others) and stress. The model is based on early work by Panksepp (1998) and Insel (e.g., Insel & Young, 2001). The work, focusing on animal models, links attachment bonds with substance dependence and opioids, suggesting that attachment might be based on the same mechanisms as addictive disorders (Burkett & Young, 2012). These mechanisms involve two neural systems, which are the same systems that Fonagy et al. focus on in their model: (1) the dopaminergic system (Ferris et al., 2005; Strathearn, Fonagy, Amico, & Montague, 2009), and (2) the oxytocinergic system (Bartels & Zeki, 2004; Champagne, Diorio, Sharma, & Meaney, 2001; Feldman, Weller, Zagoory-Sharon, & Levine, 2007). The dopaminergic system is associated with sensitivity to cues, and both the dopaminergic and oxytocinergic systems are associated with responding to social cues and with rewarding social and relational behaviors.

Tying their model to personality disorders, Fonagy et al. (2011) suggest that complex interactions among environmental, biological, and psychosocial factors affect the two neural systems, which in turn shape the attachment system, and more specifically its threshold of activation. These interactions also affect people's ability to differentiate the mental states of self and others, which decreases the sensitivity and susceptibility to contagion from other people's mental states, reduces integration of cognitive and affective aspects of mentalization, and increases dysfunctions in stress regulation systems. These, in turn, affect the ability of people to regulate their behavior. Together, the changes in threshold level and regulation or control can lead to the development of insecure or even disorganized attachment. Fonagy et al.'s model focuses on attachment and its association with mental disorders. It draws a lot of its evidence from findings relevant to mothers' behaviors in response to their offspring, which are more closely related to the activation of the caregiving system than to that of the attachment system (for similar models, see Atzil, Hendler, & Feldman, 2011; Galynker et al., 2012). Hence I turn next to Vrticka and Vuilleumier's (2012) model, which focuses less on mental disorders and the caregiving system.

Vrticka and Vuilleumier (2012) suggest that individual differences in attachment styles correlate with various affective and cognitive processes, particularly in attachment-relevant or social contexts. Their model of the influence of adult attachment on social processing, which incorporates Fonagy et al.'s (2011) model, involves two core networks: one network that is associated with affective evaluation processes (such as threat or reward), and includes approach and avoidance components; and another network that is associated with cognitive control and mentalizing abilities, and includes emotion regulation and mental state representation components). Their model is similar to the attachment model suggested by Pietromonaco and Barrett (2000) in terms of its affective and emotion regulation components, and to more general models of social cognition and emotion processing (e.g., Lieberman, 2007).

When describing the neuroscientific aspect of their model, Vrticka and Vuilleumier (2012) add the serotonergic and cortisol systems to the dopaminergic and oxytocinergic systems suggested by Fonagy et al. (2011), and discuss a set of specific brain regions for each network's component: *approach* (the ventral tegmental, hypothalamus, striatum, and ventral medial OFC), *avoidance* (the amygdala, hippocampus, insula, ACC, and anterior temporal pole), *emotion regulation* (the dorsolateral PFC and lateral OFC), and *mental state representation* (the medial PFC, posterior cingulate cortex, precuneus, posterior superior temporal sulcus, temporoparietal junction, and anterior superior temporal gyrus).

Vrticka and Vuilleumier (2012) further suggest that there is a dynamic balance between the threat-sensitive system motivating social aversion and the attachment system that promotes a sense of safety via close relationships and approach (MacDonald & MacDonald, 2011). According to this explanation, attachment bonds serve as social rewards in the approach system. Both approach and aversion are thought to be shaped by genes and the environment, and modulated by attachment avoidance and anxiety. Thus people high on attachment avoidance are thought to have weaker brain activation in areas related to both the approach and the avoidance systems, in line with their use of deactivating strategies; by contrast, people high on anxiety are thought to have stronger brain activation, but mainly with regard to the aversion system and the processing of negative social cues, in line with their use of hyperactivating strategies. People who are low on both dimensions are thought to have weaker reactions as compared with anxiously attached individuals, but due to their effective regulation rather than their deactivation of the attachment system (for a similar model and findings, see Warren et al., 2010).

Coan (2010) suggests a different model—one that focuses on the regulatory role of the attachment system via overt emotional and social

behavior. His model describes the neural systems involved in the formation and maintenance of adult attachment relationships and the way the
brain supports attachment behaviors. As Vrticka and Vuilleumier (2012)
do, Coan (2010) builds on research regarding the neural systems supporting emotion, emotion regulation, motivation, and social behavior. He also
introduces the *social baseline* model of social affect regulation. The model
integrates existing models of attachment with a neuroscientific principle—
economy of action—in the management of metabolic resources devoted to
emotional and social behavior. According to the model, adult attachment
relationships conserve brain metabolic resources, especially those of the
PFC.

Coan's (2010) model, which is an attempt to bridge the gap between
the broad animal literature on bonding and the extended work on human
attachment behavior, depicts the attachment behavioral system as a higher-
order construct. This construct includes basic behaviors, such as recognition and familiarity, proximity seeking, separation distress, soothing
behaviors, and maternal caregiving. Like Vrticka and Vuilleumier (2012)
and Fonagy et al. (2011), Coan talks about emotion and emotion regulation systems used for attachment behaviors, the relevance of threat- and
reward-related systems, and associations between attachment and cognitive
processes, such as attention and memory. However, he adds an economic
aspect above and beyond these other models. Accordingly, attachment is
tied to the brain's energy expenditure management, and being together
or feeling securely attached "saves" brain energy. Being alone is straining
and costly (Beckes & Coan, 2011), whereas interacting with others—the
default setting of human existence, according to Coan—is less effortful.
Being with others allows people to spend fewer resources on activities such
as threat detection and emotion regulation, because it involves load sharing
via familiarity, interdependence, and interpersonal conditioning.

Summary and Future Directions

The three theoretical models reviewed above have a few things in common.
They all discuss two aspects or systems underlying attachment styles, which
broadly represent (1) threshold or sensitivity and (2) regulation, and involve
both automatic and controlled processes. This is in line with both non-
neuroscientific models of attachment (e.g., Pietromonaco & Barrett, 2000),
and with non-attachment-related models in neuroscience (e.g., Lieberman,
2007). All three models also connect attachment with broader literatures,
whether these are the temperament or personality literature, or the cognitive
literature on affect regulation and thought control. The models use findings from these broader literatures to explain attachment-related processes,
and identify brain systems or genes relevant to attachment. Finally, all the

models highlight similar neurotransmitters (e.g., dopamine, oxytocin, and serotonin) and their role in animal and human attachment (although this is less central in Coan's [2010] model).

However, there are a few things still missing in current models of attachment neuroscience. First, there is a need for an integrative explanation that describes how the various aspects reviewed above (e.g., brain structure and function, genes, neurotransmitters) fit into a comprehensive model. Second, existing neuroscientific models focus on the micro level of attachment (intraindividual factors) without connecting it to the macro level (e.g., context, culture). Third, most models (and the attachment literature more broadly) focus on explaining attachment insecurity, and less attention is given to the underlying mechanisms of attachment security. Below, I suggest some solutions to start bridging these theoretical gaps.

A model of attachment neuroscience should integrate all the components reviewed above (and potentially others not reviewed here) into a comprehensive explanation that takes advantage of the unique contributions of each method or approach and integrates them into an overall picture. This idea is not unique to the neuroscience of attachment, and is related to data fusion and analytical approaches that deal with fusion (Calhoun, Liu, & Adali, 2009). For example, in many recent studies, researchers collect multiple types of imaging data from the same participants (fMRI, ERPs, etc.). Each imaging method focuses on a limited domain (e.g., near-scalp electrical activity) and provides both common and unique information about the issue being studied. For instance, ERPs reveal the exact *when*, whereas fMRIs reveal the *where* of a phenomenon. Combining them in the same study can provide a fuller picture than getting answers in different studies. Statistical approaches such as independent component analysis (ICA) allow one to put these pieces (brain imaging, electrophysiology, genetics, etc.) together. Beyond the mathematical or statistical level represented by ICA, there is also a need to provide a theoretical framework that connects all the informational dots. We (Gillath, Canterberry, & Collins, 2012) have started this task (see Figure 2.1), connecting genetics, specific brain structure/volume and functioning, connectivity between the areas of activation, and attachment behaviors. For example, attachment anxiety is associated with polymorphisms of dopamine (fewer D2 receptors); decreased hippocampal volume; higher activation of the hippocampus, ATP, dorsal ACC, and a few other areas; lower activation of the OFC; negative correlations between these activations; and higher sensitivity to attachment-related information. Conversely, avoidant attachment is associated with polymorphisms of serotonin (fewer 5HT receptors), increases in early brain waves (C1 and P1), higher activation in dorsolateral PFC, and higher ability to suppress attachment-related cues. Future research should further test the associations among the components of the framework we have suggested by including different methodologies in the *same* study, and by adding more components (or puzzle pieces) as the evidence for their role accumulates.

While neuroscience provides researchers with a preview of the micro level of attachment, combining micro-level research with the macro-level studies will be necessary for a full understanding of the attachment system (see Figure 2.2, and Gillath et al., 2012). For instance, adopting a cultural perspective can allow researchers to grasp how the brain adapts to fit better with specific contexts or demands (e.g., Wilson, 2010). Understanding the functions of attachment in the culture-ready brain (Whitehead, 2010) can position attachment at the forefront of the new domain of cultural neuroscience (Chiao, 2010). Some preliminary work in this direction already exists. For example, Eisenberg et al. (2010) describe the role of D4 dopamine receptors in pair-bonding processes across different cultures/contexts, and Ray et al. (2010) describe differences in neural representations of self and other (specifically, the mother) as a function of a specific cultural context—interdependent self-construal.

Any model that seeks to explain the neuroscience of attachment should also deal with the construct of attachment security and its underlying mechanisms. As mentioned above, we (Canterberry & Gillath, 2012) recently conducted a study focusing on this aspect, showing that security involves affective (increased positive mood and relaxation), cognitive (increased self- and emotion regulation), and behavioral (prosocial tendencies) components.

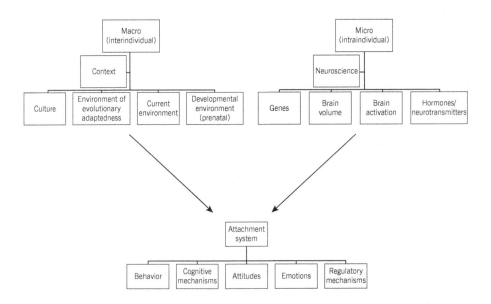

FIGURE 2.2. Combining the micro and macro levels to gain a better understanding of attachment.

In a different study (Gillath, Atchley, Imran, & El-Hodiri, 2014), using cognitive methods and ERPs, we showed that priming attachment security increased the tendency to behave generously, and affected the reactions people had to their generosity's being reciprocated or not. Examining FN (feedback negativity) and P3 ERP components, we also found that security buffers emotional reactions to loss, especially among insecurely attached people, potentially making them focus on the importance of social cues (other people) rather than financial ones (possessions). In yet another study, exposing people to an attachment security prime resulted in increased glucose levels, supporting the idea that security provides resources to people, which in turn allows them to deal with stress and react more efficiently and flexibly to threats (Gillath, Pressman, Stetler, & Moskovitz, 2014).

While providing initial information on security, these studies do not deal with the association between security and insecurity. Right now, for example, it is unclear whether the two constructs represent two different systems (i.e., attachment and security) or two sides of the same system/dimension (see Figure 2.3). More work is needed to answer such questions as "What happens when people are exposed to an insecurity prime?" We know that the attachment system is activated (Mikulincer, Gillath, & Shaver, 2002), and that people seek proximity to regain security, but what is the end result of this process with regard to the system? Is it "returning to baseline" (its zero or default state)? Or, because security is achieved or regained, are people "above baseline" in a state that is closer to how they would feel (or would experience) when primed with a security prime? Using

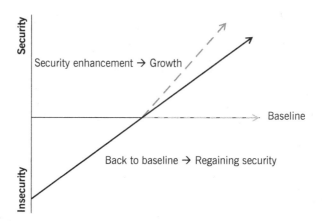

FIGURE 2.3. The relations between attachment security and insecurity. The dashed lines represent alternatives to the insecurity–security continuum, and more generally the potential for two separate processes or systems for security and insecurity.

neuroscience techniques and comparing activation when security versus insecurity is primed can help answer these important questions. From our own findings, it seems that security priming brings people into a higher state of growth or flow, each of which is associated with different brain mechanisms from those associated with insecurity. Another question has to do with state versus trait differences in attachment (e.g., Gillath, Hart, et al., 2009). For example, what happens when a dispositionally insecure person is primed with security? These issues should be tested and integrated into the suggested framework of attachment, while keeping other models of attachment in mind; for example, how does security fit into models depicting attachment (and love) as an addiction (Burkett & Young, 2012)?

In summary, the domain of attachment neuroscience, though young, is growing rapidly and continually contributing to our understanding of attachment. Although adult attachment has been studied for almost 30 years, and attachment in general has been studied for more than 50 years, there is still much to learn, and many open questions remain. Neuroscience is an essential approach to finding answers to these questions. In this chapter, I have reviewed some of the key findings obtained in research using various methods of neuroscience, have described some of the models suggested to explain the neuroscience of attachment, and have provided a few directions for future investigations. I am looking forward enthusiastically to seeing what new technologies, approaches, and models will tell us about attachment.

References

Ahern, G. L., & Schwartz, G. E. (1985). Differential lateralization for positive and negative emotion in the human brain: EEG spectral analysis. *Neuropsychologia, 23*, 745–755.

Ainsworth, M. D. S., Blehar, M. C., Waters, E., & Wall, S. (1978). *Patterns of attachment: A psychological study of the Strange Situation.* Hillsdale, NJ: Erlbaum.

Anderson, M. C., Ochsner, K. N., Kuhl, B., Cooper, J., Robertson, E., Gabrieli, S. W., et al. (2004). Neural systems underlying the suppression of unwanted memories. *Science, 303,* 232–235.

Aron, A., Fisher, H., Mashek, D. J., Strong, G., Li, H. F., & Brown, L. L. (2005). Reward, motivation, and emotion systems associated with early-stage intense romantic love. *Journal of Neurophysiology, 94,* 327–337.

Atzil, S., Hendler, T., & Feldman, R. (2011). Specifying the neurobiological basis of human attachment: Brain, hormones, and behavior in synchronous and intrusive mothers. *Neuropsychopharmacology, 36,* 2603–2615.

Bagot, R. C., van Hasselt, F. N., Champagne, D. L., Meaney, M. J., Krugers, H. J., & Joels, M. (2009). Maternal care determines rapid effects of stress mediators on synaptic plasticity in adult rat hippocampal dentate gyrus. *Neurobiology of Learning and Memory, 92,* 292–300.

Bakermans-Kranenburg, M. J., & van IJzendoorn, M. H. (2011). Differential susceptibility to rearing environment depending on dopamine-related genes: New evidence and a meta-analysis. *Development and Psychopathology, 23,* 39–52.

Bakermans-Kranenburg, M. J., & van IJzendoorn, M. H. (2014). A sociability gene?: Meta-analysis of oxytocin receptor genotype effects in humans. *Psychiatric genetics, 24,* 45–51.

Baldwin, M. W., Keelan, J. P. R., Fehr, B., Enns, V., & Koh Rangarajoo, E. (1996). Social-cognitive conceptualization of attachment working models: Availability and accessibility effects. *Journal of Personality and Social Psychology, 71,* 94–109.

Bales, K. L., Maninger, N., & Hinde, K. (2012). New directions in the neurobiology and physiology of paternal care. In O. Gillath, G. Adams, & A. Kunkel (Eds.), *Relationship science: Integrating evolutionary, neuroscience, and sociocultural approaches* (pp. 91–111). Washington, DC: American Psychological Association.

Bartels, A., & Zeki, S. (2004). The neural correlates of maternal and romantic love. *NeuroImage, 21,* 1155–1166.

Bartz, J. A., Zaki, J., Ochsner, K. N., Bolger, N., Kolevzon, A., Ludwig, N., & Lydon, J. E. (2010). Effects of oxytocin on recollections of maternal care and closeness. *Proceedings of the National Academy of Sciences USA, 107,* 21371–21375.

Beckes, L., & Coan, J. A. (2011). Social baseline theory: The role of social proximity in emotion and economy of action. *Social and Personality Psychology Compass, 5,* 976–988.

Benetti, S., McCrory, E., Arulanantham, S., De Sanctis, T., McGuire, P., & Mechelli, A. (2010). Attachment style, affective loss and gray matter volume: A voxel-based morphometry study. *Human Brain Mapping, 31*(10), 1482–1489.

Berridge, K. C. (2007). The debate over dopamine's role in reward: The case for incentive salience. *Psychopharmacology, 191,* 391–431.

Bowlby, J. (1969/1982). *Attachment and loss: Vol. 1. Attachment.* New York: Basic Books.

Brennan, K. A., Clark, C. L., & Shaver, P. R. (1998). Self-report measurement of adult romantic attachment: An integrative overview. In J. A. Simpson & W. S. Rholes (Eds.), *Attachment theory and close relationships* (pp. 46–76). New York: Guilford Press.

Bretherton, I., & Munholland, K. A. (2008). Internal working models in attachment relationships. Elaborating a central construct. In J. Cassidy & P. R. Shaver (Eds.), *Handbook of attachment: Theory, research, and clinical applications* (2nd ed., pp. 102–127). New York: Guilford Press.

Brumbaugh, C. C., & Fraley, R. C. (2006). Transference and attachment: How do attachment patterns get carried forward from one relationship to the next? *Personality and Social Psychology Bulletin, 32,* 552–560.

Buchheim, A., Erk, S., George, C., Kächele, H., Ruchsow, M., Spitzer, M., et al. (2006). Measuring attachment representation in an fMRI environment: A pilot study. *Psychopathology, 39,* 144–152.

Burkett, J. P., & Young, L. J. (2012). The behavioral, anatomical and pharmacological parallels between social attachment, love and addiction. *Psychopharmacology, 224,* 1–26.

Calhoun, V. D., Liu, J., & Adali, T. (2009). A review of group ICA for fMRI data and ICA for joint inference of imaging, genetic, and ERP data. *NeuroImage, 45,* S163–S172.

Canterberry, M., & Gillath, O. (2012). Neural evidence for a multifaceted model of attachment security. *International Journal of Psychophysiology, 88,* 232–240.

Carter, C. S., Ahnert, L., Grossmann, K. E., Hrdy, S. B., Lamb, M. E., Porges, S. W., et al. (Eds.). (2005). *Attachment and bonding: A new synthesis* (Dahlem Workshop Reports No. 92). Cambridge, MA: MIT Press.

Caspers, K. M., Paradiso, S., Yucuis, R., Troutman, B., Arndt, S., & Philibert, R. (2009). Association between the serotonin transporter promoter polymorphism (5-HTTLPR) and adult unresolved attachment. *Developmental Psychology, 45*(1), 64–76.

Cassidy, J., & Shaver, P. R. (Eds.). (2008). *Handbook of attachment: Theory, research, and clinical applications* (2nd ed.). New York: Guilford Press.

Champagne, F., Diorio, J., Sharma, S., & Meaney, M. J. (2001). Naturally occurring variations in maternal behavior in the rat are associated with differences in estrogen-inducible central oxytocin receptors. *Proceedings of the National Academy of Sciences USA, 98,* 12736–12741.

Chen, F. S., & Johnson, S. C. (2012). An oxytocin receptor gene variant predicts attachment anxiety in females and autism-spectrum traits in males. *Social Psychological and Personality Science, 3,* 93–99.

Chiao, J. Y. (2010). At the frontier of cultural neuroscience: Introduction to the special issue. *Social Cognitive and Affective Neuroscience, 5,* 109–110.

Chisholm, K. (1998). A three year follow-up of attachment and indiscriminate friendliness in children adopted from Romanian orphanages. *Child Development, 69,* 1092–1106.

Cicchetti, D., Rogosch, F. A., & Toth, S. L. (2011). The effects of child maltreatment and polymorphisms of the serotonin transporter and dopamine D4 receptor genes on infant attachment and intervention efficacy. *Development and Psychopathology, 23,* 357–372.

Coan, J. A. (2008). Toward a neuroscience of attachment. In J. Cassidy & P. R. Shaver (Eds.), *Handbook of attachment: Theory, research, and clinical applications* (2nd ed., pp. 241–265). New York: Guilford Press.

Coan, J. A. (2010). Adult attachment and the brain. *Journal of Social and Personal Relationships, 27,* 210–217.

Cohen, M. X., & Shaver, P. R. (2004). Avoidant attachment and hemispheric lateralization of the processing of attachment- and emotion-related words. *Cognition and Emotion, 18,* 799–813.

Costa, B., Pini, S., Gabelloni, P., Abelli, M., Lari, L., Cardini, A., et al. (2009). Oxytocin receptor polymorphisms and adult attachment style in patients with depression. *Psychoneuroendocrinology, 34,* 1506–1514.

Crawford, T. N., Livesley, W. J., Jang, K. L., Shaver, P. R., Cohen, P., & Ganiban, J. (2007). Insecure attachment and personality disorder: A twin study of adults. *European Journal of Personality, 21,* 191–208.

Dan, O., & Raz, S. (2012). Adult attachment and emotional processing biases: An event-related potentials (ERPs) study. *Biological Psychology, 91,* 212–220.

Dawson, G., Ashman, S. B., Hessl, D., Spieker, S., Frey, K., Panagiotides, H., et al. (2001). Autonomic and brain electrical activity in securely- and insecurely-attached infants of depressed mothers. *Infant Behavior and Development, 24*, 135–149.

De Dreu, C. K. (2012). Oxytocin modulates the link between adult attachment and cooperation through reduced betrayal aversion. *Psychoneuroendocrinology, 37*, 871–880.

DeWall, C. N., Masten, C. L., Powell, C., Combs, D., Schurtz, D. R., & Eisenberger, N. I. (2012). Do neural responses to rejection depend on attachment style?: An fMRI study. *Social Cognitive and Affective Neuroscience, 7*, 184–192.

Del Giudice, M. (2009). Sex, attachment, and the development of reproductive strategies. *Behavioral and Brain Sciences, 32*, 1–21.

Diamond, L. M., & Fagundes, C. P. (2010). Psychobiological research on attachment. *Journal of Social and Personal Relationships, 27*, 218–225.

Donnellan, M. B., Burt, S. A., Levendosky, A. A., & Klump, K. L. (2008). Genes, personality, and attachment in adults: A multivariate behavioral genetic analysis. *Personality and Social Psychology Bulletin, 34*, 3–16.

Drevets, W. C. (2000). Neuroimaging studies of mood disorders. *Biological Psychiatry, 48*, 813–829.

Eisenberg, D. T. A., Apicella, C. L., Campbell, B. C., Dreber, A., Garcia, J. R., & Lum, J. K. (2010). Assortative human pair-bonding for partner ancestry and allelic variation of the dopamine receptor D4 (DRD4) gene. *Social Cognitive and Affective Neuroscience, 5*, 194–202.

Eisenberger, N. I., & Lieberman, M. D. (2004). Why rejection hurts: A common neural alarm system for physical and social pain. *Trends in Cognitive Sciences, 8*, 294–300.

Eisenberger, N. I., Master, S. L., Inagaki, T. K., Taylor, S. E., Shirinyan, D., Lieberman, M. D., et al. (2011). Attachment figures activate a safety signal-related neural region and reduce pain experience. *Proceedings of the National Academy of Sciences USA, 108*, 11721–11726.

Elliot, A. J., & Reis, H. T. (2003). Attachment and exploration in adulthood. *Journal of Personality and Social Psychology, 85*, 317–331.

Feldman, R., Weller, A., Zagoory-Sharon, O., & Levine, A. (2007). Evidence for a neuroendocrinological foundation of human affiliation plasma oxytocin levels across pregnancy and the postpartum period predict mother–infant bonding. *Psychological Science, 18*, 965–970.

Ferris, C. F., Kulkarni, P., Sullivan, J. M., Harder, J. A., Messenger, T. L., & Febo, M. (2005). Pup suckling is more rewarding than cocaine: Evidence from functional magnetic resonance imaging and three-dimensional computational analysis. *Journal of Neuroscience, 25*, 149–156.

Fonagy, P., Luyten, P., & Strathearn, L. (2011). Borderline personality disorder, mentalization, and the neurobiology of attachment. *Infant Mental Health Journal, 32*, 47–69.

Fraley, R. C., Roisman, G. I., Booth-LaForce, C., Owen, M. T., & Holland, A. S. (2013). Interpersonal and genetic origins of adult attachment styles: A longitudinal study from infancy to early adulthood. *Journal of Personality and Social Psychology, 104*, 817–838.

Galynker, I. I., Yaseen, Z. S., Katz, C., Zhang, X., Jennings-Donovan, G., Dash-naw, S., et al. (2012). Distinct but overlapping neural networks subserve depression and insecure attachment. *Social Cognitive and Affective Neuroscience, 7*, 896–908.

Gillath, O., Atchley, R., Imran, A., & El-Hodiri, M. (2014). *Attachment, game theory, and neuroscience: Examining the enhancement and experience of generous behavior.* Manuscript submitted for publication.

Gillath, O., Bunge, S. A., Shaver, P. R., Wendelken, C., & Mikulincer, M. (2005). Attachment-style differences in the ability to suppress negative thoughts: Exploring the neural correlates. *NeuroImage, 28*, 835–847.

Gillath, O., Canterberry, M., & Collins, T. J. (2012). A multilevel multimethod interdisciplinary approach to the understanding of attachment? In O. Gillath, G. Adams, & A. D. Kunkel (Eds.), *Relationship science: Integrating evolutionary, neuroscience, and sociocultural approaches* (pp. 219–240). Washington, DC: American Psychological Association.

Gillath, O., Giesbrecht, B., & Shaver, P. R. (2009). Attachment, attention, and cognitive control: Attachment style and performance on general attention tasks. *Journal of Experimental Social Psychology, 45*, 647–654.

Gillath, O., Hart, J., Noftle, E. E., & Stockdale, G. D. (2009). Development and validation of a state adult attachment measure (SAAM). *Journal of Research in Personality, 43*, 362–373.

Gillath, O., Pressman, S., Stetler, D., & Moskovitz, J. (2014). *Attachment security and metabolic energy: Enhancement of security results with increased blood glucose.* Manuscript submitted for publication.

Gillath, O., Selcuk, E., & Shaver, P. R. (2008). Moving toward a secure attachment style: Can repeated security priming help? *Social and Personality Psychology Compass, 2*(4), 1651–1666.

Gillath, O., Sesko, A. K., Shaver, P. R., & Chun, D. S. (2010). Attachment, authenticity, and honesty: Dispositional and experimentally induced security can reduce self- and other-deception. *Journal of Personality and Social Psychology, 98*, 841–855.

Gross, C., Zhuang, X., Stark, K., Ramboz, S., Oosting, R., Kirby, L., et al. (2002). Serotonin 1A receptor acts during development to establish normal anxiety-like behavior in the adult. *Nature, 416*, 396–400.

Hellige, J. B. (1993). *Hemispheric asymmetry.* Cambridge, MA: Harvard University Press.

Hillyard, S. A., Teder-Sälejärvi, W. A., & Münte, T. F. (1998). Temporal dynamics of early perceptual processing. *Current Opinion in Neurobiology, 8*, 202–210.

Insel, T. R., & Young, L. J. (2001). The neurobiology of attachment. *Nature Reviews Neuroscience, 2*, 129–136.

Karremans, J. C., Heslenfeld, D. J., van Dillen, L. F., & Van Lange, P. A. (2011). Secure attachment partners attenuate neural responses to social exclusion: An fMRI investigation. *International Journal of Psychophysiology, 81*, 44–50.

Kennedy, P. J., & Shapiro, M. L. (2004). Retrieving memories via internal context requires the hippocampus. *Journal of Neuroscience, 24*, 6979–6985.

Lakatos, K., Nemoda, Z., Toth, I., Ronai, Z., Ney, K., Sasvari-Szekely, M., et al. (2002). Further evidence for the role of the dopamine D4 receptor (DRD4) gene in attachment disorganization: Interaction of the exon III 48-bp repeat and the 521-C/T promoter polymorphisms. *Molecular Psychiatry, 7*, 27–31.

Lemche, E., Giampietro, V. P., Surguladze, S. A., Amaro, E. J., Andrew, C. M., Williams, S. C. R., et al. (2006). Human attachment security is mediated by the amygdala: Evidence from combined fMRI and psychophysiological measures. *Human Brain Mapping, 27*, 623–635.

Levinger, G. (1994). Figure versus ground: Micro- and macro perspectives on the social psychology of personal relationships. In R. Erber & R. Gilmour (Eds.), *Theoretical frameworks for personal relationships* (pp. 1–28). Hillsdale, NJ: Erlbaum.

Lieberman, M. D. (2007). Social cognitive neuroscience: A review of core processes. *Annual Review of Psychology, 58*, 259–289.

Lim, M. M., & Young, L. J. (2006). Neuropeptidergic regulation of affiliative behavior and social bonding in animals. *Hormones and Behavior, 50*, 506–517.

MacDonald, K., & MacDonald, T. M. (2011). The peptide that binds: A systematic review of oxytocin and its prosocial effects in humans. *Harvard Review of Psychiatry, 18*, 1–21.

Main, M., & Solomon, J. (1990). Procedures for identifying infants as disorganized-disoriented during the Ainsworth Strange Situation. In M. T. Greenberg, D. Cicchetti, & E. M. Cummings (Eds.), *Attachment in the preschool years: Theory, research and intervention* (pp. 121–160). Chicago: University of Chicago Press.

Mikulincer, M., Gillath, O., & Shaver, P. R. (2002). Activation of the attachment system in adulthood: Threat-related primes increase the accessibility of mental representations of attachment figures. *Journal of Personality and Social Psychology, 83*, 881–895.

Mikulincer, M., Hirschberger, G., Nachmias, O., & Gillath, O. (2001). The affective component of the secure base schema: Affective priming with representations of attachment security. *Journal of Personality and Social Psychology, 81*, 305–321.

Mikulincer, M., & Shaver, P. R. (2007a). *Attachment in adulthood: Structure, dynamics, and change.* New York: Guilford Press.

Mikulincer, M., & Shaver, P. R. (2007b). Boosting attachment security to promote mental health, prosocial values, and inter-group tolerance. *Psychological Inquiry, 18*, 139–156.

Miller, E. K., & Cohen, J. D. (2001). An integrative theory of prefrontal cortex function. *Annual Review of Neuroscience, 24*, 167–202.

Nash, K., Prentice, M., Hirsh, J., McGregor, I., & Inzlicht, M. (2014). Muted neural response to distress among securely attached people. *Social Cognitive and Affective Neuroscience, 9*(8), 1239–1245.

Niedenthal, P. M., Brauer, M., Robin, L., & Innes-Ker, A. H. (2002). Adult attachment and the perception of facial expression of emotion. *Journal of Personality and Social Psychology 82*, 419–433.

O'Connor, T. G., & Croft, C. M. (2001). A twin study of attachment in preschool children. *Child Development, 72*, 1501–1511.

Panksepp, J. (1998). *Affective neuroscience: The foundations of human and animal emotions.* New York: Oxford University Press.

Phelps, E. A., & LeDoux, J. E. (2005). Contributions of the amygdala to emotion processing: From animal models to human behavior. *Neuron, 48,* 175–187.

Pietromonaco, P. R., & Barrett, L. F. (2000). Internal working models: What do we really know about the self in relation to others? *Review of General Psychology, 4,* 155–175.

Powers, S. I., Pietromonaco, P. R., Gunlicks, M., & Sayer, A. (2006). Dating couples' attachment styles and patterns of cortisol reactivity and recovery in response to a relationship conflict. *Journal of Personality and Social Psychology, 90,* 613–628.

Quirin, M., Gillath, O., Eggert, L., Pruessner, J., Kuestermann, E., & Kuhl, J. (2010). Attachment insecurity and cell density in the hippocampus. *Social Cognitive and Affective Neuroscience, 5,* 39–47.

Raleigh, M. J., Brammer, G. L., & McGuire, M. T. (1983). Male dominance, serotonergic systems, and the behavioral and physiological effects of drugs in vervet monkeys (*Cercopithecus aethiops sabaeus*). In K. A. Miczek (Ed.), *Ethopharmacology: Primate models of neuropsychiatric disorders* (pp. 185–197). New York: Alan R. Liss.

Ray, R. D., Shelton, A. L., Hollon, N. G., Matsumoto, D., Frankel, C. B., Gross, J. J., et al. (2010). Interdependent self-construal and neural representations of self and mother. *Social Cognitive and Affective Neuroscience, 5*(2–3), 318–323.

Redgrave, P., Prescott, T. J., & Gurney, K. (1999). The basal ganglia: A vertebrate solution to the selection problem? *Neuroscience, 89,* 1009–1023.

Rockliff, H., Karl, A., McEwan, K., Gilbert, J., Matos, M., & Gilbert, P. (2011). Effects of intranasal oxytocin on "compassion focused imagery." *Emotion, 11,* 1388–1396.

Salo, J., Jokela, M., Lehtimäki, T., & Keltikangas-Järvinen, L. (2011). Serotonin receptor 2A gene moderates the effect of childhood maternal nurturance on adulthood social attachment. *Genes, Brain and Behavior, 10,* 702–709.

Schneier, F. R., Liebowitz, M. R., Abi-Dargham, A., Zea-Ponce, Y., Lin, S. H., & Laruelle, M. (2000). Low dopamine D2 receptor binding potential in social phobia. *American Journal of Psychiatry, 157,* 457–459.

Strathearn, L., Fonagy, P., Amico, J., & Montague, P. R. (2009). Adult attachment predicts maternal brain and oxytocin response to infant cues. *Neuropsychopharmacology, 34,* 2655–2666.

Tharner, A., Herba, C. M., Luijk, M. P., van IJzendoorn, M. H., Bakermans-Kranenburg, M. J., Govaert, P. P., et al. (2011). Subcortical structures and the neurobiology of infant attachment disorganization: A longitudinal ultrasound imaging study. *Social Neuroscience, 6,* 336–347.

Troisi, A., Frazzetto, G., Carola, V., Di Lorenzo, G., Coviello, M., Siracusano, A., et al. (2012). Variation in the μ-opioid receptor gene (OPRM1) moderates the influence of early maternal care on fearful attachment. *Social Cognitive and Affective Neuroscience, 7,* 542–547.

Vrticka, P., Andersson, F., Grandjean, D., Sander, D., & Vuilleumier, P. (2008). Individual attachment style modulates human amygdala and striatum activation during social appraisal. *PLoS ONE, 3,* e2868.

Vrticka, P., & Vuilleumier, P. (2012). Neuroscience of human social interactions and adult attachment style. *Frontiers in Human Neuroscience, 6,* 212.

Warren, S. L., Bost, K. K., Roisman, G. I., Silton, R. L., Spielberg, J. M., Engels, A. S., et al. (2010). Effects of adult attachment and emotional distractors on brain mechanisms of cognitive control. *Psychological Science, 21,* 1818–1826.

Whitehead, C. (2010). The culture ready brain. *Social Cognitive and Affective Neuroscience, 5,* 168–179.

Wilson, M. (2010). The re-tooled mind: How culture re-engineers cognition. *Social Cognitive and Affective Neuroscience, 5,* 180–187.

Young, L. J., & Wang, Z. (2004). The neurobiology of pair bonding. *Nature Neuroscience, 7,* 1048–1054.

Zayas, V., & Hazan, C. (Eds.). (2015). *Bases of adult attachment: Linking brain, mind, and behavior.* New York: Springer.

Zayas, V., Shoda, Y., Mischel, W., Osterhout, L., & Takahashi, M. (2009). Neural responses to partner rejection cues. *Psychological Science, 20,* 813–821.

Zhang, X., Li, T., & Zhou, X. (2008). Brain responses to facial expressions by adults with different attachment-orientations. *NeuroReport, 19,* 437–441.

Zilber, A., Goldstein, A., & Mikulincer, M. (2007). Adult attachment orientations and the processing of emotional pictures–ERP correlates. *Personality and Individual Differences, 43,* 1898–1907.

Fooled Around and Fell in Love

The Role of Sex in Adult Romantic
Attachment Formation

Vivian Zayas
Sarah Merrill
Cindy Hazan

A central proposition of Bowlby's ethological attachment theory is that attachment is integral to human behavior throughout the lifespan, "from the cradle to the grave" (1979, p. 129). The theory provides a comprehensive and detailed account of the evolutionary roots, ontogeny, and developmental sequelae of infant–caregiver bonds. Although in adulthood individuals may be attached to multiple individuals (e.g., parents, friends, siblings; Baldwin, Keelan, Fehr, Enns, & Koh-Rangarajoo, 1996), the theory posits that *pair bonds*, or relationships between romantic partners, are the prototypical instantiation of attachment in adulthood.

Whether in infancy or adulthood, the features that distinguish attachment bonds from other types of social ties are the same (Hazan & Shaver, 1987). Specifically, attachments are characterized by *proximity seeking/ maintenance* (the tendency to stay in touch), *safe haven* (the tendency to turn to attachment figures for comfort or reassurance), *separation distress* (the tendency to resist and be upset by unwanted or prolonged separations), and *secure base* (the tendency to explore because one is emboldened by knowing that support is available when needed).

Despite these similarities in attachment relationships, infant–caregiver relationships and adult romantic relationships differ in important ways.

In particular, infant–caregiver relationships are typically complementary. That is, infants seek security and comfort from, but do not intentionally provide security or comfort to, attachment figures. In contrast, adult romantic relationships are reciprocal: Partners serve as both recipients and providers of security and comfort. In addition, and most relevant to the present chapter, adult romantic relationships are typically sexual in nature. In other words, adult attachment bonds involve the integration of three distinct behavioral systems: attachment, caregiving, and sexual mating.

It is thus somewhat surprising how very little adult attachment research has addressed the sexual mating system. Indeed, the fields of sex research and adult attachment research have progressed quite independently. Although sex can be an entirely casual or even solo activity, most sexual interactions occur within the context of an ongoing romantic relationship (Impett, Muise, & Peragine, 2013). The specific question that we address in the present chapter is what role sex may play in the formation of an adult attachment bond. For the purposes of this chapter, we are defining *sexual interactions* as any behaviors that are motivated by an urge to gratify sexual motivation, including (but not limited to) sexual touch, sexual kissing, rubbing or stimulation of the genitals, nipples, or other erogenous zones, cunnilingus, fellatio, and vaginal and anal penetration.

The process by which two individuals go from being relative strangers to having developed a full-fledged attachment bond is still not well understood (Zayas & Hazan, 2015). Nonetheless, there is good reason to think about the role of sex in adult attachment. We propose that the sexual mating system is first involved in sparking initial attraction and interest in, and promoting proximity toward, one person (over all other potential partners). But also, critically, once a relationship is under way, repeated sexual activity with the same partner is expected to condition basic physiological and endocrinological systems; this conditioning, in turn, distinguishes this relationship from others and serves to promote a pair bond.

In particular, in initial stages of relationship formation, the sexual mating system is involved in attraction, and this has important implications for attachment formation. As noted above, a defining feature of attachment is proximity seeking. Humans are an altricial species, and offspring are born in a state of extreme immaturity and dependence. As a result of evolutionary processes, human infants are born with an attachment system that promotes seeking and maintaining proximity to important others (adult caregivers) who are able to provide protection, support, and comfort (Bowlby, 1982). But what motivates mature members of the human species to seek proximity to each other? One major force is sexual attraction. Infants are drawn to conspecifics in early life because their very lives depend on seeking protection and care, but adults are motivated to seek proximity to and contact with others for reasons of sexual interest. By fostering physical intimacy and triggering associated neurochemical systems, this initial sexual attraction sets the stage for potentially developing a full-fledged attachment relationship.

Moreover, as the relationship gets under way, the sexual mating system plays a key role in transforming the relationship from one of simple attraction between two strangers to one between two attached partners. In this respect, there are two issues of central importance. First, although the sexual mating and attachment systems are distinct and independent, and have evolved to serve different functions (Diamond, 2004), there is still considerable overlap in basic structures of the two systems (Diamond & Dickenson, 2012). Second, having sex repeatedly with the same person engages these specific (and overlapping) brain structures and activates specific neurochemical systems that facilitate the formation of an adult attachment bond. In what follows, we focus specifically on the dopaminergic reward system and the oxytocinergic/opioid arousal-relieving systems. The take-home message of the extant findings, which are discussed below, is that through repeated sexual exchanges with the same person, these systems become conditioned. The effect of the conditioning is that this other person, whether physically present or just mentally conjured, can automatically activate these systems. This process of the conditioning of specific reward and relief neural systems, in our view, is the core of adult attachment formation.

First, a few caveats. Exactly how sex affects adult attachment is complicated, and is likely to vary as a function of multiple individual and group, and possibly gender, factors. We intentionally suspend commentary on these possible variations (although we return to them at the end of the chapter) in order to focus attention on a set of processes and mechanisms that have yet to be articulated or explored in the attachment literature, and that hold promise for shedding light on the role of sexual intercourse in the formation of adult attachment bonds.

The chapter is organized as follows. We begin by providing a brief summary of the behavioral, psychological, physiological, and neural correlates assumed to characterize an adult attachment bond. We then describe the basic physiological and neural processes involved in sexual intercourse, and highlight systems that overlap with the attachment system. We conclude by raising many interesting, but as yet unanswered, questions with regard to personal and situational moderators of the purported model that we hope will fuel future investigations.

The Adult Attachment System

In adulthood, long-term pair bonds confer a number of psychological and physical benefits. Partners are capable of regulating each other's physiological systems, daily mood and affective states, and eating and sleeping patterns (Selcuk, Zayas, & Hazan, 2010). There is a rich literature delineating the precise psychological and neural systems that underlie adult pair bonds and give rise to attachment-related behaviors (proximity maintenance, safe haven, secure base, and separation distress) (see Mikulincer & Shaver, 2007, for review).

These manifestations of adult pair bonds in terms of physiology, emotion, and behavior are assumed to reflect the functioning of *mental representations*, or *internal working models*. A core idea of attachment theory is that the residue of past interactions with the particular partner, as well as of interactions in other past and present relationships, is stored in memory (e.g., Bowlby, 1973, 1982; Bretherton & Munholland, 2008; Collins, Guichard, Ford, & Feeney, 2004; Pietromonaco & Barrett, 2000; Zayas, Mischel, Shoda, & Aber, 2011). Mental representations consist of detailed memories of interactions with, and conscious and nonconscious affective evaluations of, attachment figures (e.g., Zayas & Shoda, 2005, 2014), as well as strategies to regulate negative affect (e.g., turning to attachment figures to alleviate negative affect, or turning away from attachment figures and coping through other means; e.g., Zayas, Shoda, Osterhout, Takahashi, & Mischel, 2009) in stressful and threatening situations (e.g., Collins et al., 2004; Pietromonaco, Barrett, & Powers, 2006). Mental representations are impactful because they implicitly affect perceptions and expectations about likely events (e.g., "If I seek help, then I will be supported"; see, e.g., Baldwin et al., 1993; Zayas et al., 2009), which in turn affect physiology, emotion, and behavior, and may do so without a person's having any conscious awareness of the process (Günaydin, Zayas, Selcuk, & Hazan, 2012).

Dopaminergic Reward System and Proximity Seeking

People move toward (approach) aspects of their environment that are rewarding, and move away from (avoid) those aspects that are not. The extent to which mental representations are associated with positive (or negative) evaluations in memory is assumed to guide approach and avoidance behaviors. A straightforward hypothesis is that various behaviors aimed at promoting proximity seeking (i.e., preferring one's partner over others) and desire for closeness reflect underlying partner representations that are laden with positive affect and hugely rewarding. Indeed, research has found that partner representations automatically activate strong positive reactions (Zayas & Shoda, 2005), and that individual differences in the strength of the automatic evaluations predict relationship closeness, satisfaction, relationship length (Zayas & Shoda, 2005) and breakup (Lee, Rogge, & Reis, 2010), even among newlyweds (McNulty, Olson, Meltzer, & Shaffer, 2013).

Studies using functional magnetic resonance imaging (fMRI) have shown that activating the mental representations of a one's partner—for example, by viewing a photograph of the partner—recruits the dopaminergic system (Aron et al., 2005; Bartels & Zeki, 2004). Dopamine-rich neural structures, such as the ventral tegmental area (VTA) and nucleus accumbens shell (NAS), are activated by stimuli with rewarding properties (e.g., food, sex, drugs, and neutral stimuli paired with reward) and are implicated in various manifestations of appetitive motivation and approach behaviors. Specifically, encountering a rewarding stimulus leads to a release of dopamine in the VTA, which projects to other structures in the limbic system such as the NAS (Fisher, Aron, & Brown, 2005; Bartels & Zeki, 2004). The activation of this pathway has been associated with subjective feelings of elation, excitement, desire, and wanting; with promoting approach behaviors through activation of locomotion in the motor system; and with physiological changes, such as increases in heart rate and blood pressure, via activation of the sympathetic nervous system (Balfour, Yu, & Coolen, 2004). Thus findings that adult romantic partners activate this dopaminergic/reward system suggest that these individuals too are subjectively rewarding and that such neural activation promotes and maintains approach-related interpersonal behaviors, such as proximity seeking.

Oxytocinergic/Opioid Arousal-Relieving Systems and Safe-Haven Functions

Pair bonds are not simply defined by the experience of pleasure and joy they confer. One feature that distinguishes attachment figures from other personally close individuals is that they serve as a safe haven. Attachment figures provide a source of relief from distress. A person who feels distressed—as a result of appraising the environment as threatening or the self as in need of help—seeks proximity to his or her attachment figure. If the attachment figure is available and responsive, the resulting contact is expected to alleviate the distress and restore emotional and physiological balance.

What is critical in order for the distress-relieving properties to emerge is the sheer repetition of interactions. Repeated positive interactions with attachment figures during times of stress reinforce the association in long-term memory between bids for support and stress reduction (e.g., Mikulincer & Shaver, 2003, 2007; Mikulincer, Shaver, & Pereg, 2003; Sroufe & Waters, 1977). At a cognitive level, these repeated interactions are encoded in mental representations as "if–then" contingencies, such as "If I turn to my partner, then I will feel safe" (e.g., Baldwin, Fehr, Keedian, Seidel, & Thomson, 1993). At a physiological level, through processes of conditioning, the person providing the comfort eventually acquires properties that signal safety and relief (e.g., Beckes, Simpson, & Erickson, 2010). Thus, eventually, simply the mental representation of the attachment figure, even in the absence of the attachment figure's actual presence, becomes capable of activating psychological and physiological states of safety and calmness originally induced by actual interactions with the figure (e.g., Depue & Morrone-Strupinsky, 2005; Uvnäs-Moberg, 1998).

Indeed, numerous studies provide support for the proposition that partners enhance affect regulation (for reviews, see Sbarra & Hazan, 2008; Selcuk et al., 2010). For instance, intimate and supportive interactions with a romantic partner, compared to nonsupportive interactions with a partner or with being alone, lead to greater calmness while anticipating a stressor (e.g., Simpson, Rholes, & Nelligan, 1992); smaller elevations in self-reported anxiety and physiological reactivity (i.e., systolic blood pressure, diastolic blood pressure, heart rate, and cortisol level; e.g., Collins & Ford, 2010; Ditzen et al., 2007; Grewen, Anderson, Girdler, & Light, 2003); attenuation of neural threat responses while experiencing a stressor (e.g., Coan, Schaefer, & Davidson, 2006); and faster emotional recovery following a stressor (e.g., Collins & Ford, 2010). Moreover, some of the distress-relieving benefits are realized simply by activating the mental representation of the partner, even in the absence of his or her actual presence. For example, simply viewing a photograph of one's partner diminishes the experience of a mildly painful stimulus (Eisenberger et al., 2011; Master et al., 2009) and lessens the deleterious affective and cognitive consequences of relieving a distressing autobiographical memory (Selcuk, Zayas, Günaydin, Hazan, & Kross, 2012).

A growing body of research has focused on identifying the neural and endocrinological mechanisms that confer these distress-alleviating effects. This work, from both the human and animal literatures, converges on the idea that interactions with attachment figures, whether actual or symbolic, increase activity of two neurotransmitter systems: oxytocin, which promotes feelings of trust, love, security, and affiliation; and endogenous opioids such as beta-endorphins, which promote relaxation and well-being, and (most importantly) decrease the experience of physical and emotional pain (Depue & Morrone-Strupinsky, 2005; Sbarra & Hazan, 2008; Young & Wang, 2004; Zak, Kurzban, & Matzner, 2005). The release of these neurotransmitters, in turn, serves to down-regulate threat-related reactivity of the hypothalamic–pituitary–adrenocortical (HPA) axis and the autonomic nervous system (ANS) (Diamond, 2001; McCubbin, 1993; Uvnäs-Moberg, 1998).

The threat response of the HPA axis and ANS has been well documented. In response to an external or internal threat, the hippocampus, involved in memory, and the bed nucleus of the stria terminalis (BNST) of the amygdala, an important brain region in the anxiety pathway, become activated and trigger a cascade of physiological responses to signal potential danger. In particular, the BNST, which provides threat feedback to the hippocampus, produces corticotropin-releasing hormone (CRH)—a precursor to cortisol, the stress hormone (Aguilera & Liu, 2012). This activates an ANS response by releasing cortisol (a glucocorticoid) into the bloodstream.

This pathway occurs in a feedback loop that causes enduring hyperexcitability until the potential danger passes.

Oxytocin and mu-opiates serve as an anxiolytic and essentially downregulate this HPA activation (Scantamburlo et al., 2007; Taylor et al., 2006; Wiedenmayer & Barr, 2000; Windle, Shanks, Lightman, & Ingram, 1997). Both neurotransmitters are released in response to various affiliative and social cues. For example, oxytocin is released in response to hugging, physical touch, sexual interactions, and orgasm (Insel, 1992), and mu-opiates are released in response to caressing touch, ventro-ventral contact, and sexual activity, especially genital stimulation (Insel, 1997; Nelson & Panksepp. 1998; Silk, Alberts, & Altmann, 2003). To the extent that past experiences with partners involved these interactions, these physiological states are encoded into the mental representation of the current partner; eventually, simply bringing the representation of the partner to mind, even in his or her physical absence, is sufficient to trigger their release (Carter, 1992).

Once released, oxytocin and opiates serve to down-regulate the HPA threat response. Oxytocin circulates centrally through the paraventricular nucleus (PVN) of the hypothalamus and has a negative influence on a number of areas involved in the detection and processing of threat—such as the anterior cingulate cortex (ACC), which is implicated in stress and emotional processing, as well as the BNST, amygdala, and hippocampus. The negative influence on the BNST subsequently reduces the amount of CRH produced, and thus cortisol, effectively reducing the duration of the stress response (Liberzon & Young, 1997; Oliet, Oliva, Castro, & Pérez-Segarra, 2007; Aguilera & Liu, 2012).

The Sexual Mating System

The sexual mating and attachment systems are distinct and independent, and have evolved to serve different functions (Diamond, 2004). Nonetheless, we propose that sexual intercourse activates several physiological and neural systems that overlap considerably with the attachment behavioral system. One correlate of our argument is that if sex is repeated with the same partner over time, neural and physiological states of sexual activity will become conditioned to the partner, and to the extent that these processes overlap with those underlying the attachment system, sex is expected to promote feelings of attachment security and facilitate the formation of the pair bond.

In what follows, we briefly describe the neural and hormonal systems associated with two constituent parts of sexual activity: the incentive/motivation reward system implicated in the *appetitive phase* (also known as the *approach phase*), which regulates sexual motivation, sexual desire, sexual arousal, and courtship behavior (Woolley, Sakata, Gupta, & Crews, 2001); and the consummatory system implicated in the *consummatory phase*, which is involved in feelings of satiation and sedation following attainment of the goal (Hinde, 1970).

To illustrate the basic activation of the sexual mating system (and later how it may promote adult attachment) in the sections that follow, we refer to a hypothetical scenario in which two individuals, Sam and Alex, meet for the first time and experience sexual attraction. A number of cues, such as facial shape and appearance, scent, body posture, and so on, will affect whether Sam will find Alex attractive.

The Appetitive Phase

The Role of the Dopaminergic Reward System

The appetitive phase in initial attraction and romantic interest is governed by the same incentive/motivation reward system active in many other fundamental behaviors, such as eating, sleeping, and drinking (Depue & Collins, 1999; Gray, 1973; Panksepp. 1986). This system is active in sexual motivation and the anticipation of sexual interaction. Moreover, both the incentive/motivation reward system and the consummatory system (discussed next) play prominent roles during actual sexual intercourse. The two systems overlap during intercourse, so that once distal cues (the possibility of sex) give way to proximal cues, as well as the incentive and possible anticipatory release of dopaminergic reward that precedes various sexual behaviors (e.g., orgasm) during the sexual encounter.

Similar to other approach behaviors, the incentive/reward motivation system is involved in the appetitive phase of sexual activity involving sexual desire and motivation. Sexual desire characterizes the myriad of behaviors that can be referred to as "courtship" and lead up to the goal of actually having sex. Thus approach behaviors range in their proximity to the goal, from seemingly distal behaviors, such as a phone call, glance of the eyes, or touch of the hand, to more proximal actions such as kissing, undressing the partner, and foreplay. All of these phases are considered appetitive in that they still involve approaching actual sexual interaction, but not having them.

In all varied aspects of these approach-related behaviors, the incentive/motivation system is at work and reflects the dopaminergic reaction in the mesolimbic reward centers of the brain (e.g., VTA, NAS) triggered in response to a rewarding stimuli. When Sam meets Alex for the first time, a number of cues, such as facial shape and appearance, scent, body posture, and so on, will affect whether Sam will find Alex attractive. Research shows not only that initial evaluations of attraction based on a photograph activate dopaminergic reward areas, but that initial evaluations of interest are strong predictors of actual behavioral intentions to date the person later (in a speed-dating paradigm; Cooper, Dunne, Furey, & O'Doherty, 2012). So, for Sam, cues associated with Alex—someone Sam inherently finds physically attractive—serve to activate the appetitive neural and behavioral systems. Subjectively, Sam's simply seeing Alex is likely to elicit an ecstatic high from dopamine release, which is a subjective high associated with stimuli that are the most rewarding. This actually occurs *before* Sam reaches Alex, in anticipation of the reward Sam will receive by interacting, possibly successfully, with an attractive potential mate. Behaviorally, this anticipatory dopaminergic reward occurs in order to propel an individual toward a rewarding stimulus, not to receive the reward itself (Depue & Collins, 1999). Sam will probably desire to engage in a number of approach-oriented behaviors, such as physically get closer to, talk with, and maintain eye contact with Alex (Breiter, Aharon, Kahneman, Dale, & Shizgal, 2001; Aharon et al., 2001).

Magnitude of Affiliative Reward

Although the reward system is involved in the processing of a wide range of rewarding stimuli, one difference in processing underlying affiliative interactions with a potential partner as compared to the processing of other rewarding stimuli (e.g., food) is in the magnitude of the neural activation and subsequent response (Meston & Frohlich, 2000). The incentive/motivation system responds proportionally to the magnitude of the perceived reward (Depue & Morrone-Strupinsky, 2005). For example, the amount of dopamine released by the VTA is directly dependent on how rewarding the experience is expected to be, as the appetitive reward is of an anticipatory nature. If the stimulus is more or less rewarding when experienced, then the incentive/motivation system adjusts, through feedback from the consummatory opioid reward system, to this difference and adjusts the expected reward accordingly (Depue & Collins, 1999). In this regard, sex (or the possibility of it) is one of the most powerful rewarding stimuli (Meston & Buss, 2007; Pfaff, 1999), triggering a large amount of dopaminergic action in the NAS (Pfaus, Damsma, Wenkstern, & Fibiger, 1995). To return to Sam and Alex, the appetitive phase is characterized by a highly excited state as they approach one another and engage in a variety of sexual behaviors. Moreover, the highest dopaminergic release during sexual activity happens approximately 2 minutes before the point of orgasm, when a large amount of dopamine is released in expectation of the impending reward stimulus (Young & Wang, 2004). Therefore, there is a dopaminergic reward delivered in anticipation of achieving the goal of sexual activity, as well as a separate dopaminergic reward delivered in anticipation of achieving the separate goal of orgasm.

Potentiation of Reward Processing via Oxytocin Activation

Relatedly, a second way in which the processing of affiliative stimuli differs from the processing of rewarding stimuli in other domains is due to the interactions between dopamine system functioning and oxytocin, vasopressin, and mu-opiates (Depue & Morrone-Strupinsky, 2005). Dopamine in the NAS may increase sexual arousal and penile erections, through the release of increasing central oxytocinergic activity when presented within the behavioral context of responding to a sociosexual stimulus (Argiolas, 1999). Similarly, oxytocin increases the dopamine release in VTA to the NAS, which leads to increased dopaminergic activity and increased sexual motivation (Melis, Enrico, Peana, & Diana, 2007). Studies in mice, rats, and prairie voles have found that oxytocin's ability to innervate dopamine neurons in the VTA sensitizes the reward system to dopamine (Kovács, Sarnyai, & Szabó, 1998; Shahrokh, Zhang, Diorio, Gratton, & Meaney, 2010). This makes the incentive reward of sexual stimuli greater in magnitude, since the amount of dopamine being released in the brain increases.

One important implication of the interactions between oxytocin and dopamine is with the formation and development of mental representations. It has been hypothesized that these interactions during the appetitive phase enhance the encoding of social contextual ensemble (e.g., partner scent, touch, facial structure) and reward associations that are defining features of mental representations (Argiolas, 1999). Subsequently, this may be one pathway by which sex facilitates the process of transforming representations of a stranger to the representation of a partner, and thus creating a lasting pair bond (Lim & Young, 2006).

The Consummatory Phase

If dopamine is released *prior* to the reward (during goal pursuit), this raises a question: What happens once Sam and Alex have actually reached their goal of sexual activity? That is, in this example, what happens neurologically to Sam and Alex, beginning during their sexual encounter and continuing once they have finished copulating and their orgasms have (ideally) taken place? The answer is that now that they are in close proximity to their goal—in this case, a sexual interaction with a sexually desirable mate—the appetitive reward phase moves on to the consummatory reward phase (Herbert, 1993). Some examples of what constitute a proximal cue, as opposed to a distal cue, that signals the consummatory phase would be sexual touch, gentle stroking, and running one's hands through the partner's hair, as well as genital stimulation and orgasm. Essentially, whereas appetitive reward is delivered *before* and *during* sex, consummatory reward is delivered *during* and *after* sex.

While appetitive reward is characterized by desire and arousal, consummatory reward is characterized by feelings of liking, pleasure, and gratification (Smillie, 2013). Similarly, whereas appetitive reward triggers approach-oriented action, consummatory reward triggers a cessation of approach behavior—namely, sedation and rest (Hilliard, Domjan, Nguyen, & Cusato, 1998). Thus consummatory reward reinforces the behaviors initiated and sustained by appetitive reward (Porges, 1998, 2001).

In the case of Sam and Alex, the consummatory reward system becomes active once they have become proximal to their goal, which is in this case to engage in sexual touch and activity with one another. During the sexual encounter, the consummatory reward overlaps with the incentive/motivation system. This is because the incentive/motivation system is still driving Sam and Alex toward orgasm, which is a separate, though often associated, reward goal (Berridge, 1999). At the end of this sexual interaction, Sam and Alex should feel gratified, calm, satiated, and lethargic.

Opioid System and Consummatory Phase

Consummatory reward is characterized by endogenous endorphin and opioid action in the brain. The involvement of this system in pair-bond maintenance in nonhuman primates has been confirmed, and it may be even more important in humans (Machin & Dunbar, 2011). In the case of sociosexual interactions, beta-endorphins are released and interact preferentially with mu-opioid receptors (Keverne, Martensz, & Tuite, 1989). Beta-endorphins are actually the most potent endogenous opioid peptides, with 80 times the analgesic potency of morphine, which also binds to the mu-opioid receptors. Regardless of the potency of beta-endorphins, the number of mu-opioid receptors directly affects the subjective experience of consummatory reward, and the prevalence of these receptors in the brain is affected by age and early life experiences (Machin & Dunbar, 2011). Activation of these mu-opioid receptors in the central nervous system causes a decrease in heart rate and blood pressure, as well as feelings of euphoria and sedation, all of which are mediated by increases in inhibitory parasympathetic activity (Irnaten et al., 2003). This opiate receptor activity also increases pain thresholds, and may be responsible for the elevated pain thresholds that are seen in concert with romantic relationships and during orgasm (Younger, Aron, Parke, Chatterjee, & Mackey, 2010; Whipple & Komisaruk, 1985). The magnitude of opiate receptor activation, which is the incentive value of the stimuli, is encoded along with the sensory cues of the immediate surrounds, associated feelings, and distinct characteristics of the sexual stimuli (usually the partner) in frontal cortex and hippocampus. This information is then used to determine the expected magnitude of the reward the next time this contextual ensemble takes place, and the subsequent appropriate anticipatory reward to incentivize individuals toward the sexual stimulus (Depue & Morrone-Strupinsky, 2005).

With regard to the consummatory phase, when the potential reward is proximal to the person, beta-endorphin-related opiate peptides (mostly mu-opiates, but also sometimes delta-opiates) are released in response to introceptive (internal cues, such as emotions, feelings, or arousal) and proximal exteroceptive (external cues, such as physical manifestations of a close reward goal or objective) stimuli (Hilliard et al., 1998; Depue & Morrone-Strupinsky, 2005).

Beta-endorphin-related opiate peptides are also active in the VTA and NAS pathway, similar to dopamine. People who were given an opiate antagonist reported that their orgasms were less *pleasurable* than those of participants on a placebo (Murphy, Checkley, Seckl, & Lightman, 1990). Essentially, the role of opiates in sexual experiences is to enhance the subjective experience of pleasure, satiation, and calm arousal relief. After sexual activity, mu-opiates are activated—especially in an important area for sexual reward processing, the medial preoptic area—within about 30 minutes after coitus, and are internalized continuously for approximately 6 hours (Coolen, Fitzgerald, Yu, & Lehman, 2004). However, in high doses, mu-opiates have an inhibitory effect on the appetitive process and lead to reduced sexual desire, making it more difficult (along with prolactin) to have consecutive, repeated sexual encounters. This is because it is very unusual for both the appetitive and consummatory reward processes to be active at the same time, just by virtue of their respective functions, with the exception of the crossover during sexual activity. Therefore, the interneurons in the dopaminergic pathway between the VTA and NAS are regulated by mu-opioid receptor activation that can inhibit dopamine receptors from firing (Balfour et al., 2004).

Oxytocin during the Consummatory Phase

Murphy et al. (1990) also suggest that mu-opiates are related to its interaction with the release of oxytocin. An important interaction that can be found between oxytocin and the endogenous opiate/endorphin system is that oxytocin inhibits the development of a tolerance to opiates (Machin & Dunbar, 2011; Kovács et al., 1998). This has the *very* important effect of preventing the magnitude of the consummatory reward from decreasing over time. Whereas the incentive motivation dopaminergic reward is sensitized by oxytocin and then habituates over time, the consummatory opioid reward stays constant due to the effects of oxytocin.

Cantor, Binik, and Pfaus (1999) found that oxytocin is necessary for ejaculation to take place. This is not surprising, given that orgasm, often associated with ejaculation in both men and women, causes an increase in oxytocin from around the time of orgasm until about 5 minutes afterward (Carmichael et al., 1987). Though the exact role, magnitude, and longevity of oxytocin release during and after orgasm have been matters of debate in the literature, especially in regard to male participants (Kruger et al., 2003; Murphy, Seckl, Burton, Checkley, & Lightman, 1987), there is general agreement that oxytocin levels do increase due to orgasm in men and women (Blaicher et al., 1999; Caldwell, 2002). However, it is also true that oxytocin is released throughout most sexual activity due to the physical intimacy of sexual intercourse (Meston & Frohlich, 2000).

The Role of Sex in Adult Attachment Formation

We propose that the sexual mating system, which governs attraction, flirting, desire, and sexual behavior, plays a critical role in adult attachment formation. Specifically, we argue that through repeated sexual interactions with the same partner, the physiological and endocrinological states that sex engenders become encoded into the mental representation of the partner. By doing so, it promotes the development of this mental representation from one of an attractive but unknown stranger to one that is rewarding and complex, and that ultimately underlies a full-fledged attachment bond.

There are multiple social, cognitive, behavioral, and neural pathways through which sex may affect attachment processes. Here we focus on the overlap between attachment and sexual mating system in the dopaminergic and oxytocinergic/opioid mechanisms, and how via shared neural mechanisms, sexual activity may promote the formation of an adult attachment bond. We focus specifically on two aspects of the sexual mating system that are likely to have profound effects on the development of the attachment bond: (1) the reward-related dopaminergic and opioid activity associated with sexual activity; and (2) the negative reinforcement properties associated with sexual interactions.

Reward-Related Dopaminergic and Opioid Activity Associated with Sex

Sex is a powerful reward. Not surprisingly, individuals who are perceived as sexually attractive (and thus as potential future sexual partners) or have been sexual partners in the past are associated with rewards, and thus trigger dopaminergic reward processing (as described in the previous section). The sheer magnitude of the reward response triggered by sexual partners (future or actual) has several implications for the development of an attachment bond.

First, such reward processing promotes proximity seeking and maintenance. Not only is proximity an important factor contributing to initial attraction (Berscheid & Walster, 1969), but sustained proximity is necessary for the *formation* of pair bonds (Hazan & Zeifman, 1994). Given that aspects of the environment (e.g., certain groups or particular people, objects, and places) that are highly positive and associated with reward lead to more approach behavior, it is self-evident that the promise of sexual reward is a motivator for initiating and promoting proximity-seeking behaviors early in a relationship. Indeed, physical attractiveness has long been identified as a key factor in initial attraction and relationship initiation, motivating individuals to approach certain persons (those who are attractive) and desire to spend time with them.

Second, the combination of dopaminergic, oxytocinergic, and opioid activity during sex has implications for memory and encoding, and specifically for building a robust, context-independent, chronically accessible mental representation of the partner, which is a defining cognitive feature of an attachment bond (Zayas, Günaydin, & Shoda, 2015). In this manner, partner representations can be easily activated in a number of situations and used to guide behaviors and color experience.

Specifically, dopamine, oxytocin, glutamate, and mu-opioid activation (especially in the brain's reward pathway and medial orbital 13 region) during sex plays critical roles in encoding information about the partner (e.g., the partner's smell, touch, sound, and appearance) into an ensemble of cues (Luu & Malenka, 2008; Depue & Morrone-Strupinsky, 2005). The strong activation of the dopaminergic, oxytocinergic, and mu-opioid systems by sex and a sexual partner suggests a neural pathway by which mental representations may become richer and more elaborated more quickly than if the sexual mating system were not activated. It also provides a neural mechanism for how the representation of the partner may become chronically accessible (always on one's mind or brought to mind with little effort) and contextually independent. To return to our hypothetical scenario, the high dopaminergic, oxytoncergic, and opioid activity during sex makes it likely that Sam and Alex will readily encode each other's cues into their respective mental representations.

Another way in which attachment representations may develop more quickly is through behavioral mechanisms differentially triggered by neural activity. That is, positive, rewarding stimuli are more salient, and more likely to grab attention, than less positive or neutral stimuli. Thus, behaviorally, an individual is more likely to form richer representations of any information involving a potential sexual partner, simply because the potential partner is the most rewarding and salient aspect of the environment. Indeed, in parent–child and sexual relationships, individual characteristics (e.g. scent, facial features), are very closely investigated (Del Cerro, 1998).

Negative Reinforcement Properties Associated with Sexual Interactions

There are certainly important differences between the cognitive and behavioral components of distress-relieving processes and those associated with relieving arousal during sexual activity. Still, there are a number of similarities.

First, negative reinforcement is common in both. In distress relief, a person feels anxiety, and another person who provides comfort will eventually become associated via conditioning with relaxation. Thus, later, even in the absence of actual physical comfort, the mere thought of the partner gives rise to feeling and physiological states of security. Likewise, during sexual encounters there is a period of sustained positive arousal during the appetitive phase (occurring before and during sexual activity), which is then followed by relief and satiation during the consummatory phase (occurring during and after sexual activity). The arousal associated with the appetitive phase is excitatory and anticipatory—activating the ANS and thus increasing heart rate and vasocongestion, and even activating the BNST of the extended amygdala, which releases extracellular dopamine (Phillips-Farfán & Fernández-Guasti, 2007; Eiler et al., 2007). However, after sex (and orgasm) there is a large release of oxytocin and mu-opiates that signals sexual satiety. In this state, the BNST is not activated and a peaceful, almost lethargic, state of calm sets in (Phillips-Farfán & Fernández-Guasti, 2007). This deactivation of the ANS is also evident in poistcoital bradycardia, when the heart drops below 60 beats per minute (Carter, 1992). Thus sexual encounters mimic distress relief in this respect.

Moreover, the neural and hormonal systems underlying distress relief and those underlying the arousal relief characteristic of sexual encounters show considerable overlap. Most important, both distress relief and sex involve the release of oxytocin. In distress relief, oxytocin receptors in the hippocampus are regulated by the release of glucocorticoids. Specifically, the feedback of glucocorticoids, such as cortisol, released by stress increases oxytocin receptor binding (Liberzon & Young, 1997). Increased glucocorticoid receptors in the hippocampus are associated with increased oxytocin receptor binding in that area, which, through the action of gamma-aminobutyric acid, has an excitatory effect on the paramedial BNST, which in turn reduces the release of PVN CRH and, through that action, cortisol. Therefore, it is through the release of stress hormones that oxytocin receptors are up-regulated, which in turn enhances the action of oxytocin released through physical touch, such as ventro-ventral contact, eye contact, or the accessing of a mental representation. In sexual interactions, a powerful release of oxytocin is associated with breast and genital stimulation, uterine contractions, contractions of the reproductive tract, sexual arousal, the act of coitus, and, most potently, orgasm (Carter,

1992). The other acts that release comparable amounts of oxytocin are lactation, parturition, and regulation of maternal behavior (Carter, 1992).

Given the large role that oxytocin plays in sexual functioning and release, along with its interaction with dopamine in the NAS, it is reasonable to hypothesize that the anxiolytic and intimacy-promoting effect of oxytocin is amplified during positive sexual encounters—especially ones resulting in orgasm for one or both of the partners. This continued distress relief and increase in trust and intimacy from repeated sexual encounters may then act to create the adult attachment bond, much as distress relief does in infancy.

Ingredients Necessary for an Attachment Relationship: Dopamine, Opioids, and Oxytocin

Thus far, we have discussed dopamine, oxytocin, and opioids as functioning relatively independently. However, it is possible that a true bond cannot be formed without a combination of these neurochemicals. Studies done by Young and Wang (2004) with prairie voles have found that blocking *either* the dopamine *or* the oxytocin receptors in prairie voles prevented their ability to form a pair. Even when a D2 receptor agonist was used to induce partner preferences in the prairie voles, no preferences were formed when there was also a blockade of oxytocin receptors.

Various findings suggest that the formation of pair bonds involves the presence of both dopamine and oxytocin (as well as vasopressin). Specifically, the release of oxytocin in the dopaminergic pathway, primarily oxytocin in the NAS and vasopressin in the ventral palladium, appears to enhance the reward processing and memory formation needed for acquiring mate preferences (Argiolas & Gessa, 1991; Sarnyai & Kovács, 1994). Consistent with this proposition, in mammals (sheep, voles, and rats), oxytocin antagonists and PVN lesions prevent the formation of partner preferences, as well as the onset of maternal behaviors (Ostrowski, 1988). Interestingly, they do not stop sexual or maternal behaviors after these behaviors have already been established.

This work suggests that oxytocin (as well as vasopressin) affects the formation of mate preferences and the development of mental representations by acting as a catalyst in the appetitive reward system. Specifically, oxytocin increases sensitivity to the huge release of dopamine that anticipates and accompanies sexual behavior, making sex more rewarding than food or cocaine (Kovács et al., 1998; Shahrokh et al., 2010). This interaction between oxytocin and dopamine also characterizes the infatuation phase of relationship development.

However, it is important to note that the relative potency of neurohormones varies as the relationship progresses. Over time, as a result of habituation, the dopaminergic response associated with sex is expected to decrease. Critically, however, even though dopaminergic reward becomes less and less intense, the opiate release associated with consummatory reward during and after sex does not lessen, as oxytocin, importantly, inhibits the development of tolerance to these opiates (Kovács et al., 1998). This opiate-consummatory release, coupled with the tolerance-inhibiting effects of oxytocin, is what is expected to maintain feelings of attachment even after the dopaminergic high elicited by the sexual system declines.

Unanswered Questions and Future Directions

When does having sex hinder the formation of an attachment bond?: Integration with the relationship literature findings

We have proposed that sexual interactions with the same partner over time are likely to promote the formation of an attachment bond. But are there instances in which sex might impede the formation of pair bonds? Just as there is an absence of theorizing on the broader issue of the role of sex in adult attachment formation, there is no work directly examining the question of whether sex may hinder attachment formation. However, the relationship literature looking at the role of sex in relationship outcomes (e.g., satisfaction vs. breakup) may shed some light.

The extant, and relatively recent, findings in the relationship literature suggest that the timing of sex during relationship formation is a critical factor in determining whether sex predicts positive or negative relationship outcomes. In a national sample of 2,035 married individuals, Busby, Carroll, and Willoughby (2010) found that spouses who waited until marriage to have sex, compared to those who started having sex early in their relationship, reported higher marital satisfaction, better communication patterns, fewer thoughts of divorce, and better sexual quality. Spouses who became sexually involved later when dating, but prior to marriage, fell somewhere in between—showing better relationship outcomes than those who had sex early in the relationship, but worse outcomes than those who waited until marriage. Moreover, these results held even when the researchers statistically controlled for several other variables (e.g., number of sexual partners, relationship length, religiosity, education). Another study by Busby and colleagues (Willoughby, Carroll, & Busby, 2014) reported similar findings. However, before we draw any conclusions, it is important to keep in mind that relationship stability, which is typically the focus of relationship researchers, is not the same as the quality of an attachment bond (Selcuk et al., 2010). That is, behaviors that characterize the attachment bond—such as partners' providing each other with a subjective sense of felt security, regulating each other's affective and physiological states, and facilitating each other's functioning outside the relationship—occur independently of the level of satisfaction experienced in the marriage. Indeed, such attachment behaviors may even occur when the marital relationship itself is not very satisfying. Thus the specific question of whether timing of sex plays a role in moderating the hypothesized effect of sex on adult attachment formation requires empirical investigation. Future work, ideally using a longitudinal framework, should be used to examine more precisely how the timing of sexual intercourse affects subsequent components of the attachment bond (e.g., alleviation distress).

How do attachment bonds differ as a function of whether a relationship is sexual or platonic?

This model effectively describes the formation of any affiliative bond; however, the key difference made by the contribution of sex is twofold: the magnitude of the dopaminergic and opiate rewards, and the administration of oxytocin. While platonic affiliative bonds and social-contextual ensembles can be created without sex by this approach–consummatory reward system, the presence of sex and sexual motivation is what makes a traditional, sexual pair bond so special. It would take a great magnitude of reinforcement (both positive in the form of reward, and negative in the form of arousal and distress alleviation) for a peer to replace one's caregiver in the attachment hierarchy. Therefore, it is possible—with the inclusion of soft touch, mutual eye gaze, and ventro-ventral contact, in order to release mu-opioids and oxytocin—for platonic bonds to be formed. However, it is far more likely, given the unconditioned reward that sexual pleasure presents and the vast differences in the magnitude of reward coupled with oxytocin-ergic activity elicited by sexual encounters, that an adult's primary attachment relationship will be with a sexual partner.

Does the proposed model work for people who engage in casual sex or who are serial monogamists?

We speculate that both people who engage in casual sex or who are serial monogamists may find the incentive motivation dopaminergic reward to be more valuable than the consummatory opioid reward. A preference for dopamine-related activities over opioid-related ones may reflect individual differences. For example, people who prefer casual sex or the beginning of relationships may be more sensitive to dopaminergic (vs. opioid) rewards, which would promote a preference for high-dopaminergic activities, such as sex, compared to high-opioid activities associated with longer relationships. Additionally, they may have fewer mu-opioid receptors due to early life experiences. In fact, people who prefer casual or brief encounters may be the neurochemical opposites of people who identify as asexual—that is, who experience consummatory reward, but have no sexual incentive motivation.

Moreover, those who prefer casual sex or who are serial monogamists may have a preference for dopamine-related activities over opioid-related ones because of the release of oxytocin. Although oxytocin is released by touch, orgasm, sexual intercourse, nipple stimulation, and similar intimate behaviors, sexual encounters consisting of fewer of these actions will trigger less oxytocin release. For example, perhaps people who prefer casual sex also tend to have less nipple stimulation, less ventro-ventral contact, less consistent orgasms, less soft touch, and so on. If this is the case, less oxytocin will be released, and while the dopaminergic reward will not be as sensitized, there will also be less inhibiting of opioid habituation. If that is the case, then once they have habituated to the dopaminergic reward, they will also have habituated to the opioid reward, thus receiving what subjectively feels like, and what neuroendocrinologically is, less reward. Instead of moving from an exciting, sexually motivating reward to a peaceful, gratifying reward, these people may be feeling very little reward. Examining the role of sex and attachment formation for people who prefer almost exclusively causal sex or who are only interested in the infatuation stage of a relationship would be a promising way of examining the function of sex in attachment formation.

Does the proposed model work for asexual individuals?

Asexual individuals do not experience sexual attraction to others. On a sexual orientation (romantic/erotic response) spectrum with "attracted to women" on one end and "attracted to men" on the other, asexuality rests at the midpoint along with bisexuality and pansexuality. Approximately 1% of the population self-identifies as asexual. Among asexual persons, there is a further distinction between a romantic and an aromantic orientation. Romantic asexuals enjoy the physical intimacy of nonsexual touch, whereas aromantic asexuals typically find even nonsexual physical intimacy aversive. Given our theorizing, we predict that adult attachment formation among asexual persons would be driven primarily or exclusively by the oxytocinergic and opioid systems, and *not* the dopaminergic (wanting, desiring, sexual motivation) system.

Orgasm and Gender Differences

It is well documented that when men and women have sex, men are far more likely than women to achieve sexual orgasm, especially in the form of sexual intercourse. Does this mean that women's attachments to their partners form more slowly, less strongly, and/or less often? There is also evidence that female same-sex couples are less sexually active but cuddle more than male same-sex couples. Does this mean that lesbians are less or differently attached to their partners than gay males are attached to theirs? On the basis of these findings and our theorizing, we hypothesize that the primary difference in the relationship between sex and attachment in women versus men is the balance of dopaminergic to oxytocinergic rewards. In other words, men on average tend to enjoy sexual novelty more than do women, and women on average tend to enjoy sexual intimacy more than do men. We can see this sex difference in interactions with sexual stimuli in a study by Festjens, Bruyneel, and Dewitte (2013), in which heterosexual men and women were presented with underwear or a t-shirt of the opposite sex and were allowed either to touch or only to look at them. Men exhibited more reward seeking after both visual and tactile cues of women's underwear. However, women only exhibited reward seeking after being allowed to touch the men's underwear, as visual cues alone were unable to elicit an appetitive response. This sex difference is perhaps due to a difference in the dopaminergic threshold that is required to experience sexual motivation; that is, perhaps having an additional sensory experience was necessary for the women in the study to reach this threshold. Alternatively, given the behavioral conditioning response associated with the reward system, perhaps the majority of women in this study had experientially learned not to associate male undergarments with the magnitude of anticipatory reward that men had learned in regard to female undergarments. This experiential learning could stem from the saturation of sexualization of women and women's underwear in mainstream culture, or even from an antiquated yet still pervasive view of women not acting as sexual aggressors.

Another possibility for the sex differences we find between men and women's sexual inclinations toward novelty versus intimacy, respectively, may be due to the gender difference in internal hormonal milieu. The *steroid/peptide theory of social bonds* (van Anders, Goldey, & Kuo, 2011) calls attention to the seemingly opposing processes of oxytocin and testosterone in social bonding: Whereas oxytocin promotes trust, testosterone inhibits it; whereas oxytocin promotes empathy, testosterone inhibits it; whereas oxytocin inhibits stress, testosterone promotes it (Bos, Panksepp, Bluthé, & Honk, 2012). van Anders et al. (2011) even go so far as to say that testosterone and oxytocin seem to act as hormonal antagonists to one another. From this antagonistic relationship between testosterone and oxytocin presented in the steroid/peptide theory, it would be reasonable to extrapolate that because men have more testosterone than women do, men may need a larger amount of oxytocin in order for the neurotransmitter to have the same effect in promoting pair bonding as it does in women. This may be one reason why, separate from social-constructionist viewpoints, it is more common for men to reach orgasm during a sexual experience than women, as it may allow for a more equitable action of oxytocin in the two partners. Future research might investigate sex differences in hormone and neurotransmitter interactions and their effects on attachment formation.

Individual Differences in Sex and Attachment

There will be, of course, individual differences in how sex affects attachment formation and maintenance. To name only a few, these include individual differences in thresholds for experiencing incentive dopaminergic reward or opioid consummatory reward, in the number of oxytocin and glucocorticoid receptors in the hippocampus, or in the attachment styles that shape individuals' expectations and behaviors within relationships. Most relevant is empirical work by Gurit Birnbaum and her colleagues (Birnbaum, 2007, 2010; Birnbaum, Reis, Mikulincer, Gillath, & Orpaz, 2006; Birnbaum & Reis, 2012) investigating how individual differences in adult attachment relate to the experience of sex. For example, securely attached people prefer their sexual interactions to be committed romantic relationships, and find these sexual experiences with their partners mutually satisfying and intimate. Avoidantly attached individuals tend to engage in less frequent sexual activities with relationship partners (Birnbaum, 2010), dislike and are uncomfortable with the physical and emotional intimacy that accompanies sex in relationships, and prefer to detach the physical intimacy of sex from the its psychological intimacy implications (Mikulincer & Shaver, 2007). Not surprisingly, then, avoidant people feel disconnected from their partners during sexual experiences and display less physical affection (Birnbaum & Reis, 2006). Finally, anxiously attached individuals look to sex in particular to fulfill other deficits in attachment-related needs, leading to a promotion of attachment-related reasons for engaging in sexual activity, and of the paramount importance of the affection-related aspects of sex over even the sex itself (Birnbaum, 2010).

On the basis of this literature, we speculate that it may be difficult for people with an avoidant attachment style to receive the same magnitude of oxytocin release associated with physical touch, as well as psychological trust and intimacy, in their relationships as securely attached people receive. If so, this should subsequently affect the formation and maintenance of attachment bonds on both a neurological and a cognitive level for people who are avoidantly attached.

With respect to anxiously attached persons, we predict that the relationship-based anxieties that such individuals feel may lead them to deny their own sexual desires and needs in order to please their partners. If so, this should prevent them from getting the magnitude and type of neural/endocrinological rewards that they desire (and possibly need to feel secure in their attachment); it should also increase their anxiety in general (Birnbaum et al., 2006).

Conclusion

Although it is the norm that romantic partners function as attachment figures *and* sex partners, and pair bonds in theory are characterized by an integration of the attachment and sexual mating systems, sex has largely been ignored by researchers focusing on adult romantic attachment. Birnbaum and colleagues' (Birnbaum & Reis, 2006; Birnbaum, 2010) work, though its focus is on individual differences and not the role of sex in attachment formation, is a notable exception.

From the evidence reviewed above, it is clear that the neural and physiological systems operating during sexual exchanges overlap significantly with those underlying attachment bonds. Notably, oxytocin is released most strongly in the context of the two types of interpersonal relationships that typically function as primary attachments—that is, infant–caregiver bonds in early life (including parturition and lactation) and romantic/sexual bonds in adulthood.

The neural systems that motivate us to engage in sexual interactions and then reward us so intensely for doing so appear to play a central role in adult attachment formation. Specifically, repeated sexual contact with the same individual over time conditions these systems to a rich mental representation of this individual that includes facial and bodily features, voice, smell, touch, and so forth. In the normal course of romantic relationship development, the dopaminergic reward declines in intensity—but, thanks to oxytocin, the opiate reward does not. Indeed, the point of "clearcut" attachment in adulthood (i.e., the marker of a qualitative change from infatuation to full-blown attachment) may be when an opioid-based sense of calm and satiety overtakes dopamine-driven feelings of desire. Furthermore, the action of oxytocin in preventing habituation to the rewarding effects of opioids is what helps maintain pair bonds over the long term.

We hope the ideas presented in this chapter will inspire adult attachment researchers to tackle the many fascinating and empirically testable questions that the proposed model suggests, and thereby help move the field of adult attachment theory forward.

References

Aguilera, G., & Liu, Y. (2012). The molecular physiology of CRH neurons. *Frontiers in Neuroendocrinology, 33*, 67–84.

Aharon, I., Etcoff, N., Ariely, D., Chabris, C. F., O'Connor, E., & Breiter, H. C. (2001). Beautiful faces have variable reward value: fMRI and behavioral evidence, *Neuron, 3*(8), 537–551.

Argiolas, A. (1999). Neuropeptides and sexual behaviour. *Neuroscience and Biobehavioral Reviews, 23*, 1127–1142.

Argiolas, A., & Gessa, G. L. (1991). Central functions of oxytocin. *Neuroscience and Biobehavioral Reviews, 15*, 217–231.

Aron, A., Fisher, H., Mashek, D., Strong, G., Li, H., & Brown, L. (2005). Reward, motivation and emotion systems associated with early-stage intense romantic love. *Journal of Neurophysiology, 93*, 327–337.

Baldwin, M. W., Fehr, B., Keedian, E., Seidel, M., & Thomson, D. W. (1993). An exploration of the relational schemata underlying attachment styles: Self-report and lexical decision approaches. *Personality and Social Psychology Bulletin, 19*, 746–754.

Baldwin, M. W., Keelan, J. P. R., Fehr, B., Enns, V., & Koh-Rangarajoo, E. (1996). Social-cognitive conceptualization of attachment working models: Availability and accessibility effects. *Journal of Personality and Social Psychology, 71*, 94–109.

Balfour, M. E., Yu, L., & Coolen, L. M. (2004). Sexual behavior and sex-associated environmental cues activate the mesolimbic system in male rats. *Neuropsychopharmacology, 29*, 718–730.

Bartels, A., & Zeki, S. (2004). The neural correlates of maternal and romantic love. *NeuroImage, 21*, 1155–1166.

Beckes, L., Simpson, J. A., & Erickson, A. (2010). Of snakes and succor: Learning secure attachment associations with novel faces via negative stimulus pairings. *Psychological Science, 21*, 721–728.

Berridge, K. C. (1999). Pleasure, pain, desire, and dread: Hidden core processes of emotion. In D. Kahneman, E. Diener, & N. Schwarz (Eds.), *Well-being: The foundations of hedonic psychology* (pp. 525–557). New York: Russell Sage Foundation.

Berscheid, E., & Walster, E. H. (1969). *Interpersonal attraction.* Reading, MA: Addison-Wesley.

Birnbaum, G. E. (2007). Attachment orientations, sexual functioning, and relationship satisfaction in a community sample of women. *Journal of Social and Personal Relationships, 24*, 21–35.

Birnbaum, G. E. (2010). Bound to interact: The divergent goals and complex interplay of attachment and sex within romantic relationships. *Journal of Social and Personal Relationships, 27*, 245–252.

Birnbaum, G. E., & Reis, H. T. (2006). Women's sexual working models: An evolutionary-attachment perspective. *Journal of Sex Research, 43*, 328–342.

Birnbaum, G. E., & Reis, H. T. (2012). When does responsiveness pique sexual interest?: Attachment and sexual desire in initial acquaintanceships. *Personality and Social Psychology Bulletin, 38*, 946–958.

Birnbaum, G. E., Reis, H. T., Mikulincer, M., Gillath, O., & Orpaz, A. (2006). When sex is more than just sex: Attachment orientations, sexual experience, and relationship quality. *Journal of Personality and Social Psychology, 91*, 929–943.

Blaicher, W., Gruber, D., Bieglmayer, C., Blaicher, A. M., Knogler, W., & Huber, J. C. (1999). The role of oxytocin in relation to female sexual arousal. *Gynecologic and Obstetric Investigation, 47*, 125–126.

Bos, P. A., Panksepp, J., Bluthé, R. M., & Honk, J. V. (2012). Acute effects of steroid hormones and neuropeptides on human social–emotional behavior: A review of single administration studies. *Frontiers in Neuroendocrinology, 33*, 17–35.

Bowlby, J. (1973). *Attachment and loss: Vol. 2. Separation: Anxiety and anger.* New York: Basic Books.

Bowlby, J. (1979). *The making and breaking of affectional bonds.* London: Tavistock.

Bowlby, J. (1982). Attachment and loss: Retrospect and prospect. *American Journal of Orthopsychiatry, 52*, 664–678.

Breiter H. C., Aharon, I., Kahneman, D., Dale, A., & Shizgal, P. (2001). Functional imaging of neural responses to expectancy and experience of monetary gains and losses. *Neuron, 30*(2), 619–639.

Bretherton, I., & Munholland, K. A. (2008). Internal working models in attachment relationships: Elaborating a central construct in attachment theory. In J. Cassidy & P. R. Shaver (Eds.), *Handbook of attachment: Theory, research, and clinical applications* (2nd ed., pp. 102–127). New York: Guilford Press.

Busby, D. M., Carroll, J. S., & Willoughby, B. J. (2010). Compatibility or restraint: The effects of sexual timing on marriage relationships. *Journal of Family Psychology, 24*, 766–774.

Caldwell, J. D. (2002). A sexual arousability model involving steroid effects at the plasma membrane. *Neuroscience and Biobehavioral Reviews, 26*, 13–30.

Cantor, J. M., Binik, Y. M., & Pfaus, J. G. (1999). Chronic fluoxetine inhibits sexual behavior in the male rat: Reversal with oxytocin. *Psychopharmacology, 144*, 355–362.

Carmichael, M. S., Humbert, R., Dixen, J., Palmisano, G., Greenleaf, W., & Davidson, J. M. (1987). Plasma oxytocin increases in the human sexual response. *Journal of Clinical Endocrinology and Metabolism, 64*, 27–31.

Carter, C. S. (1992). Oxytocin and sexual behavior. *Neuroscience and Biobehavioral Reviews, 16*, 131–144.

Coan, J. A., Schaefer, H. S., & Davidson, R. J. (2006). Lending a hand: Social regulation of the neural response to threat. *Psychological Science, 17*, 1032–1039.

Collins, N. L., & Ford, M. (2010). Responding to the needs of others: The interplay of the attachment and caregiving systems in adult intimate relationships. *Journal of Social and Personal Relationships, 27*, 235–244.

Collins, N. L., Guichard, A. C., Ford, M. B., & Feeney, B. C. (2004). Working models of attachment: New developments and emerging themes. In W. S. Rholes & J. A. Simpson (Eds.), *Adult attachment: Theory, research, and clinical implications* (pp. 196–239). New York: Guilford Press.

Coolen, L. M., Fitzgerald, M. E., Yu, L., & Lehman, M. N. (2004). Activation of μ opioid receptors in the medial preoptic area following copulation in male rats. *Neuroscience, 124*, 11–21.

Cooper, J. C., Dunne, S., Furey, T., & O'Doherty, J. P. (2012). Dorsomedial prefrontal cortex mediates rapid evaluations predicting the outcome of romantic interactions. *Journal of Neuroscience, 32*, 15647–15656.

Del Cerro, C. R. (1998). Role of the vomeronasal input in maternal behavior. *Psychoneuroendocrinology, 23*, 905–926.

Depue, R. A., & Collins, P. F. (1999). Neurobiology of the structure of personality: Dopamine, facilitation of incentive motivation, and extraversion. *Behavioral and Brain Sciences, 22*, 491–517.

Depue, R. A., & Morrone-Strupinsky, J. V. (2005). A neurobehavioral model of affiliative bonding: Implications for conceptualizing a human trait of affiliation. *Behavioral and Brain Sciences, 28*, 313–349.

Diamond, L. M. (2001). Contributions of psychophysiology to research on adult attachment: Review and recommendations. *Personality and Social Psychology Review, 5*, 276–295.

Diamond, L. M. (2004). Emerging perspectives on distinctions between romantic love and sexual desire. *Current Directions in Psychological Science, 13*, 116–119.

Diamond, L. M., & Dickenson, J. (2012). The neuroimaging of love and desire: Review and future directions. *Clinical Neuropsychiatry, 9*, 39–46.

Ditzen, B., Neumann, I. D., Bodenmann, G., von Dawans, B., Turner, R. A., Ehlert, U., et al. (2007). Effects of different kinds of couple interaction on cortisol and heart rate responses to stress in women. *Psychoneuroendocrinology, 32*, 565–574.

Eiler, W. J., Hardy, L., Goergen, J., Seyoum, R., Mensah-Zoe, B., & June, H. L. (2007). Responding for brain stimulation reward in the bed nucleus of the stria terminalis in alcohol-preferring rats following alcohol and amphetamine pretreatments. *Synapse, 61*, 912–924.

Eisenberger, N. I., Master, S. L., Inagaki, T. K., Taylor, S. E., Shirinyan, D., Lieberman, M. D., et al. (2011). Attachment figures activate a safety signal-related neural region and reduce pain experience. *Proceedings of the National Academy of Sciences USA, 108*, 11721–11726.

Festjens, A., Bruyneel, S., & Dewitte, S. (2013). What a feeling!: Touching sexually laden stimuli makes women seek rewards. *Journal of Consumer Psychology, 24*(3), 387–393.

Fisher, H., Aron, A., & Brown, L. L. (2005). Romantic love: An fMRI study of a neural mechanism for mate choice. *Journal of Comparative Neurology, 493*, 58–62.

Gray, J. A. (1973). Causal theories of personality and how to test them. In J. R. Royce (Ed.), *Multivariate analysis and psychological theory* (pp. 409–463). New York: Academic Press.

Grewen, K. M., Anderson, B. J., Girdler, S. S., & Light, K. C. (2003). Warm partner contact is related to lower cardiovascular reactivity. *Behavioral Medicine, 29*, 123–130.

Günaydin, G., Zayas, V., Selcuk, E., & Hazan, C. (2012). I like you but I don't know why: Objective facial resemblance to significant others influences snap judgments. *Journal of Experimental Social Psychology, 48*, 250–353.

Hazan, C., & Shaver, P. (1987). Romantic love conceptualized as an attachment process. *Journal of Personality and Social Psychology, 52*, 511–524.

Hazan, C., & Zeifman, D. (1994). Sex and the psychological tether. In K. Bartholomew & D. Perlman (Eds.), *Advances in personal relationships: Vol. 5. Attachment processes in adulthood* (pp. 151–178). London: Jessica Kingsley.

Herbert, J. (1993). Peptides in the limbic system: Neurochemical codes for co-ordinated adaptive responses to behavioural and physiological demand. *Progress in Neurobiology, 41*, 723–791.

Hilliard, S., Domjan, M., Nguyen, M., & Cusato, B. (1998). Dissociation of conditioned appetitive and consummatory sexual behavior: Satiation and extinction tests. *Animal Learning and Behavior, 26*, 20–33.

Hinde, R. A. (1970). *Animal behaviour: A synthesis of ethology and comparative psychology.* New York: McGraw-Hill.

Impett, E. A., Muise, A., & Peragine, D. (2014). Sexuality in the context of relationships. In L. M. Diamond & D. L. Tolman (Eds.), *APA handbook of sexuality and psychology* (Vol. 1, pp. 269–316). Washington, DC: American Psychological Association.

Insel, T. R. (1992). Oxytocin—a neuropeptide for affiliation: Evidence from behavioral, receptor autoradiographic, and comparative studies. *Psychoneuroendocrinology, 17*, 3–35.

Insel, T. R. (1997). A neurobiological basis of social attachment. *American Journal of Psychiatry*, *154*, 726–735.

Irnaten, M., Aicher, S. A., Wang, J., Venkatesan, P., Evans, C., Baxi, S., et al. (2003). μ-opioid receptors are located postsynaptically and endomorphin-1 inhibits voltage-gated calcium currents in premotor cardiac parasympathetic neurons in the rat nucleus ambiguus. *Neuroscience*, *116*, 573–582.

Keverne, E. B., Martensz, N. D., & Tuite, B. (1989). Beta-endorphin concentrations in cerebrospinal fluid of monkeys are influenced by grooming relationships. *Psychoneuroendocrinology*, *14*, 155–161.

Kovács, G., Sarnyai, Z., & Szabó, G. (1998). Oxytocin and addiction: A review. *Psychoneuroendocrinology*, *23*, 945–962.

Kruger, T. H., Haake, P., Chereath, D., Knapp, W., Janssen, O. E., Exton, M. S., et al. (2003). Specificity of the neuroendocrine response to orgasm during sexual arousal in men. *Journal of Endocrinology*, *177*, 57–64.

Lee, S., Rogge, R. D., & Reis, H. T. (2010). Assessing the seeds of relationship decay: Using implicit evaluations to detect the early stages of disillusionment. *Psychological Science*, *21*, 857–864.

Liberzon, I., & Young, E. A. (1997). Effects of stress and glucocorticoids on CNS oxytocin receptor binding. *Psychoneuroendocrinology*, *22*, 411–422.

Lim, M. M., & Young, L. J. (2006). Neuropeptidergic regulation of affiliative behavior and social bonding in animals. *Hormones and Behavior*, *50*, 506–517.

Luu, P., & Malenka, R. C. (2008). Spike timing-dependent long-term potentiation in ventral tegmental area dopamine cells requires PKC. *Journal of Neurophysiology*, *100*, 533–538.

Machin, A. J., & Dunbar, R. I. M. (2011). The brain opioid theory of social attachment: A review of the evidence. *Behaviour*, *148*, 9–10.

Master, S. L., Eisenberger, N. I., Taylor, S. E., Naliboff, B. D., Shirinyan, D., & Lieberman, M. D. (2009). A picture's worth: Partner photographs reduce experimentally induced pain. *Psychological Science*, *20*, 1316–1318.

McCubbin, J. A. (1993). Stress and endogenous opioids: Behavioral and circulatory interactions. *Biological Psychology*, *35*, 91–122.

McNulty, J. K., Olson, M. A., Meltzer, A. L., & Shaffer, M. J. (2013). Though they may be unaware, newlyweds implicitly know whether their marriage will be satisfying. *Science*, *342*, 1119–1120.

Melis, M., Enrico, P., Peana, A. T., & Diana, M. (2007). Acetaldehyde mediates alcohol activation of the mesolimbic dopamine system. *European Journal of Neuroscience*, *26*, 2824–2833.

Meston, C. M., & Buss, D. M. (2007). Why humans have sex. *Archives of Sexual Behavior*, *36*, 477–507.

Meston, C. M., & Frohlich, P. F. (2000). The neurobiology of sexual function. *Archives of General Psychiatry*, *57*, 1012–1030.

Mikulincer, M., & Shaver, P. R. (2003). The attachment behavioral system in adulthood: Activation, psychodynamics, and interpersonal processes. In M. P. Zanna (Ed.), *Advances in experimental social psychology* (Vol. 35, pp. 53–152). San Diego, CA: Academic Press.

Mikulincer, M., & Shaver, P. R. (2007). *Attachment in adulthood: Structure, dynamics, and change*. New York: Guilford Press.

Mikulincer, M., Shaver, P. R., & Pereg, D. (2003). Attachment theory and affect regulation: The dynamics, development, and cognitive consequences of attachment-related strategies. *Motivation and Emotion, 27*, 77–102.

Murphy, M. R., Checkley, S. A., Seckl, J. R., & Lightman, S. L. (1990). Naloxone inhibits oxytocin release at orgasm in men. *Journal of Clinical Endocrinology and Metabolism, 71*, 1056–1058.

Murphy, M. R., Seckl, J. R., Burton, S., Checkley, S. A., & Lightman, S. L. (1987). Changes in oxytocin and vasopressin secretion during sexual activity in men. *Journal of Clinical Endocrinology and Metabolism, 65*, 738–741.

Nelson, E. E., & Panksepp, J. (1998). Brain substrates of infant–mother attachment: Contributions of opioids, oxytocin, and norepinephrine. *Neuroscience and Biobehavioral Reviews, 22*, 437–452.

Oliet, C., Oliva, A., Castro, J., & Pérez-Segarra, C. D. (2007). Parametric studies on automotive radiators. *Applied Thermal Engineering, 27*, 2033–2043.

Ostrowski, N. L. (1998). Oxytocin receptor mRNA expression in rat brain: Implications for behavioral integration and reproductive success. *Psychoneuroendocrinology, 23*, 989–1004.

Panksepp, J. (1986). The anatomy of emotions. In R. Plutchik & D. Kellerman (Eds.), *Emotion: Theory, research and experience* (Vol. 3, pp. 91–124). New York: Academic Press

Pfaff, D. W. (1999). *Drive: Neurobiological and molecular mechanisms of sexual motivation*. Cambridge, MA: MIT Press.

Pfaus, J. G., Damsma, G., Wenkstern, D., & Fibiger, H. C. (1995). Sexual activity increases dopamine transmission in the nucleus accumbens and striatum of female rats. *Brain Research, 693*(1), 21–30.

Phillips-Farfán, B. V., & Fernández-Guasti, A. (2009). Endocrine, neural and pharmacological aspects of sexual satiety in male rats. *Neuroscience and Biobehavioral Reviews, 33*, 442–455.

Pietromonaco, P. R., & Barrett, L. F. (2000). The internal working models concept: What do we really know about the self in relation to others? *Review of General Psychology, 4*, 155–175.

Pietromonaco, P. R., Barrett, L. F., & Powers, S. I. (2006). Adult attachment theory and affective reactivity and regulation. In D. K. Snyder, J. A. Simpson, & J. N. Hughes (Eds.), *Emotion regulation in families and close relationships: Pathways to dysfunction and health* (pp. 57–74). Washington, DC: American Psychological Association.

Porges, S. W. (1998). Love: An emergent property of the mammalian autonomic nervous system. *Psychoneuroendocrinology, 23*, 837–861.

Porges, S. W. (2001). The polyvagal theory: Phylogenetic substrates of a social nervous system. *International Journal of Psychophysiology, 42*, 123–146.

Sarnyai, Z., & Kovács, G. L. (1994). Role of oxytocin in the neuroadaptation to drugs of abuse. *Psychoneuroendocrinology, 19*, 85–117.

Sbarra, D. A., & Hazan, C. (2008). Coregulation, dysregulation, self-regulation: An integrative analysis and empirical agenda for understanding adult attachment, separation, loss, and recovery. *Personality and Social Psychology Review, 12*, 141–167.

Scantamburlo, G., Hansenne, M., Fuchs, S., Pitchot, W., Maréchal, P., Pequeux,

C., et al. (2007). Plasma oxytocin levels and anxiety in patients with major depression. *Psychoneuroendocrinology*, *32*, 407–410.

Selcuk, E., Zayas, V., Günaydin, G., Hazan, C., & Kross, E. (2012). Mental representations of attachment figures facilitate emotional recovery following upsetting autobiographical memory recall. *Journal of Personality and Social Psychology*, *103*, 362–378.

Selcuk, E., Zayas, V., & Hazan, C. (2010). Beyond satisfaction: The role of attachment in marital functioning. *Journal of Family Theory and Review*, *2*, 258–279.

Shahrokh, D. K., Zhang, T. Y., Diorio, J., Gratton, A., & Meaney, M. J. (2010). Oxytocin–dopamine interactions mediate variations in maternal behavior in the rat. *Endocrinology*, *151*, 2276–2286.

Silk, J. B., Alberts, S. C., & Altmann, J. (2003). Social bonds of female baboons enhance infant survival. *Science*, *302*, 1231–1234.

Simpson, J. A., Rholes, W. S., & Nelligan, J. S. (1992). Support seeking and support giving within couples in an anxiety-provoking situation: The role of attachment styles. *Journal of Personality and Social Psychology*, *62*, 434–446.

Smillie, L. D. (2013). Extraversion and reward processing. *Current Directions in Psychological Science*, *22*, 167–172.

Sroufe, L. A., & Waters, E. (1977). Attachment as an organizational construct. *Child Development*, *48*, 1184–1199.

Taylor, S. E., Gonzaga, G. C., Klein, L. C., Hu, P., Greendale, G. A., & Seeman, T. E. (2006). Relation of oxytocin to psychological stress responses and hypothalamic–pituitary–adrenocortical axis activity in older women. *Psychosomatic Medicine*, *68*, 238–245.

Uvnäs-Moberg, K. (1998). Antistress pattern induced by oxytocin. *Physiology*, *13*(1), 22–25.

van Anders, S. M., Goldey, K. L., & Kuo, P. X. (2011). The steroid/peptide theory of social bonds: Integrating testosterone and peptide responses for classifying social behavioral contexts. *Psychoneuroendocrinology*, *36*, 1265–1275.

Whipple, B., & Komisaruk, B. R. (1985). Elevation of pain threshold by vaginal stimulation in women. *Pain*, *21*, 357–367.

Wiedenmayer, C. P., & Barr, G. A. (2000). Mu opioid receptors in the ventrolateral periaqueductal gray mediate stress-induced analgesia but not immobility in rat pups. *Behavioral Neuroscience*, *114*, 125–136.

Willoughby, B. J., Carroll, J. S., & Busby, D. M. (2014). Differing relationship outcomes when sex happens before, on, or after first dates. *Journal of Sex Research*, *51*, 52–61.

Windle, R. J., Shanks, N., Lightman, S. L., & Ingram, C. D. (1997). Central oxytocin administration reduces stress-induced corticosterone release and anxiety behavior in rats: 1. *Endocrinology*, *138*, 2829–2834.

Woolley, S. C., Sakata, J. T., Gupta, A., & Crews, D. (2001). Evolutionary changes in dopaminergic modulation of courtship behavior in Cnemidophorus whiptail lizards. *Hormone and Behavior*, *40*, 483–489.

Young, L. J., & Wang, Z. (2004). The neurobiology of pair bonding. *Nature Neuroscience*, *7*, 1048–1054.

Younger, J., Aron, A., Parke, S., Chatterjee, N., & Mackey, S. (2010). Viewing pictures of a romantic partner reduces experimental pain: Involvement of neural reward systems. *PLoS ONE, 5*, e13309.

Zak, P. J., Kurzban, R., & Matzner, W. T. (2005). Oxytocin is associated with human trustworthiness. *Hormones and Behavior, 48*, 522–527.

Zayas, V., Günaydin, G., & Shoda, Y. (2015). From an unknown other to an attachment figure: How do mental representations change with attachment formation? In V. Zayas & C. Hazan (Eds.), *Bases of adult attachment: Linking brain, mind, and behavior* (pp. 157–183). New York: Springer.

Zayas, V., & Hazan, C. (Eds.). (2015). *Bases of adult attachment: Linking brain, mind, and behavior.* New York: Springer.

Zayas, V., Mischel, W., Shoda, Y., & Aber, J. L. (2011). Roots of adult attachment: Maternal caregiving at 18 months predicts adult attachment to peers and partners. *Social Psychological and Personality Science, 2*, 289–297.

Zayas, V., & Shoda, Y. (2005). Do automatic reactions elicited by thoughts of romantic partner, mother, and self relate to adult romantic attachment? *Personality and Social Psychology Bulletin, 31*, 1011–1025.

Zayas, V., & Shoda, Y. (2014). Love you? hate you? maybe it's both: Evidence that significant others trigger bivalent-priming. *Social Psychological and Personality Science.* Epub ahead of print.

Zayas, V., Shoda, Y., Osterhout, L., Takahashi, M. M., & Mischel, W. (2009). Neural responses to partner rejection cues. *Psychological Science, 20*, 813–821.

4

Stress and Attachment

Lisa M. Diamond

Although attachment theory is often considered a theory of interpersonal functioning, Bowlby (1977) placed considerable emphasis on the role of the attachment system in governing overall responses to danger and threat, given that its evolutionary function is infant survival. Hence researchers investigating both infant and adult attachment have devoted increasing attention to understanding how the attachment system relates to individuals' affective, behavioral, and physiological responses to stress (Hostinar & Gunnar, 2013b; Nolte, Guiney, Fonagy, Mayes, & Luyten, 2012; Simpson & Rholes, 2012). Much of this research focuses on the underlying biological mechanisms of stress reactivity, given that the processes by which attachment figures regulate their infants' ongoing emotional experiences are now understood to play a central role in "tuning" stress regulatory systems in the orbitofrontal cortex (Schore, 2001; Siegel, 2001).

The goal of this chapter is to review this body of research, focusing specifically on the implications of attachment for stress reactivity in the autonomic nervous system (ANS) and the hypothalamic–pituitary–adrenocortical (HPA) axis of the endocrine system. I first provide a brief review of these systems, followed by evidence for the critical role of early caregiving in establishing enduring reactivity profiles. I then consider whether the quality of infant–caregiver attachment influences the development of these systems independently of other known contextual influences, such as infant adversity, poverty, maltreatment, and neglect, and I discuss the implications of this question for our basic understanding of links between attachment and stress regulation. The final part of the chapter is devoted to exploring links between attachment theory and the adaptive calibration model outlined by Del Giudice, Ellis, and Shirtcliff (2011), which argues that children with exaggerated physiological stress reactivity, engendered by early exposure to adversity, may show disproportionate *benefits* when exposed later to conditions of high nurturance and support. I consider the implications of this model for considering stress-related plasticity and adaptation in attachment insecurity over the life course.

The HPA Axis

Our bodies regulate responses to psychological stress through two primary pathways: the HPA axis, characterized by activation of the pituitary gland and release of adrenocorticotropic hormone (ACTH) and cortisol, and the sympathetic–adrenal medullary (SAM) axis, characterized by activation of the adrenal medulla (which is part of the ANS), release of catecholamines (such as norepinephrine and epinephrine), and immediate effects on cardiovascular functioning. Hence both HPA and ANS activation are markers of stress reactivity, but they represent distinct "channels" through which stress is regulated in the body, with different antecedents, different effects on other stress-induced biological processes (such as cellular immune function), and different long-term consequences for physical and mental health (Cacioppo, 1994). Research has found that the manner in which individuals appraise the stressor at hand shapes the degree to which their physiological response is characterized by combined SAM–HPA activation as opposed to SAM activation alone (Cacioppo, 1994).

In cases where stressors are primarily appraised as challenges (i.e., in which one's resources are viewed as adequate for meeting the demand), the hypothalamus activates the adrenal medulla to release catecholamines, which activate the sympathetic nervous system (SNS) and inhibit the parasympathetic nervous system (PNS), producing increased heart rate, blood pressure, and respiration. In cases where stressors are primarily appraised as threats (i.e., in which one's resources are not viewed as adequate for meeting the demand), the hypothalamus activates the anterior pituitary in addition to the adrenal medulla. The pituitary is then signaled to release ACTH, which in turn triggers the release of glucocorticoid hormones (primarily cortisol) into the bloodstream. The release of cortisol facilitates the body's response to stress by regulating glucose metabolism, inflammatory responses, localized blood flow, and the maturation of lymphocytes. Although most responses to stress involve combined patterns of HPA and SAM activation, the differences between the antecedents and consequences of these two different stress pathways make it important to discuss each system separately.

Studies examining patterns of HPA reactivity to stress have generally followed two different approaches. The first involves measurement of increases in cortisol in response to a standard laboratory stress task, relative to a pretask baseline (for a comprehensive review of published research using such paradigms, and a synthesis of the task characteristics most strongly associated with reactivity, see Dickerson & Kemeny, 2004). Yet studies have also investigated how acute and chronic stressors influence sustained patterns of cortisol release over 1 day or more. Cortisol release follows a diurnal pattern in most people, peaking in the first half hour after waking and then declining over the rest of the day.

Extensive research has found that exposure to major and minor stress can produce both transient and lasting alterations in this pattern of secretion (see Miller, Chen, & Zhou, 2007). Importantly, whereas laboratory studies of momentary HPA reactivity typically detect transient *increases* in cortisol in response to psychological stress, studies of longer-term patterns of cortisol release have found that sustained exposure to stress can elicit chronic increases *or* decreases in cortisol. Hence stress-related dysregulation of the HPA axis appears to take two forms: exaggerated cortisol release (hyperreactivity), paralleling the transient increases found in laboratory studies; and dampened or blunted cortisol release (hyporeactivity), in which the pattern of diurnal secretion lacks the pronounced morning rise or the evening fall that characterizes normal HPA functioning.

Exaggerated HPA activity is believed to result from stress-related disruption of the normal feedback processes through which HPA activation is typically "shut down" once sufficient levels of cortisol are present in the bloodstream to meet environmental demands. Flattened or blunted HPA activity, in contrast, has been interpreted as a potentially adaptive mechanism for protecting the brain from the detrimental effects of sustained stress-related exposure to cortisol. Awareness of both patterns of dysregulation is important, given that both patterns have been linked to early stress and caregiving experiences (Miller, Chen, & Parker, 2011).

The Autonomic Nervous System

The classic "fight-or-flight" response to stress, with its well-known manifestations of increased heart rate, blood pressure, and sweat production, is part of a larger syndrome of physiological changes produced by the ANS, including increased cardiac output, widespread vasoconstriction, and changes in blood flow to the skeletal muscles, myocardium, brain, kidneys, gastrointestinal tract, and skin. All of these changes serve the purpose of redistributing metabolic energy throughout the body so that the organism can either "fight" or "flee" threats.

The ANS has two branches, the PNS and the SNS, which have antagonistic effects on autonomic functioning. Heightened activation of the SNS produces the physiological changes most commonly associated with fight-or-flight responses (acceleration in heart rate, increased blood pressure, increased sweating, etc.). In contrast, the PNS is responsible for maintaining normal growth and restoration of internal organs—processes that are suspended in times of intense stress. Thus stress-induced activation of the SNS is usually accompanied by some degree of "withdrawal" or "suppression" in the PNS, which functions to redistribute metabolic resources to cope with the external threat. Poststress reengagement of the PNS channels metabolic energy back toward normal maintenance of internal organs and reestablishes homeostasis. Thus PNS engagement produces the types of physiological changes associated with relaxation rather than arousal, such as decreased heart rate and blood pressure.

PNS activity is typically indexed by measuring the degree of heart rate variability that occurs in response to respiration (known as respiratory sinus arrhythmia, or RSA). To explain briefly, heart rate accelerates slightly with each inhalation and decelerates slightly with each exhalation. This regular oscillation reflects the repeated withdrawal and subsequent reinstatement of parasympathetic influence. The greater the parasympathetic regulation of metabolic activity, the more the heart rate will accelerate and decelerate in response to inhalation and exhalation, producing an RSA waveform with a larger amplitude. Baseline-to-task changes in RSA reflect task-related changes in PNS activity. SNS activity is commonly assessed with measures of electrodermal activity (also called skin conductance), although assessments of preejection period (PEP) provided through impedance cardiography provide a more specific (although less common) measure.

Each and every stress-related change in ANS activity reflects changes in both parasympathetic and sympathetic influence, but the specific balance of changes (activation of the SNS, withdrawal of the PNS, or some combination of the two) varies across stressors (Berntson, Cacioppo, & Fieldstone, 1996) and persons (Cacioppo, Uchino, & Berntson, 1994). ANS stress responses that involve a greater degree of PNS withdrawal than SNS activation appear to be more rapid, more flexible, and easier to disengage than SNS-dominated responses (Saul, 1990; Spear, Kronhaus, Moore, & Kline, 1979). As a result, individuals who have more parasympathetically mediated patterns of cardiovascular reactivity are conceptualized as having nervous systems that more flexibly react to and recover from environmental stressors than those with sympathetically mediated patterns (Calkins, 1997; Porges, 1992; Porges, Doussard-Roosevelt, & Maiti, 1994). Consistent with this view, studies suggest that individuals who have greater reductions in RSA during stress have more adaptive patterns of emotional and interpersonal functioning (El-Sheikh & Whitson, 2006; Hessler & Katz, 2007; Moore & Calkins, 2004).

Yet it is not quite appropriate to characterize stress-related reductions in

PNS as "the" singular adaptive pattern of PNS activity during stress, given that an increasing body of research has found that PNS activity sometimes *increases* during stress, especially in tasks that call for active regulatory effort (Beauchaine, 2001; Segerstrom & Nes, 2007; Thayer & Lane, 2000). It has been theorized that this pattern of increased PNS activity may serve to facilitate attention and vigilance to environmental demands by slowing down cardiovascular activity. Hence both PNS increases and decreases in response to stress can be viewed as adaptive responses, depending on the conditions, and researchers have not yet identified a stable set of criteria by which we might view one pattern or the other as "more appropriate."

In addition to situational variation in PNS responses to stress, there also appear to be individual differences. Katz (2007) has argued that individuals exposed to *chronically* stressful environments may develop an enduring pattern of PNS engagement during stress, which may help them to monitor their environment and maintain control over their emotions and behavior. Although such a pattern may prove adaptive in the short term, it may prove taxing over the long term. Many researchers have begun to conceptualize regulatory capacity as being relatively finite, analogous to a muscle that tires upon repeated use (Muraven & Baumeister, 2000). Hence individuals who show chronic patterns of increased RSA in response to stress may experience chronic regulatory "fatigue," leaving them vulnerable to frequent failures of self-control (Vohs, Baumeister, & Ciarocco, 2005). This may explain why individuals who show heightened RSA during stress also show multiple indicators of emotion dysregulation, such as depression, anxiety, and hostility (Hessler & Katz, 2007; Neumann, Sollers, Thayer, & Waldstein, 2004).

Early Caregiving and HPA and ANS Reactivity

Multiple studies of animals and humans have documented stable individual differences in both HPA and ANS stress reactivity that appear to have both genetic and environmental determinants (Kirschbaum, Wust, Faig, & Hellhammer, 1992; Snieder, Boomsma, Van Doornen, & De Geus, 1997). For both systems, one of the major environmental determinants is the quality of early caregiving. With respect to HPA functioning, inadequate parental care appears to have enduring detrimental effects on HPA regulation and broader neurodevelopment (Buss et al., 2007; Heim & Nemeroff, 1999; Heim, Newport, Mletzko, Miller, & Nemeroff, 2008)—particularly during the earliest years of life, when brain systems such as the hippocampus and prefrontal cortex, which play key roles in the regulation of the HPA axis, undergo major development (Sanchez, Ladd, & Plotsky, 2001; Teicher et al., 2003). Notably, significant effects have been detected for *both* maternal and paternal care. Recent studies have found that paternal negativity is associated with heightened cortisol release to stress in infancy (Mills-Koonce, Garrett-Peters, et al., 2011) and with heightened basal and reactive cortisol (in response to peer interactions) in adolescence (Byrd-Craven, Auer, Granger, & Massey, 2012). Maltreatment and prolonged foster care have been associated with blunted cortisol levels, suggesting dysregulation of the normal diurnal cycle of HPA activity (see Hostinar & Gunnar, 2013c). In contrast to the detrimental effects of inadequate parental care, high levels of physical affection and warmth between a caregiver and his or her infant during stressful circumstances have been tied to normal HPA activation profiles in response to environmental demands (Gunnar, 1998; Spangler, Schieche, Ilg, Maier, & Ackerman, 1994), which are thought to promote overall biobehavioral regulation and well-being (Gunnar & Donzella, 2002).

Regarding ANS activity, studies have found that individual differences in PNS reactivity to stress in children are associated with the quality of parenting practices (Blandon, Calkins, Keane, & O'Brien, 2010; Calkins, Smith, Gill, & Johnson, 1998). In infants, PNS reactivity is associated with the degree of synchrony and symmetric responsiveness of mother–infant interaction (Moore & Calkins, 2004) and with the quality of maternal emotional support (Perry et al., 2013). Foster children who have experienced extreme neglect show heightened SNS stress reactivity to separations from their caregivers (Oosterman, De Schipper, Fisher, Dozier, & Schuengel, 2010), and children who have experienced caregiver maltreatment show lower PNS regulation (Skowron et al., 2011). Other aspects of the home environment, such as marital conflict, are also significantly associated with PNS functioning (Porter, Wouden-Miller, Silva, & Porter, 2003). Links between early caregiving and ANS functioning appear to be preserved into adolescence and adulthood. For example, Luecken (1998) found elevated blood pressure reactivity in young adults who had undergone the loss of a parent as children (coupled with poor relationship quality in the family), and other work has documented interaction effects between parental loss and parental caring in predicting adult blood pressure reactivity and recovery (Luecken, Rodriguez, & Appelhans, 2005).

Early Adversity and HPA and ANS Reactivity

Paralleling the findings on early caregiving, numerous studies have documented associations between individuals' HPA and ANS functioning and their exposure to environmental stress and adversity in early life. (Many of these studies include caregiving deficits as a form of adversity, but I consider them separately because of their differential relevance in the context of attachment processes.) Hunter, Minnis, and Wilson (2011) recently reviewed the literature linking early adversity to HPA functioning, focusing specifically on evidence for HPA dysregulation observed within the first 5 years of life. Of the 30 studies they identified that measured infants' exposure to stress (including conditions such as maternal anxiety and depression, maternal history of childhood abuse, low income, psychosocial risk, placement in foster care, maternal attachment insecurity, and maternal insensitivity) and the infants' HPA reactivity to stress between 0 and 5 years of age, 27 studies found significant associations between exposure to adversity and children's baseline or stress-induced HPA functioning. However, the effects were relatively heterogeneous across different types of stressors and different types of HPA responses. For example, although 13 studies found that children exposed to infant adversity had heightened HPA stress reactivity, 3 studies found that children exposed to infant adversity had significantly dampened HPA stress reactivity (paralleling similar patterns in adults, in which chronic stress is sometimes associated with hyperreactivity in the HPA axis and sometimes associated with hyporeactivity; see Miller et al., 2007). Hunter and colleagues also found that 3 studies reported elevated baseline HPA activity in children exposed to infant adversity, whereas 2 studies reported lowered baseline HPA activity in such children.

Hunter et al. (2011) concluded that the accumulated evidence clearly supports an influence of early adversity on the development and functioning of the HPA axis between birth and 5 years. They also emphasized the correspondence between their findings and those of studies focusing on HPA functioning during later childhood, adolescence, and adulthood (Hostinar & Gunnar, 2013b; Miller et al., 2007). Yet they also pointed out that the correspondence between the findings of studies focusing on different stages of the lifespan does not provide reliable evidence that adversity-related disruptions in HPA functioning are permanent. Rather, different types of adversity, experienced at different points during infancy and childhood, may have differential effects on HPA functioning and different time courses for expression (see also Glover, O'Connor, & O'Donnell, 2010; Gunnar, Frenn, Wewerka, & Van Ryzin, 2009). For example, severe child abuse appears to consistently predict a flattening of the overall cortisol cycle as opposed to hyperreactivity in responses to stress (Cicchetti, Rogosch, Gunnar, & Toth, 2010). Hunter and colleagues also noted the possibility that early adversity may "prime" the HPA system to be differentially sensitive to later-occurring stressors, so that the strongest alterations of the HPA response may be observed in children who have experienced repeated or sustained stressors over time. This is consistent with research showing that preschoolers in foster care who had experienced the greatest degree of previous neglect had the greatest HPA dysregulation, in the form of blunted morning levels (Bruce, Fisher, Pears, & Levine, 2009).

There is less evidence for links between infant/child exposure to poverty and subsequent ANS functioning, but the pattern of results is consistent with that regarding the HPA axis: Early adversity predicts poorer stress-related regulation in the PNS (Lengua, 2012; Propper, 2012) as well as heightened SNS stress reactivity (Gunnar et al., 2009; Oosterman et al., 2010), and the specific postnatal neural mechanisms underlying these associations have been well elaborated by Rinaman, Banihashemi, and Koehnle (2011). It also bears noting that there is extensive evidence for links between ANS stress reactivity and early child health indicators, such as low birth weight, poor maternal nutrition, preterm birth, and poor rate of growth (see Kajantie & Räikkönen, 2010), suggesting that health-related correlates of adversity may prove particularly important for tuning the ANS.

What Does Attachment Contribute?

The literature linking early stress exposure to later physiological stress reactivity has focused on a broad range of early stressors, such as poverty, marital conflict, parental mental health, abuse, neglect, early illness, and inadequate parental care. Many of these stressors occur in tandem, but not uniformly so. Hence it is worth considering whether "attachment-relevant" forms of stress such as maternal insensitivity have appreciably different consequences from those of "environmental" stressors such as poverty and household disruption. Even when focusing solely on caregiving-related adversity, such as parental neglect, researchers have questioned whether attachment insecurity influences stress dysregulation independently of other basic caregiving deficits. In other words, does insecure attachment (or, more specifically, the poor caregiving that leads to insecure attachment) constitute a unique form of childhood burden that has independent effects on a child's developing profile of stress regulation, or is it simply another form of overall adversity that has only incremental importance?

According to Gunnar and colleagues (see Gunnar, 2005), there is currently insufficient evidence to conclude that attachment relationships have regulating influences on the development of stress regulation that are independent of the overall effects of other social relationships, which are likely to include other environmental stressors. Other studies, however, have found independent contributions of *disorganized* attachment, rather than attachment insecurity. Disorganized attachment represents a breakdown of the infant's capacity for dyadic stress regulation (Main & Solomon, 1990). It is thought to result from cases in which the attachment figure is a source of fear as well as distress alleviation (Hesse & Main, 2006; Madigan et al., 2006), which explains why there are associations with caregiver maltreatment (Stronach et al., 2011). One study of foster children found that those who had disorganized patterns of attachment to their foster caregivers showed elevated SNS reactivity and poorer PNS regulation during and after brief separations from the foster caregivers (Oosterman et al., 2010). Notably, one large-scale study of 450 mother–infant dyads found that disorganized attachment moderated the association between early caregiving deficits and later PNS functioning. Specifically, infants who had depressed mothers showed low levels of tonic PNS regulation only if they also exhibited a disorganized pattern of attachment (Tharner et al., 2013).

The best way to examine the unique contribution of attachment security to physiological stress regulation is to examine children who show varying levels of correspondence between early adversity and attachment insecurity longitudinally. Such variation has in fact been documented: Although many forms of childhood adversity (such as poverty, household conflict, maternal depression, or maternal stress) can strain caregivers' ability to provide consistently sensitive, responsive care (Mills-Koonce, Appleyard, et al., 2011), children exposed to such stressors do not always develop insecure attachments. Numerous studies have found that household poverty does not consistently predict either maternal insensitivity or infant insecurity (Mills-Koonce, Appleyard, et al., 2011; Susman Stillman, Kalkose, Egeland, & Waldman, 1996). Rather, it appears to be the *combination* of poverty with other simultaneous stressors that predicts infant insecurity, reflecting a cumulative risk model (Cicchetti, Rogosch, & Toth, 1998; Shaw & Vondra, 1993). Hence, whereas economically disadvantaged infants may not uniformly develop attachment insecurity, those for whom the stress of economic disadvantage is combined with maltreatment face heightened risk for insecurity (Stronach et al., 2011). It is not entirely clear whether this reflects the impact of cumulative risk on an infant's need for security, the effect of cumulative risk on a mother's ability to provide security, or (most likely) both.

Attachment Insecurity and HPA–ANS Functioning

If sensitive and responsive caregiving is responsible *both* for the development of attachment security *and* for the calibration of the stress regulation functions of the HPA axis and the ANS, one might expect that individual differences in attachment styles relate directly to the functioning of these systems from childhood into adulthood. Research increasingly supports this view. Children who have insecure patterns of attachment show heightened HPA responses to acute stress (Nachmias, Gunnar, Mangelsdorf, Parritz, & Buss, 1996; van Bakel & Riksen-Walraven, 2004). A recent study found that attachment insecurity in adolescence is also linked to heightened basal levels of cortisol (Oskis, Loveday, Hucklebridge, Thorn, & Clow, 2011). As for adults, Quirin, Pruessner, and Kuhl (2008) found that adults' attachment anxiety was associated with heightened HPA reactivity to a standardized laboratory stressor, and both attachment anxiety and avoidance have been found to be associated with lower vagal tone (Diamond & Hicks, 2005; Maunder, Lancee, Nolan, Hunter, & Tannenbaum, 2006).

One shortcoming of this body of research is that few studies assess or control for childhood exposure to adversity, which (as noted above) may partially explain the shared variance between attachment insecurity and stress dysregulation. One exception is a study by Pierrehumbert, Torrisi, Ansermet, Borghini, and Halfon (2012), which evaluated HPA stress reactivity by using the Trier Social Stress Test in a sample of adults, more than half of whom had experienced some form of childhood adversity (such as abuse, trauma, or life-threatening illness). Independently of adversity exposure, those who had been classified as dismissing according to the Adult Attachment Interview (AAI)—an interview method for discerning individuals' childhood attachment security on the basis of their narrative recollections and reconstructions in adulthood (Hesse, 1999; Main, Kaplan, & Cassidy, 1985)—reported moderate levels of subjective stress but significantly elevated levels of HPA activity, whereas those classified as preoccupied on the AAI did not show elevated HPA activity. Notably, those classified as unresolved on the AAI (a pattern often associated with childhood trauma) reported significantly *elevated* levels of subjective stress and *dampened* levels of HPA activity.

A number of studies have investigated links between attachment insecurity and HPA or ANS stress reactivity in adulthood. For example, Powers, Pietromonaco, Gunlicks, and Sayer (2006) found that insecurely attached individuals showed greater HPA reactivity to laboratory-induced romantic conflict than did securely attached individuals. Specifically, attachment avoidance in female participants was related to increased HPA reactivity to couple conflict, whereas men showed elevated reactivity if they had high levels of anxiety combined with high avoidance. Individuals who had high attachment anxiety also showed poorer recovery of HPA levels after the conflict (Laurent & Powers, 2007). Dewitte, De Houwer, Goubert, and Buysse (2010) led participants to believe that each was going to have to watch a tape of his or her partner being interviewed about previous sexual and romantic relationships by an attractive opposite-sex experimenter. Participants who had higher attachment anxiety showed heightened HPA reactivity while anticipating this stressful event, with the largest increases found in women who were highly anxious *and* avoidant. Finally, during an *actual* 4- to 7-day physical separation from their romantic partners, individuals who had high attachment anxiety showed tonically elevated levels of cortisol (Diamond, Hicks, & Otter-Henderson, 2008).

All of these findings are consistent with the notion that anxiety is associated with a lower threshold for attachment-related threats (conflict, partner unavailability, jealousy, etc.; see Simpson & Rholes, 1994), which manifests itself in heightened physiological response. Yet it is also possible that insecurely attached individuals possess a *generalized* predisposition for heightened HPA or ANS stress reactivity (to both relationship-specific as well as other stressors), and that this heightened reactivity contributes to the development of their attachment insecurity over the course of their social development. This interpretation is consistent with the limited body of findings cited above on associations between attachment security and overall patterns of ANS and HPA functioning (Diamond & Hicks, 2005; Maunder et al., 2006; Oskis et al., 2011; Quirin et al., 2008), but considerably more research is needed. In particular, future research should conduct comprehensive comparisons between anxious and avoidant individuals' physiological, cognitive, and emotional reactivity to relationship-related stressors *as well as* generalized stressors at multiple time points, to determine the degree to which patterns of reactivity reflect stable features of *individuals* (which "travel" from relationship to relationship and from situation to situation) versus the degree to which they reflect features of individuals' current relationship experiences (i.e., the degree of hostility or avoidance or support in *this particular* interaction with the current partner).

Another important area for future research concerns *plasticity* in both stress reactivity and attachment insecurity. The degree to which changes in a child's caregiving environment or in the quality of an adult's romantic ties can produce corresponding changes in attachment styles has long been a topic of theoretical debate and empirical research (see Davila, Karney, & Bradbury, 1999; Fraley, 2007; Hamilton, 2000; Lopez & Gormley, 2002; Mitchell, 2007; Roisman, Collins, Sroufe, & Egeland, 2005; Waters, Merrick, Treboux, Crowell, & Albersheim, 2000; Weinfield, Sroufe, & Egeland, 2000; Zhang & Labouvie-Vief, 2004). Similarly, the stability of individual differences in HPA and ANS reactivity, and the potential sensitivity of these patterns to developmental change and environmental influence, have also received significant attention (see Alkon, Boyce, Davis, & Eskenazi, 2011; Diamond & Cribbet, 2013; Hinnant, Elmore-Staton, & El-Sheikh, 2011; Salomon, 2005; Vasilev, Crowell, Beauchaine, Mead, & Gatzke-Kopp. 2009). One intriguing new direction in this line of inquiry comes from the *adaptive calibration* model proposed by Del Giudice et al. (2011), which is an extension of related models of *biological sensitivity to context* (Boyce & Ellis, 2005) and *differential susceptibility* (Belsky & Pluess, 2009). What is novel about this perspective is its contention that adversity-related profiles of stress hyperreactivity, which have been shown to augment children's vulnerability to social and environmental deficits, simultaneously augment children's sensitivity to social and environmental *strengths*. In other words, heightened stress reactivity may be better conceptualized as heightened susceptibility to social–environmental influence, whether that influence is positive or negative. In recasting "vulnerability" factors as potential sources of resilience, this model offers provocative new ways of framing the implications of early stress exposure for long-term social and emotional development. The implications of the adaptive calibration model for conceptualizing links between stress exposure and *attachment* processes have been largely unexplored. I consider these implications below after briefly outlining the key features of the model.

Differential Susceptibility and Adaptive Calibration

Historically, research on links between individual differences in ANS and HPA functioning and socioemotional development has adopted a diathesis–stress perspective, positing that children with heightened ANS and HPA responses to stress are disproportionately vulnerable to stressful rearing environments because of their deficits in stress regulation (see Boyce & Ellis, 2005). Yet differential susceptibility models (Belsky, Bakermans-Kranenburg, & van IJzendoorn, 2007; Belsky & Pluess, 2009; Del Giudice et al., 2011; Ellis, Boyce, Belsky, Bakermans-Kranenburg, & van IJzendoorn, 2011) posit that the same factors that render children highly reactive to negative environments also render them highly reactive to positive and nurturant environments. Hence, whereas both the diathesis–stress perspective and the differential susceptibility perspective predict that children who have exaggerated ANS and HPA stress reactivity will show disproportionately negative outcomes in negative environmental contexts (as shown by Boyce, Chesney, Alkon, & Tschann, 1995; Bubier, Drabick, & Breiner, 2009; Cummings, El-Sheikh, Kouros, & Keller, 2007; El-Sheikh et al., 2009; Katz, 2007), the differential susceptibility perspective additionally predicts that such children will show disproportionately positive outcomes in positive environments (see Belsky et al., 2007; Belsky & Pluess, 2009), and should be more likely to benefit socioemotionally if their general environment or the quality of their caregiving drastically improves.

The theoretical basis for this prediction of heightened benefit *and* risk is the premise that the early "programming" of the ANS and PNS by early adversity and early caregiving is evolutionarily adaptive, acting to calibrate individuals' stress response systems to "match" their local environments. As set forth in the adaptive calibration model (hereafter abbreviated as ACM; Del Giudice et al., 2011), humans evolved to encode critical features of the local environment at an early age (e.g., its adversity, danger, unpredictability, and nurturance), and these features trigger the development of specific patterns of stress responsivity (interacting with genetic predispositions, as shown by Frigerio et al., 2009; Gilissen, Bakermans-Kranenburg, van IJzendoorn, & Linting, 2008), which in turn maximize an individual's survival in that particular environment.

Both early adversity and poor caregiving serve as indicators to the infant's developing stress regulation system that the local environment is harsh and/or unpredictable. In such conditions, survival is facilitated by a stress response system that responds quickly and robustly to potential sources of threat, given that (1) the local environment contains many such threats, and (2) caregivers may not be reliable protectors. Hence a hyper-vigilant, hyperreactive profile of stress reactivity (entailing both cognitive sensitivity to signs of threat and robust physiological response to these signs) should facilitate quick and effective self-defense. Although this heightened defensiveness has cumulative psychological and physiological costs over the long run, and although it may prove maladaptive in benign environments, it proves protective and survival-enhancing in harsh and threatening contexts.

The notion that early life experiences "program" the developing organism in an adaptive, environmentally tailored fashion is commonly referred to as *developmental plasticity*, which is presumed to operate via multiple mechanisms through which information about the external environment is internalized and shapes the developing organism (Bateson et al., 2004). The ACM proposes that there may be several developmental periods of heightened plasticity. Though the initial calibration of HPA and ANS functioning may take place during infancy, this process is not wholly deterministic. Rather, Del Giudice and colleagues propose that the stress response system may undergo several subsequent periods of heightened plasticity, such as middle childhood and puberty, during which individuals' stress response systems are recalibrated to current threats and resources to maintain an optimal "match" to current conditions.

What Counts as Adaptive?

The ACM represents a notable departure from the classic diathesis–stress model, which posits heightened stress reactivity as a uniform risk factor for maladjustment. As outlined by Hostinar and Gunnar (2013a), it also diverges from the *allostatic load* model (ALM), which posits that early adversity leads to long-term health problems because heightened stress reactivity creates chronic "wear and tear" on the stress regulatory systems (McEwen, 1998; McEwen & Stellar, 1993). According to the ALM, early deficits in caregiving set in motion a chain of stress-regulating patterns that engender chronic social deficits and maladaptive overactivation of the HPA axis and ANS (Repetti, Taylor, & Seeman, 2002). As summarized by Hostinar and Gunnar (2013a), these models focus on the proximal processes linking early adversity to stress regulation through which early adversity confers disadvantage. According to the ACM, early deficits in caregiving set in motion a chain of stress-regulating patterns that are adaptive in an adverse environment, but maladaptive in a benign one. Hence, whereas the ALM frames the problem as cumulative overload, the ACM poses the problem as a mismatch between the individual and his or her current context.

Thus the very features of HPA and ANS functioning that have historically been viewed as risk factors from the perspective of the ALM are viewed as *either* risk or resiliency factors from the perspective of the ACM. This implies that we can no longer casually use the word *adaptive*: *Adaptive* is a fundamentally relative construct, defined with respect to the challenges and environments at hand.

Scholars considering these two models generally concur that there is insufficient empirical evidence to determine whether the effects of early adversity are best conceptualized in terms of cumulative risk or adaptive calibration (Hostinar & Gunnar, 2013a; O'Connor & Spagnola, 2009). However, a growing body of findings suggests that heightened physiological stress reactivity is associated with differential risk in adverse conditions, but (in some cases and for some outcomes) differential benefit in highly nurturant conditions (see Belsky et al., 2007; Conradt, Measelle, & Ablow, 2013; Del Giudice, Hinnant, Ellis, & El-Sheikh, 2012; Diamond, Fagundes, & Cribbet, 2012; Pluess & Belsky, 2009, 2010, 2013). Overall, the pattern of findings of differential risk is more robust than the pattern of findings of differential benefit (Belsky & Pluess, 2012; Boyce et al., 1995; Cummings et al., 2007; Diamond et al., 2012; El-Sheikh et al., 2009; Katz, 2007); this difference is partially attributable to the fact that most studies examining stress reactivity as a moderator of children's vulnerability to environmental deficits have not even tested whether stress reactivity simultaneously moderates the benefits of enhanced environments.

Is Attachment Insecurity a Form of Adaptive Calibration?

The ACM suggests two intriguing reframings of the association between stress exposure and attachment security, both of which warrant future study. First, just as physiological hyperreactivity may represent a beneficial adaptation to harsh and/or predictable environments, attachment insecurity (i.e., high anxiety or high avoidance) may also be reframed as survival-promoting adaptations to caregiver insensitivity, rather than uniform risk factors for mental and interpersonal shortcomings. This is not a new idea (see Chisholm, Quinlivan, Petersen, & Coall, 2005; Crittenden, 2000; Hinde & Stevenson-Hinde, 1990; Main, 1981; Simpson & Belsky, 2008), but over the years the negative ramifications of attachment insecurity for stress regulation and socioemotional functioning over the life course have received substantially more attention than their potential adaptive consequences under adverse conditions. As summarized by Crittenden (2000), a prototypically secure attachment strategy of open emotional experience and interpersonal trust should prove beneficial only in relatively safe and nurturant environments in which stressors are manageable and reliable caregiving is available. In adverse and dangerous environments, in which caregivers cannot be relied upon to provide adequate protection, both the anxious strategy of hypervigilance to threat and the avoidant strategy of excessive self-reliance should prove to be more effective and adaptive.

Of course, these strategies entail a cost, as extensively documented by decades of research on the detrimental psychosocial correlates of attachment insecurity (see Mikulincer & Florian, 2004; Shaver & Mikulincer, 2007). Hence we must take care to make determinations of "adaptation" in the appropriate context. As noted by Frankenhuis and Del Giudice (2012), traits or behaviors that are adaptive from the perspective of natural selection (i.e., promoting survival and reproduction) may not be adaptive from the perspective of developmental psychology (i.e., promoting subjective well-being, emotional stability, and social competence). Although "strategies" such as attachment anxiety or avoidance may have a range of detrimental psychosocial "side effects" in benign environments, they should successfully promote infant survival and protection *in stressful environments*. Humans evolved in environments that varied widely with respect to environmental danger and caregiver availability, and the attachment system should have evolved to respond flexibly to such variation, directing an infant's development along the path most likely to ensure safety and survival. As Crittenden (2000) has argued, "There are many ways to do it right. But in all cases 'it' is the same: to protect self and progeny. The appropriate strategy depends on the context and the individual's maturation" (p. 383).

What remains unknown, however, is whether the ACM's key prediction of heightened *benefit* in nurturant environments applies to the case of attachment insecurity. There is currently no evidence suggesting that insecure children, upon making a transition into extremely nurturant environments in which caregiver insensitivity is completely supplanted by caregiver responsiveness and attentiveness, differentially "absorb" these positive features and show enhanced subsequent functioning. One of the reasons this is a difficult question to answer is that most caregiving environments are relatively stable. Hence it is unlikely that an insecure child's caregiver suddenly becomes unusually responsive. Studies of children in foster care show that children who have been exposed to extreme adversity can in fact manifest notable benefits when the caregiving environment is radically improved (see Hostinar & Gunnar, 2013c), but it is not known whether such children respond to such improvements significantly more strongly than children whose early rearing has provided more security.

The time course for such sensitivity is also unknown. The ACM predicts that there may be several postinfancy periods of heightened sensitivity to environmental influence, such as middle childhood and puberty; this suggests that insecure children may be most likely to benefit from enhanced caregiving during these periods. One possibility is that such caregiving could be provided outside the home, perhaps by nurturant teachers, athletic coaches, or relatives. The possibility that insecurely attached children may benefit disproportionately from nurturance provided by such nonfamilial sources is worth exploring.

Does Stress Reactivity Render Some Children More Susceptible to Attachment Insecurity?

A second possible implication of the ACM for attachment theory casts attachment security as the *outcome* of a child's differential sensitivity, rather than as one of the *sources* of differential sensitivity. In other words, it may not be the case that insecure children are differentially likely to show links between caregiving quality and later socioemotional adjustment. Rather, it may be that highly stress-reactive children are differentially likely to show links between caregiving quality and *attachment security*. Accordingly, perhaps children who have reactive HPA and ANS functioning are more likely to show changes in attachment security when the caregiving context changes.

This possibility may help to explain the considerable variation observed in links between childhood maltreatment and later attachment disturbances. As reviewed by O'Connor and Spagnola (2009), studies of institutionalized, neglected, and maltreated children reliably find that they have higher rates of attachment disorders—but there are sizable individual differences in this link, so that only a minority of neglected and maltreated children show severe disturbances in attachment. O'Connor and Spagnola (2009) note that an important emerging direction in this area of research is investigating specific "phenotypes" that confer high susceptibility to the attachment-related consequences of early caregiving deficits, potentially manifested in biological profiles of stress response. Yet they also raise important cautions about whether research on links between child maltreatment and attachment disorders can be generalized to nonclinical populations of children who show normative variation in both caregiving and attachment security. As they point out, in the case of maltreated, neglected, or institutionalized children, the key issue may not be attachment insecurity, but the formation of *any* functional attachment bond, and the relative roles of these two scenarios for long-term stress regulation remain unknown.

Another pressing question concerns change in attachment security between infancy/childhood and adulthood. Bowlby's (1973) "prototype hypothesis" specified that early attachment security lays the foundation for adult romantic security by fundamentally shaping individuals' expectations and beliefs about love relationships. This claim has been called the "boldest assertion of attachment theory," serving as "a lightning rod of controversy" among developmental psychologists (Roisman, Collins, Sroufe, & Egeland, 2005, p. 105). The strictest, most "trait-like" version of the prototype hypothesis maintains that infant–caregiver attachment patterns are laid down during the first year of life and largely "grow up" into adult romantic attachment styles, establishing robust working models of adult love dynamics before an individual has even had his or her first romantic relationship. From this perspective, subsequent romantic experiences usually strengthen and confirm the individual's initial attachment style because working models function as self-fulfilling prophecies, reliably altering individuals' selection of romantic partners and their ongoing appraisals of partners' responsiveness and availability.

The evidence for this "strong trait" perspective is mixed, given that longitudinal studies have detected varying degrees of continuity in attachment styles from childhood to adulthood (Hamilton, 2000; Lewis, Feiring, & Rosenthal, 2000; Roisman et al., 2005; Waters et al., 2000; Weinfield et al., 2000) and over adulthood from relationship to relationship (Baldwin & Fehr, 1995; Davila, Burge, & Hammen, 1997; Davila et al., 1999; Fraley, 2007; Klohnen & Bera, 1998; Lopez & Gormley, 2002; Mitchell, 2007; Scharfe & Bartholomew, 1995; Zhang & Labouvie-Vief, 2004). Many researchers have sidestepped this debate by gravitating toward a "two-pronged" conceptualization of adult attachment styles, in which individuals have *both* a global working model (which is carried forward from childhood) that provides a general, trait-like template for an individual's relationship expectations, and *also* a relationship-specific model based on *particular* attachment figures, such as current or recent romantic partners (Baldwin & Fehr, 1995; Baldwin, Keelan, Fehr, Enns, & Koh-Rangarajoo, 1996; La Guardia, Ryan, Couchman, & Deci, 2000). This perspective takes more seriously the phenomenon of reciprocal influence between prior and current attachment expectations and experiences, and hence it holds more promise for the development of lifespan models of attachment that take into account an individual's entire cumulative trajectory of attachment-relevant experiences.

The unique contribution of the ACM is the notion that cumulative trajectories of attachment-relevant experiences may be more influential for some individuals than others due to individual differences in stress reactivity, which render certain individuals disproportionately sensitive to environmental and interpersonal threats *and* resources. Hence an intriguing direction for future research involves longitudinal assessment of individual differences in stress reactivity as predictors of the correspondence between changes in social–environmental conditions and concurrent changes in psychosocial functioning.

Conclusion

The increasing body of psychobiological research on attachment and stress regulation underscores the critical role of attachment relationships in fostering psychological, physical, and interpersonal functioning at all stages of the life course. Understanding the role of early attachment relationships in calibrating critical stress-regulating systems, and the long-term implications of these systems for well-being, provides important new ways to understand the fundamental functions of attachment over the life course. The development of integrative, lifespan, biobehavioral models of the attachment system remains a priority for future research. The quality of an individual's parental attachments clearly has critical implications for subjective and physiological aspects of stress regulation as well as for long-term social and psychological functioning, opening up a host of fascinating questions regarding our inherently social nature. Future research on the mutual, cascading relations between stress exposure and attachment processes from childhood to adulthood will contribute to our increasingly sophisticated understanding of the fundamental role of attachment relationships for psychological and physical well-being over the life course.

References

Alkon, A., Boyce, W. T., Davis, N. V., & Eskenazi, B. (2011). Developmental changes in autonomic nervous system resting and reactivity measures in Latino children from 6 to 60 months of age. *Journal of Developmental and Behavioral Pediatrics, 32,* 668–677.

Baldwin, M. W., & Fehr, B. (1995). On the instability of attachment style ratings. *Personal Relationships, 2,* 247–261.

Baldwin, M. W., Keelan, J. P. R., Fehr, B., Enns, V., & Koh-Rangarajoo, E. (1996). Social-cognitive conceptualization of attachment working models: Availability and accessibility effects. *Journal of Personality and Social Psychology, 71,* 94–109.

Bateson, P., Barker, D., Clutton-Brock, T., Deb, D., D'Udine, B., Foley, R. A., et al. (2004). Developmental plasticity and human health. *Nature, 430,* 419–421.

Beauchaine, T. P. (2001). Vagal tone, development, and Gray's motivational theory: Toward an integrated model of autonomic nervous system functioning in psychopathology. *Development and Psychopathology, 13,* 183–214.

Belsky, J., Bakermans-Kranenburg, M. J., & van IJzendoorn, M. H. (2007). For better and for worse: Differential susceptibility to environmental influences. *Current Directions in Psychological Science, 16,* 300–304.

Belsky, J., & Pluess, M. (2009). Beyond diathesis stress: Differential susceptibility to environmental influences. *Psychological Bulletin, 135,* 885–908.

Belsky, J., & Pluess, M. (2012). Differential susceptibility to long-term effects of quality of child care on externalizing behavior in adolescence? *International Journal of Behavioral Development, 36,* 2–10.

Berntson, G. G., Cacioppo, J. T., & Fieldstone, A. (1996). Illusions, arithmetic, and the bidirectional modulation of vagal control of the heart. *Biological Psychology, 44,* 1–17.

Blandon, A. Y., Calkins, S. D., Keane, S. P., & O'Brien, M. (2010). Contributions of child's physiology and maternal behavior to children's trajectories of temperamental reactivity. *Developmental Psychology, 46,* 1089–1102.

Bowlby, J. (1973). *Attachment and loss: Vol. 2. Separation: Anxiety and anger.* New York: Basic Books.

Bowlby, J. (1977). The making and breaking of affectional bonds: I. Aetiology and psychopathology in the light of attachment theory. *British Journal of Psychiatry, 130,* 201–210.

Boyce, W. T., Chesney, M., Alkon, A., & Tschann, J. M. (1995). Psychobiologic reactivity to stress and childhood respiratory illnesses: Results of two prospective studies. *Psychosomatic Medicine, 57,* 411–422.

Boyce, W. T., & Ellis, B. J. (2005). Biological sensitivity to context: I. An evolutionary-developmental theory of the origins and functions of stress reactivity. *Development and Psychopathology, 17,* 271–301.

Bruce, J., Fisher, P. A., Pears, K. C., & Levine, S. (2009). Morning cortisol levels in preschool-aged foster children: Differential effects of maltreatment type. *Developmental Psychobiology, 51,* 14–23.

Bubier, J. L., Drabick, D. A. G., & Breiner, T. (2009). Autonomic functioning moderates the relations between contextual factors and externalizing behaviors among inner-city children. *Journal of Family Psychology, 23,* 500–510.

Buss, C., Lord, C., Wadiwalla, M., Hellhammer, D. H., Lupien, S. J., Meaney, M. J., & Pruessner, J. C. (2007). Maternal care modulates the relationship between prenatal risk and hippocampal volume in women but not in men. *Journal of Neuroscience, 27,* 2592–2595.

Byrd-Craven, J., Auer, B. J., Granger, D. A., & Massey, A. R. (2012). The father–daughter dance: The relationship between father–daughter relationship quality and daughters' stress response. *Journal of Family Psychology, 26,* 87–94.

Cacioppo, J. T. (1994). Social neuroscience: Autonomic, neuroendocrine, and immune responses to stress. *Psychophysiology, 31,* 113–128.

Cacioppo, J. T., Uchino, B. N., & Berntson, G. G. (1994). Individual differences in the autonomic origins of heart rate reactivity: The psychometrics of respiratory sinus arrhythmia and preejection period. *Psychophysiology, 31,* 412–419.

Calkins, S. D. (1997). Cardiac vagal tone indices of temperamental reactivity and behavioral regulation in young children. *Developmental Psychobiology, 31,* 125–135.

Calkins, S. D., Smith, C. L., Gill, K. L., & Johnson, M. C. (1998). Maternal interactive style across contexts: Relations to emotional, behavioral, and physiological regulation during toddlerhood. *Social Development, 7,* 350–369.

Chisholm, J. S., Quinlivan, J. A., Petersen, R. W., & Coall, D. A. (2005). Early stress predicts age at menarche and first birth, adult attachment, and expected lifespan. *Human Nature, 16,* 233–265.

Cicchetti, D., Rogosch, F. A., Gunnar, M. R., & Toth, S. L. (2010). The differential impacts of early physical and sexual abuse and internalizing problems on daytime cortisol rhythm in school-aged children. *Child Development, 81,* 252–269.

Cicchetti, D., Rogosch, F. A., & Toth, S. L. (1998). Maternal depressive disorder and contextual risk: Contributions to the development of attachment insecurity and behavior problems in toddlerhood. *Development and Psychopathology, 10,* 283–300.

Conradt, E., Measelle, J., & Ablow, J. C. (2013). Poverty, problem behavior, and promise: Differential susceptibility among infants reared in poverty. *Psychological Science, 24,* 235–242.

Crittenden, P. M. (2000). A dynamic-maturational exploration of the meaning of security and adaptation. In P. M. Crittenden & A. H. Claussen (Eds.), *The organization of attachment relationships: Maturation, culture, and context* (pp. 358–383). New York: Cambridge University Press.

Cummings, E. M., El-Sheikh, C. D., Kouros, C. D., & Keller, P. S. (2007). Children's skin conductance reactivity as a mechanism of risk in the context of parental depressive symptoms. *Journal of Child Psychology and Psychiatry, 48,* 436–445.

Davila, J., Burge, D., & Hammen, C. (1997). Why does attachment style change? *Journal of Personality and Social Psychology, 73,* 826–838.

Davila, J., Karney, B. R., & Bradbury, T. N. (1999). Attachment change processes in the early years of marriage. *Journal of Personality and Social Psychology, 76,* 783–802.

Del Giudice, M., Ellis, B. J., & Shirtcliff, E. A. (2011). The adaptive calibration model of stress responsivity. *Neuroscience and Biobehavioral Reviews, 35,* 1562–1592.

Del Giudice, M., Hinnant, J. B., Ellis, B. J., & El-Sheikh, M. (2012). Adaptive patterns of stress responsivity: A preliminary investigation. *Developmental Psychology, 48,* 775–790.

Dewitte, M., De Houwer, J., Goubert, L., & Buysse, A. (2010). A multi-modal approach to the study of attachment-related distress. *Biological Psychology, 85,* 149–162.

Diamond, L. M., & Cribbet, M. R. (2013). Links between adolescent sympathetic and parasympathetic nervous system functioning and interpersonal behavior over time. *International Journal of Psychophysiology, 88,* 339–348.

Diamond, L. M., Fagundes, C. P., & Cribbet, M. R. (2012). Individual differences in adolescent sympathetic and parasympathetic functioning moderate associations between family environment and psychosocial adjustment. *Developmental Psychology, 48,* 918–931.

Diamond, L. M., & Hicks, A. M. (2005). Attachment style, current relationship security, and negative emotions: The mediating role of physiological regulation. *Journal of Social and Personal Relationships, 22,* 499–518.

Diamond, L. M., Hicks, A. M., & Otter-Henderson, K. A. (2008). Every time you go away: Changes in affect, behavior, and physiology associated with travel-related separations from romantic partners. *Journal of Personality and Social Psychology, 95,* 385–403.

Dickerson, S. S., & Kemeny, M. E. (2004). Acute stressors and cortisol responses: A theoretical integration and synthesis of laboratory research. *Psychological Bulletin, 130,* 355–391.

El-Sheikh, M., Kouros, C. D., Erath, S., Cummings, E. M., Keller, P., Staton, L., et al. (2009). Marital conflict and children's externalizing behavior: Interactions between parasympathetic and sympathetic nervous system activity. *Monographs of the Society for Research in Child Development, 74*(1, Serial No. 292), 1–79.

El-Sheikh, M., & Whitson, S. A. (2006). Longitudinal relations between marital conflict and child adjustment: Vagal regulation as a protective factor. *Journal of Family Psychology, 20*, 30–39.

Ellis, B. J., Boyce, W. T., Belsky, J., Bakermans-Kranenburg, M. J., & van IJzendoorn, M. H. (2011). Differential susceptibility to the environment: An evolutionary-neurodevelopmental theory. *Development and Psychopathology, 23*, 7–28.

Fraley, R. C. (2007). A connectionist approach to the organization and continuity of working models of attachment. *Journal of Personality, 75*, 1157–1180.

Frankenhuis, W. E., & Del Giudice, M. (2012). When do adaptive developmental mechanisms yield maladaptive outcomes? *Developmental Psychology, 48*, 628–642.

Frigerio, A., Ceppi, E., Rusconi, M., Giorda, R., Raggi, M. E., & Fearon, P. (2009). The role played by the interaction between genetic factors and attachment in the stress response in infancy. *Journal of Child Psychology and Psychiatry, 50*, 1513–1522.

Gilissen, R., Bakermans-Kranenburg, M. J., van IJzendoorn, M. H., & Linting, M. (2008). Electrodermal reactivity during the Trier Social Stress Test for Children: Interaction between the serotonin transporter polymorphism and children's attachment representation. *Developmental Psychobiology, 50*, 615–625.

Glover, V., O'Connor, T. G., & O'Donnell, K. (2010). Prenatal stress and the programming of the HPA axis. *Neuroscience and Biobehavioral Reviews, 35*, 17–22.

Gunnar, M. R. (1998). Quality of early care and buffering of neuroendocrine stress reactions: Potential effects on the developing human brain. *Preventive Medicine, 27*, 208–211.

Gunnar, M. R. (2005). Attachment and stress in early development: Does attachment add to the potency of social regulators of infant stress? In C. S. Carter, L. Ahnert, K. E. Grossmann, S. B. Hrdy, M. E. Lamb, S. W. Porges, et al. (Eds.), *Attachment and bonding: A new synthesis* (pp. 245–255). Cambridge, MA: MIT Press.

Gunnar, M. R., & Donzella, B. (2002). Social regulation of cortisol levels in early human development. *Psychoneuroendocrinology, 27*, 199–220.

Gunnar, M. R., Frenn, K., Wewerka, S. S., & Van Ryzin, M. J. (2009). Moderate versus severe early life stress: Associations with stress reactivity and regulation in 10–12-year-old children. *Psychoneuroendocrinology, 34*, 62–75.

Hamilton, C. E. (2000). Continuity and discontinuity of attachment from infancy through adolescence. *Child Development, 71*, 690–694.

Heim, C., & Nemeroff, C. B. (1999). The impact of early adverse experiences on brain systems involved in the pathophysiology of anxiety and affective disorders. *Biological Psychiatry, 46*, 1509–1522.

Heim, C., Newport, D. J., Mletzko, T., Miller, A. H., & Nemeroff, C. B. (2008). The link between childhood trauma and depression: Insights from HPA axis studies in humans. *Psychoneuroendocrinology, 33*, 693–710.

Hesse, E. (1999). The Adult Attachment Interview: Historical and current perspectives. In J. Cassidy & P. R. Shaver (Eds.), *Handbook of attachment: Theory, research, and clinical applications* (pp. 395–433). New York: Guilford Press.

Hesse, E., & Main, M. (2006). Frightened, threatening, and dissociative parental behavior in low-risk samples: Description, discussion, and interpretations. *Development and Psychopathology, 18*, 309–343.

Hessler, D. M., & Katz, L. F. (2007). Children's emotion regulation: Self-report and physiological response to peer provocation. *Developmental Psychology, 43*, 27–38.

Hinde, R. A., & Stevenson-Hinde, J. (1990). Attachment: Biological, cultural and individual desiderata. *Human Development, 33*, 62–72.

Hinnant, J. B., Elmore-Staton, L., & El-Sheikh, M. (2011). Developmental trajectories of respiratory sinus arrythmia and preejection period in middle childhood. *Developmental Psychobiology, 53*, 59–68.

Hostinar, C. E., & Gunnar, M. R. (2013a). The developmental effects of early life stress: An overview of current theoretical frameworks. *Current Directions in Psychological Science, 22*, 400–406.

Hostinar, C. E., & Gunnar, M. R. (2013b). The developmental psychobiology of stress and emotion in childhood. In I. B. Weiner (Series Ed.) & R. M. Lerner, M. A. Easterbrooks, & J. Mistry (Vol. Eds.), *Handbook of psychology: Vol. 6. Developmental psychology* (2nd ed., pp. 121–141). Hoboken, NJ: Wiley.

Hostinar, C. E., & Gunnar, M. R. (2013c). Future directions in the study of social relationships as regulators of the HPA axis across development. *Journal of Clinical Child and Adolescent Psychology, 42*, 564–575.

Hunter, A. L., Minnis, H., & Wilson, P. (2011). Altered stress responses in children exposed to early adversity: A systematic review of salivary cortisol studies. *Stress: International Journal on the Biology of Stress, 14*, 614–626.

Kajantie, E., & Räikkönen, K. (2010). Early life predictors of the physiological stress response later in life. *Neuroscience and Biobehavioral Reviews, 35*, 23–32.

Katz, L. F. (2007). Domestic violence and vagal reactivity to peer provocation. *Biological Psychology, 74*, 154–164.

Kirschbaum, C., Wust, S., Faig, H. G., & Hellhammer, D. H. (1992). Heritability of cortisol responses to human corticotropin-releasing hormone, ergometry, and psychological stress in humans. *Journal of Clinical Endocrinology and Metabolism, 75*, 1526–1530.

Klohnen, E. C., & Bera, S. (1998). Behavioral and experiential patterns of avoidantly and securely attached women across adulthood: A 31-year longitudinal perspective. *Journal of Personality and Social Psychology, 74*, 211–223.

La Guardia, J. G., Ryan, R. M., Couchman, C. E., & Deci, E. L. (2000). Within-person variation in security of attachment: A self-determination theory perspective on attachment, need fulfillment, and well-being. *Journal of Personality and Social Psychology, 79*, 367–384.

Laurent, H., & Powers, S. (2007). Emotion regulation in emerging adult couples: Temperament, attachment, and HPA response to conflict. *Biological Psychology, 76*, 61–71.

Lengua, L. J. (2012). Poverty, the development of effortful control, and children's academic, social, and emotional adjustment. In V. Maholmes & R. B. King (Eds.), *The Oxford handbook of poverty and child development* (pp. 491–511). New York: Oxford University Press.

Lewis, M., Feiring, C., & Rosenthal, S. (2000). Attachment over time. *Child Development, 71*, 707–720.

Lopez, F. G., & Gormley, B. (2002). Stability and change in adult attachment style over the first-year college transition: Relations to self-confidence, coping, and distress patterns. *Journal of Counseling Psychology, 49,* 355–364.

Luecken, L. J. (1998). Childhood attachment and loss experiences affect adult cardiovascular and cortisol function. *Psychosomatic Medicine, 60,* 765–772.

Luecken, L. J., Rodriguez, A. P., & Appelhans, B. M. (2005). Cardiovascular stress responses in young adulthood associated with family-of-origin relationship experiences. *Psychosomatic Medicine, 67,* 514–521.

Madigan, S., Bakermans-Kranenburg, M. J., van IJzendoorn, M. H., Moran, G., Pederson, D. R., & Benoit, D. (2006). Unresolved states of mind, anomalous parental behavior, and disorganized attachment: A review and meta-analysis of a transmission gap. *Attachment and Human Development, 8,* 89–111.

Main, M. (1981). Avoidance in the service of attachment: A working paper. In K. Immelmann, G. Barlow, L. Petrinovich, & M. Main (Eds.), *Behavioral development: The Bielefeld interdisciplinary project* (pp. 651–693). New York: Cambridge University Press.

Main, M., Kaplan, N., & Cassidy, J. (1985). Security in infancy, childhood, and adulthood: A move to the level of representation. In I. Bretherton & E. Waters (Eds.), Growing points of attachment theory and research. *Monographs of the Society for Research in Child Development, 50*(1–2, Serial No. 209), 66–104.

Main, M., & Solomon, J. (1990). Procedures for identifying infants as disorganized/disoriented during the Ainsworth Strange Situation. In M. T. Greenberg, D. Cicchetti, & E. M. Cummings (Eds.), *Attachment in the preschool years: Theory, research, and intervention* (pp. 121–160). Chicago: University of Chicago Press.

Maunder, R. G., Lancee, W. J., Nolan, R. P., Hunter, J. J., & Tannenbaum, D. W. (2006). The relationship of attachment insecurity to subjective stress and autonomic function during standardized acute stress in healthy adults. *Journal of Psychosomatic Research, 60,* 283–290.

McEwen, B. S. (1998). Stress, adaptation, and disease: Allostasis and allostatic load. *Annals of the New York Academy of Sciences, 840,* 33–44.

McEwen, B. S., & Stellar, E. (1993). Stress and the individual: Mechanisms leading to disease. *Archives of Internal Medicine, 153,* 2093–2101.

Mikulincer, M., & Florian, V. (2004). Attachment style and affect regulation: Implications for coping with stress and mental health. In M. B. Brewer & M. Hewstone (Eds.), *Applied social psychology* (pp. 28–49). Malden, MA: Blackwell.

Miller, G. E., Chen, E., & Parker, K. J. (2011). Psychological stress in childhood and susceptibility to the chronic diseases of aging: Moving toward a model of behavioral and biological mechanisms. *Psychological Bulletin, 137,* 959–997.

Miller, G. E., Chen, E., & Zhou, E. S. (2007). If it goes up, must it come down?: Chronic stress and the hypothalamic–pituitary–adrenocortical axis in humans. *Psychological Bulletin, 133,* 25–45.

Mills-Koonce, W. R., Appleyard, K., Barnett, M., Deng, M., Putallaz, M., & Cox, M. (2011). Adult attachment style and stress as risk factors for early maternal sensitivity and negativity. *Infant Mental Health Journal, 32,* 277–285.

Mills-Koonce, W. R., Garrett-Peters, P., Barnett, M., Granger, D. A., Blair, C., &

Cox, M. J. (2011). Father contributions to cortisol responses in infancy and toddlerhood. *Developmental Psychology, 47*, 388–395.

Mitchell, V. (2007). Earning a secure attachment style: A narrative of personality change in adulthood. In R. Josselson, A. Lieblich, & D. P. McAdams (Eds.), *The meaning of others: Narrative studies of relationships* (pp. 93–116). Washington, DC: American Psychological Association.

Moore, G. A., & Calkins, S. D. (2004). Infants' vagal regulation in the still-face paradigm is related to dyadic coordination of mother–infant interaction. *Developmental Psychology, 40*, 1068–1080.

Muraven, M., & Baumeister, R. F. (2000). Self-regulation and depletion of limited resources: Does self-control resemble a muscle? *Psychological Bulletin, 126*, 247–259.

Nachmias, M., Gunnar, M. R., Mangelsdorf, S., Parritz, R. H., & Buss, K. (1996). Behavioral inhibition and stress reactivity: The moderating role of attachment security. *Child Development, 67*, 508–522.

Neumann, S. A., Sollers, J. J., Thayer, J. F., & Waldstein, S. R. (2004). Alexithymia predicts attenuated autonomic reactivity, but prolonged recovery to anger recall in young women. *International Journal of Psychophysiology, 53*, 183–195.

Nolte, T., Guiney, J., Fonagy, P., Mayes, L. C., & Luyten, P. (2012). Interpersonal stress regulation and the development of anxiety disorders: An attachment-based developmental framework. *Frontiers in Behavioral Neuroscience, 5*, 1–21.

O'Connor, T. G., & Spagnola, M. E. (2009). Early stress exposure: Concepts, findings, and implications, with particular emphasis on attachment disturbances. *Child and Adolescent Psychiatry and Mental Health, 3*, 24.

Oosterman, M., De Schipper, J. C., Fisher, P., Dozier, M., & Schuengel, C. (2010). Autonomic reactivity in relation to attachment and early adversity among foster children. *Development and Psychopathology, 22*, 109–118.

Oskis, A., Loveday, C., Hucklebridge, F., Thorn, L., & Clow, A. (2011). Anxious attachment style and salivary cortisol dysregulation in healthy female children and adolescents. *Journal of Child Psychology and Psychiatry, 52*, 111–118.

Perry, N. B., Nelson, J. A., Swingler, M. M., Leerkes, E. M., Calkins, S. D., Marcovitch, S., et al. (2013). The relation between maternal emotional support and child physiological regulation across the preschool years. *Developmental Psychobiology, 55*, 382–394.

Pierrehumbert, B., Torrisi, R., Ansermet, F., Borghini, A., & Halfon, O. (2012). Adult attachment representations predict cortisol and oxytocin responses to stress. *Attachment and Human Development, 14*, 453–476.

Pluess, M., & Belsky, J. (2009). Differential susceptibility to rearing experience: The case of childcare. *Journal of Child Psychology and Psychiatry, 50*, 396–404.

Pluess, M., & Belsky, J. (2010). Differential susceptibility to parenting and quality child care. *Developmental Psychology, 46*, 379–390.

Pluess, M., & Belsky, J. (2013). Vantage sensitivity: Individual differences in response to positive experiences. *Psychological Bulletin, 139*, 901–916.

Porges, S. W. (1992). Autonomic regulation and attention. In B. A. Campbell, H.

Hayne, & R. Richardson (Eds.), *Attention and information processing in infants and adults* (pp. 201–223). Hillsdale, NJ: Erlbaum.

Porges, S. W., Doussard-Roosevelt, J. A., & Maiti, A. K. (1994). Vagal tone and the physiological regulation of emotion. In N. Fox (Ed.), The development of emotion regulation: Biological and behavioral considerations. *Monographs of the Society for Research in Child Development, 59*(2–3, Serial No. 240), 167–186.

Porter, C. L., Wouden-Miller, M., Silva, S. S., & Porter, A. E. (2003). Marital harmony and conflict: Linked to infants' emotional regulation and cardiac vagal tone. *Infancy, 4*, 297–307.

Powers, S. I., Pietromonaco, P. R., Gunlicks, M., & Sayer, A. (2006). Dating couples' attachment styles and patterns of cortisol reactivity and recovery in response to a relationship conflict. *Journal of Personality and Social Psychology, 90*, 613–628.

Propper, C. (2012). The early development of vagal tone: Effects of poverty and elevated contextual risk. In V. Maholmes & R. B. King (Eds.), *The Oxford handbook of poverty and child development* (pp. 103–123). New York: Oxford University Press.

Quirin, M., Pruessner, J. C., & Kuhl, J. (2008). HPA system regulation and adult attachment anxiety: Individual differences in reactive and awakening cortisol. *Psychoneuroendocrinology, 33*, 581–590.

Repetti, R. L., Taylor, S. E., & Seeman, T. E. (2002). Risky families: Family social environments and the mental and physical health of offspring. *Psychological Bulletin, 128*, 330–366.

Rinaman, L., Banihashemi, L., & Koehnle, T. J. (2011). Early life experience shapes the functional organization of stress-responsive visceral circuits. *Physiology and Behavior, 104*, 632–640.

Roisman, G. I., Collins, W. A., Sroufe, L. A., & Egeland, B. (2005). Predictors of young adults' representations of and behavior in their current romantic relationship: Prospective tests of the prototype hypothesis. *Attachment and Human Development, 7*, 105–121.

Salomon, K. (2005). Respiratory sinus arrhythmia during stress predicts resting respiratory sinus arrhythmia three years later in a pediatric sample. *Health Psychology, 24*, 68–76.

Sanchez, M. M., Ladd, C. O., & Plotsky, P. M. (2001). Early adverse experience as a developmental risk factor for later psychopathology: Evidence from rodent and primate models. *Development and Psychopathology, 13*, 419–449.

Saul, J. P. (1990). Beat-to-beat variations of heart rate reflect modulation of cardiac autonomic outflow. *News in Psychological Science, 5*, 32–37.

Scharfe, E., & Bartholomew, K. (1995). Accommodation and attachment representations in young couples. *Journal of Social and Personal Relationships, 12*, 389–401.

Schore, A. N. (2001). Effects of a secure attachment relationship on right brain development, affect regulation, and infant mental health. *Infant Mental Health Journal, 22*, 7–66.

Segerstrom, S. C., & Nes, L. S. (2007). Heart rate variability reflects self-regulatory strength, effort, and fatigue. *Psychological Science, 18*, 275–281.

Shaver, P. R., & Mikulincer, M. (2007). Attachment theory and research: Core concepts, basic principles, conceptual bridges. In A. W. Kruglanski & E. T. Higgins (Eds.), *Social psychology: Handbook of basic principles* (2nd ed., pp. 650–677). New York: Guilford Press.

Shaw, D. S., & Vondra, J. I. (1993). Chronic family adversity and infant attachment security. *Child Psychology and Psychiatry, 34,* 1205–1215.

Siegel, D. J. (2001). Toward an interpersonal neurobiology of the developing mind: Attachment relationships, "mindsight," and neural integration. *Infant Mental Health Journal, 22,* 67–94.

Simpson, J. A., & Belsky, J. (2008). Attachment theory within a modern evolutionary framework. In P. R. Shaver & J. Cassidy (Eds.), *Handbook of attachment: Theory, research, and clinical applications* (2nd ed., pp. 131–157). New York: Guilford Press.

Simpson, J. A., & Rholes, W. S. (1994). Stress and secure base relationships in adulthood. *Advances in Personal Relationships, 5,* 181–204.

Simpson, J. A., & Rholes, W. S. (2012). Adult attachment orientations, stress, and romantic relationships. In P. Devine & A. Plant (Eds.), *Advances in experimental social psychology* (Vol. 45, pp. 279–328). San Diego, CA: Academic Press.

Skowron, E. A., Loken, E., Gatzke-Kopp, L. M., Cipriano-Essel, E. A., Woehrle, P. L., Van Epps, J. J., et al. (2011). Mapping cardiac physiology and parenting processes in maltreating mother–child dyads. *Journal of Family Psychology, 25,* 663–674.

Snieder, H., Boomsma, D. I., Van Doornen, L. J. P., & De Geus, E. J. C. (1997). Heritability of respiratory sinus arrhythmia: Dependency on task and respiration rate. *Psychophysiology, 34,* 317–328.

Spangler, G., Schieche, M., Ilg, U., Maier, U., & Ackerman, C. (1994). Maternal sensitivity as an external organizer for biobehavioral regulation in infancy. *Developmental Psychobiology, 27,* 425–437.

Spear, J. F., Kronhaus, K. D., Moore, E. N., & Kline, R. P. (1979). The effect of brief vagal stimulation on the isolated rabbit sinus node. *Circulation Research, 44,* 75–88.

Stronach, E. P., Toth, S. L., Rogosch, F., Oshri, A., Manly, J. T., & Cicchetti, D. (2011). Child maltreatment, attachment security, and internal representations of mother and mother–child relationships. *Child Maltreatment, 16,* 137–145.

Susman Stillman, A., Kalkose, M., Egeland, B., & Waldman, I. (1996). Infant temperament and maternal sensitivity as predictors of attachment security. *Infant Behavior and Development, 19,* 33–47.

Teicher, M. H., Andersen, S. L., Polcari, A., Anderson, C. M., Navalta, C. P., & Kim, D. M. (2003). The neurobiological consequences of early stress and childhood maltreatment. *Neuroscience and Biobehavioral Reviews, 27,* 33–44.

Tharner, A., Dierckx, B., Luijk, M. P. C. M., van IJzendoorn, M. H., Bakermans-Kranenburg, M. J., van Ginkel, J. R., et al. (2013). Attachment disorganization moderates the effect of maternal postnatal depressive symptoms on infant autonomic functioning. *Psychophysiology, 50,* 195–203.

Thayer, J. F., & Lane, R. D. (2000). A model of neurovisceral integration in emotion regulation and dysregulation. *Journal of Affective Disorders, 61,* 201–216.

van Bakel, H. J. A., & Riksen-Walraven, J. M. (2004). Stress reactivity in 15-month-old infants: Links with infant temperament, cognitive competence, and attachment security. *Developmental Psychobiology, 44,* 157–167.

Vasilev, C. A., Crowell, S. E., Beauchaine, T. P., Mead, H. K., & Gatzke-Kopp, L. M. (2009). Correspondence between physiological and self-report measures of emotion dysregulation: A longitudinal investigation of youth with and without psychopathology. *Journal of Child Psychology and Psychiatry, 50,* 1357–1364.

Vohs, K. D., Baumeister, R. F., & Ciarocco, N. J. (2005). Self-regulation and self-presentation: Regulatory resource depletion impairs impression management and effortful self-presentation depletes regulatory resources. *Journal of Personality and Social Psychology, 88,* 632–657.

Waters, E., Merrick, S., Treboux, D., Crowell, J., & Albersheim, L. (2000). Attachment security in infancy and early adulthood: A twenty-year longitudinal study. *Child Development, 71,* 678–683.

Weinfield, N. S., Sroufe, L. A., & Egeland, B. (2000). Attachment from infancy to early adulthood in a high-risk sample: Continuity, discontinuity, and their correlates. *Child Development, 71,* 695–702.

Zhang, F., & Labouvie-Vief, G. (2004). Stability and fluctuation in adult attachment style over a 6-year period. *Attachment and Human Development, 6,* 419–437.

5

Boosting Attachment Security in Adulthood

The "Broaden-and-Build" Effects of Security-Enhancing Mental Representations and Interpersonal Contexts

Mario Mikulincer
Phillip R. Shaver

Attachment theory conceptualizes the effects of experiences in close relationships on the development of both favorable and (in the case of non-optimal relationships) unfavorable personality characteristics. In his exposition of attachment theory, John Bowlby (1969/1982, 1973, 1980, 1988) explained why the availability of caring, supportive relationship partners, beginning in infancy, is so important to developing a sense of attachment security—confidence that one is competent and lovable, and that caregivers will be responsive and supportive when needed. This sense of security is a resilience resource in times of need and a building block of mental health and social adjustment. Adult attachment researchers have found that a person's sense of attachment security is associated with self-esteem, emotional stability, constructive coping strategies, and mutually satisfying relationships throughout life (Mikulincer & Shaver, 2003, 2007a; Shaver & Mikulincer, 2002).

In this chapter, we move beyond the well-researched correlates of dispositional measures of attachment security (which attachment researchers call attachment *styles* or *orientations*) to review what has been learned during the last decade about the causal effects of contextually boosting a person's sense of security in laboratory experiments as well as field studies. The chapter begins with a brief account of attachment theory and then explains our model of attachment processes in adulthood (Mikulincer & Shaver, 2007a), which is an extension of Bowlby's theory, now supported by over 25 years of research by personality and social psychologists. Next, we focus on the anchoring of attachment security in expectations concerning relationship partners' sensitivity and responsiveness (expectations organized within a *secure-base script*), and review findings from laboratory studies showing that experimentally augmented security (based on priming mental representations of security) has positive effects on emotion regulation, appraisals of self and others, mental health, and prosocial behavior. Finally, we review findings from laboratory and field studies showing that real-life interpersonal contexts that strengthen a person's sense of attachment security (e.g., being in a relationship with a responsive and supportive partner) bring about beneficial changes in psychological functioning. The findings provide strong support for Bowlby's ideas about the plasticity of the attachment system across the lifespan and the growth-enhancing consequences of secure attachments.

Attachment Theory: Basic Concepts

Bowlby (1969/1982) began with the observation that human infants are unusually vulnerable because of their prematurity (compared with other mammalian offspring) but are born with a repertoire of *attachment behaviors*, selected during evolution because they assured proximity to supportive others (*attachment figures*) as a means of protection (from predation, starvation, injuries, etc.). When attachment behaviors repeatedly achieve their psychobiological goal of safety and security, they contribute to a general sense of *felt security* (Sroufe & Waters, 1977), which makes exploration, learning, and participation in social relationships easier and more successful.

Security-promoting attachment behaviors are organized by an innate *attachment behavioral system*, which Bowlby (1969/1982) characterized as a cybernetic program that includes detection of threats, the ability to signal a need for help from attachment figures, and actions to establish contact with these figures and allow reliance on them for reassurance and safety. Although the attachment system is most important early in life, Bowlby (1988) viewed it as active across the human lifespan, as indicated by emotional bonds with close friends and romantic partners, and by intense grief reactions when an emotional bond is broken due to separation, divorce, or the death of a close other.

Bowlby (1973) also described important individual differences in attachment system functioning. In his view, these individual differences are rooted in the reactions of one's relationship partners to bids for proximity and support in times of need, and in the incorporation of such reactions into working models of self and relationships. Interactions with attachment figures who are available, sensitive, and supportive in times of need facilitate the smooth, normative functioning of the attachment system; promote a sense of connectedness and security; and contribute to positive working models of self and others. When a person's attachment figures are not reliably available and supportive, however, a pervasive, dispositional sense of security is not attained; worries about one's social value and others' intentions are strengthened; and strategies of affect regulation other than normal proximity seeking are adopted (these are termed *secondary attachment strategies*, characterized by *anxiety* or defensive *avoidance*).

When studying individual differences in attachment system functioning in adults, attachment researchers have focused on attachment orientations or styles—patterns of relational expectations, emotions, and behaviors that result from internalizing a particular history of attachment experiences (Shaver & Mikulincer, 2002). Research, beginning with Ainsworth, Blehar, Waters, and Wall (1978) and continuing through scores of more recent studies by social and personality psychologists (reviewed by Mikulincer & Shaver, 2007a), indicates that attachment styles are located in a two-dimensional space defined by roughly orthogonal factors that we call attachment-related *anxiety* and *avoidance* (Brennan, Clark, & Shaver, 1998; Fraley & Waller, 1998). The avoidance dimension reflects the extent to which a person distrusts relationship partners' goodwill and defensively strives to maintain behavioral and emotional independence and distance. The anxiety dimension reflects the extent to which a person worries that a partner will not be available in times of need, partly because of the person's self-doubts about his or her worthiness. People who score low on both dimensions are relatively secure with respect to attachment. A person's location in the two-dimensional space can be measured with reliable and valid self-report scales (e.g., Brennan et al., 1998) and is associated in theoretically predictable ways with a wide variety of measures of relationship quality and psychological adjustment (see Mikulincer & Shaver, 2007a, for a review).

Although attachment orientations are initially formed during childhood in relationships with parents and other early caregivers (Cassidy & Shaver, 2008), Bowlby (1988) believed that important interactions with relationship partners beyond childhood can alter a person's working models and move him or her from one region of the two-dimensional anxiety × avoidance space to another. Moreover, although a person's attachment style is often conceptualized as a single global orientation toward relationships (which can be measured as such and has been shown to have reliable, predictable correlates), it is an emergent property of a complex network of cognitive and affective processes, which include many episodic, context-relative, and relationship-specific memories and schemas (Bowlby, 1988; Mikulincer & Shaver, 2003). Many studies indicate that a person's attachment orientation can change, depending on context and recent experiences

(Mikulincer & Shaver, 2007b); this makes it possible to study the causal effects of an experimentally primed sense of security within the confines of a social psychological laboratory, or to examine the long-term effects of real-life security-enhancing interpersonal contexts.

We (Mikulincer & Shaver, 2007a) have proposed that individuals' location in the two-dimensional anxiety × avoidance space reflects both their sense of attachment security and the way they deal with threats and stressors. People who score low on the two insecurity dimensions are generally secure, hold positive working models of self and others, and tend to employ constructive and effective affect regulation strategies. Those who score high on either attachment anxiety or avoidance suffer from attachment insecurities, worries about self-worth, or distrust of others' goodwill and responsiveness in times of need. Moreover, insecure people tend to use secondary attachment strategies that we, following Cassidy and Kobak (1988), characterize as attachment system *hyperactivation* or *deactivation* when coping with threats, frustrations, rejections, and losses. People who score high on attachment anxiety rely on hyperactivating strategies—energetic attempts to achieve support and love, combined with lack of confidence that these resources will be provided and with feelings of anger and despair when they are not provided (Cassidy & Kobak, 1988). In contrast, people who score high on attachment-related avoidance tend to use deactivating strategies— trying not to seek proximity to others when threatened, denying vulnerability and needs for other people, and avoiding closeness and interdependence in relationships.

With these ideas in mind, we can provide an overview of the cognitive, affective, and relational outcomes associated with attachment system functioning in adulthood. On the one hand, interactions with security-enhancing attachment figures contribute to a stable and solid sense of attachment security, which is an important aspect of healthy personality development, favorable psychological functioning, and good social and personal adjustment (see Mikulincer & Shaver, 2007a, for a review). On the other hand, adoption of hyperactivating or deactivating strategies influences the specific defenses used by insecure people to regulate distress and manage doubts about their self-worth and others' availability, sensitivity, and responsiveness. Adoption of a particular insecure strategy also shapes the different emotional and relational problems that result from anxious and avoidant forms of attachment. In the next section, we summarize the positive effects of attachment security and related mental representations on a person's social motives, cognitions, and behaviors.

Mental Representations of Attachment Security

According to our model of adult attachment system functioning (Mikulincer & Shaver, 2003, 2007a), appraisal of the availability and supportiveness of an attachment figure in times of need automatically activates mental representations of attachment security. These representations include both declarative and procedural knowledge organized around a relational prototype or *secure-base script* (Waters & Waters, 2006), which contains something like the following "if–then" propositions: "If I encounter an obstacle and/or become distressed, I can approach a significant other for help; he or she is likely to be available and supportive; I will experience relief and comfort as a result of proximity to this person; I can then return to other activities." Having many experiences that contribute to the construction of this script makes it easier for a person to confront stressful situations with optimistic expectations, which in turn helps the person maintain relative calm and optimistic hope while coping with problems.

There is evidence for the psychological reality of the secure-base script in young adults. For example, we and our colleagues (Mikulincer, Shaver, Sapir-Lavid, & Avihou-Kanza, 2009) found that people who scored lower on self-report scales tapping attachment anxiety or avoidance (i.e., more secure participants) were more likely than those who scored higher to include elements of the secure-base script (e.g., support seeking, support provision, distress relief) when writing about projective test pictures of a troubled person. Moreover, the two kinds of insecurity—anxiety and avoidance—were associated with different types of gaps in the script. People who scored relatively high on the anxiety scale tended to omit or deemphasize the final step in the script (relief and return to other activities), whereas those who scored relatively high on the avoidance scale tended to omit the part about seeking and benefiting from others' support. That is, anxious participants more often wrote about an injured protagonist who was seeking support and not achieving relief, whereas avoidant participants more often wrote about a person achieving relief without seeking or receiving support. These results were not explained by alternative predictor variables, such as neuroticism, extraversion, or verbal ability.

Attachment figure availability also fosters what we, following Fredrickson (2001), call a *broaden-and-build* cycle of attachment security, which increases a person's resilience and expands his or her perspectives, coping flexibility, and skills and capabilities. The most immediate psychological effects of attachment figure availability are effective management of distress and restoration of emotional equanimity. According to attachment theory, interactions with available and supportive attachment figures, by imparting a pervasive sense of safety, assuage distress and elicit positive emotions such as relief, satisfaction, and gratitude. Secure people can therefore remain relatively unperturbed in times of stress and experience longer periods of positive affect, which in turn contribute to their sustained emotional well-being and mental health.

Experiences of attachment figure availability also contribute to a reservoir of core cognitive representations, which play a central role in maintaining emotional stability and personal adjustment. During positive interactions with sensitive and available attachment figures, individuals learn that distress is manageable, that external obstacles can be overcome, and that the course and outcome of most threatening events are at least partially controllable. Adult attachment studies provide extensive evidence that secure individuals, as identified by self-report measures, appraise a wide variety of stressful events in less threatening terms than insecure people (either anxious or avoidant) do, and that they hold more optimistic expectations about their ability to cope with stressors (e.g., Berant, Mikulincer, & Florian, 2001; Mikulincer & Florian, 1995; Radecki-Bush, Farrell, & Bush, 1993).

In addition, during interactions with supportive attachment figures, individuals learn about others' potential sensitivity, responsiveness, and goodwill. They also learn to view themselves as active, strong, and competent because they can effectively mobilize a partner's support and overcome threats that activate attachment behavior. Moreover, they perceive themselves as valuable, lovable, and special, thanks to being valued, loved, and regarded as special by caring attachment figures. Research has consistently shown that such positive mental representations of self and others are characteristic of secure persons (e.g., Baldwin, Fehr, Keedian, Seidel, & Thomson, 1993; Collins, 1996; Collins & Read, 1990; Cooper, Shaver, & Collins, 1998; Mickelson, Kessler, & Shaver, 1997; Mikulincer, 1995; Simpson, 1990).

The broaden-and-build cycle of attachment security is renewed every time a person notices that an actual or imaginary caring and loving attachment figure is available in times of stress. To examine the psychological reality of this cycle, we cannot rely solely on correlational studies examining cross-sectional or even prospective longitudinal associations between dispositional measures of attachment orientations and measures of psychological functioning and mental health. Rather, we need to test whether momentary or more prolonged experiences with actual or imaginary responsive and supportive attachment figures, which we expect to increase a person's sense of security even if he or she is dispositionally insecure, can activate the broaden-and-build cycle of attachment security and its positive effects on psychological functioning. In the following sections of this chapter we review studies that examined the psychological effects of momentary or more prolonged boosts in attachment security. We first review findings from laboratory experiments in which the security-enhancing mental representations were primed in various ways. We then review findings from both laboratory and field studies that have examined the effects of security-heightening interpersonal experiences.

Evidence for the Effects of Security-Enhancing Mental Representations

In several laboratory experiments, we and other attachment researchers have examined the psychological effects of temporarily activating mental representations of security by exposing people to security-related stimuli (a process known as *security priming*). These experiments use well-validated social-cognitive research techniques to activate mental representations of security and measure their psychological effects. These techniques include presentation (either explicit/supraliminal or implicit/subliminal presentation) of pictures suggesting attachment figure availability (e.g., a Picasso drawing of a mother cradling an infant in her arms; a couple holding hands and gazing into each other's eyes); presentation of the names of actual people designated by participants as security-enhancing attachment figures; guided imagery concerning the availability and supportiveness of an attachment figure; visualization of the faces of security-enhancing attachment figures; and viewing the photograph of an attachment figure. The effects of these primes have usually been compared with the effects of emotionally positive but attachment-unrelated stimuli (e.g., pictures of a large amount of money, the names or faces of acquaintances who are not attachment figures) or emotionally neutral stimuli (e.g., pictures of furniture, neutral words, faces, or names).

With regard to the emotional effects of experimentally induced security primes, research consistently indicates that portrayals of attachment figure availability improve participants' moods, and that they do so more reliably and powerfully than other positive stimuli (e.g., Mikulincer, Hirschberger, Nachmias, & Gillath, 2001; Mikulincer, Gillath, et al., 2001; Mikulincer et al., 2003; Mikulincer & Shaver, 2001). Mikulincer, Hirschberger, et al. (2001) also found that priming representations of supportive attachment figures infused neutral stimuli with more positive affect, even when the priming was done subliminally. For example, subliminal presentation of the names of people who were designated by participants as security-enhancing attachment figures, compared with the names of close others or mere acquaintances who were not nominated as attachment figures, led to greater liking of previously unfamiliar Chinese ideographs. Moreover, subliminally priming mental representations of available attachment figures induced more positive evaluations of neutral stimuli even in threatening contexts, and eliminated the detrimental effects that threats otherwise had on liking for neutral stimuli. Thus temporary priming of mental representations of security-enhancing attachment figures appears to have a calming, soothing effect.

There is also evidence that the symbolic presence of a responsive attachment figure is a modulator of emotional responses to specific distress-eliciting experiences. For example, Selcuk, Zayas, Günaydin, Hazan, and Kross (2012) found that both explicit and implicit priming of attachment figure representations speeded up emotional recovery and reduced negative thoughts after participants recalled an upsetting experience. Eisenberger and colleagues (Eisenberger et al., 2011; Master et al., 2009) found that viewing a photograph of a romantic partner (vs. a stranger or an object) reduced participants' subjective experience and neural representation of pain in response to heat stimuli. Younger, Aron, Parke, Chatterjee, and Mackey (2010) replicated these findings in a functional magnetic resonance imaging (fMRI) study, finding that greater analgesia while viewing pictures of a romantic partner was associated with increased activity in several reward-processing brain regions, such as the nucleus accumbens, lateral orbitofrontal cortex, and dorsolateral prefrontal cortex.

Along with these findings, we (Mikulincer, Shaver, & Horesh, 2006) examined whether the soothing effects of security priming mitigate the emotional damage caused by traumatic experiences, such as war, acts of terrorism, hurricanes, rape, and witnessing violent domestic disputes. In this study, we focused on a well-known cognitive manifestation of posttraumatic responses—longer reaction times when naming the colors in which trauma-related words were printed (Emilien et al., 2000). The participants were Israeli undergraduates who reported high or low levels of posttraumatic stress disorder (PTSD) symptoms related to terrorist attacks. They performed a computerized Stroop color-naming task that included, among other words, 10 terror-related words. During the task, the students were subliminally primed with an attachment security word (the Hebrew word for "being loved"), a positively valenced but attachment-unrelated word, or a neutral word. The results showed that a higher level of PTSD symptoms was associated with longer color-naming latencies for terror-related words, indicating greater automatic accessibility of the words. However, this association was significant only when participants were subliminally primed with a neutral or positive word. The effect was not significant following the priming of an attachment security representation. That is, symbolic mobilization of attachment security representations ("being loved") during the Stroop task had a soothing effect, lowering the accessibility of trauma-related thoughts.

Laboratory experiments have also provided support for the hypothesized effects of security priming on mental representations of self and others. For example, Baccus, Baldwin, and Packer (2004) showed that experimental priming with loving and accepting faces automatically increased the primed persons' sense of self-worth, even when they were unaware of the faces. Two other experimental studies showed that security priming can instill a sense of self-worth that renders defensive self-inflation unnecessary (Arndt, Schimel, Greenberg, & Pyszczynski, 2002; Schimel, Arndt, Pyszczynski, & Greenberg, 2001). In these studies, thoughts about either attachment figure availability (e.g., thinking about an accepting and loving other) or neutral thoughts were encouraged, and participants' use of particular self-enhancement strategies was then assessed. These strategies included self-enhancing biases in social comparison (Schimel et al., 2001) and defensive self-handicapping (Arndt et al., 2002). In both studies, momentary strengthening of mental representations of attachment figure availability weakened the tendency to make self-enhancing social comparisons or self-handicapping attributions.

Attachment researchers have also found that security priming has beneficial effects on expectations of a partner's behavior (Carnelley & Rowe, 2007; Pierce & Lydon, 1998; Rowe & Carnelley, 2003). In Rowe and Carnelley's (2003) study, for example, participants who were primed with representations of attachment figure availability (writing for 10 minutes about a past relationship in which they felt secure) reported more positive expectations for the current relationship than those who were primed with insecure representations. In Pierce and Lydon's (1998) study, young women who were subliminally exposed to security-related words (compared to those exposed to neutral words) were more likely to rely on support seeking as a way of coping with a hypothetical scenario in which they unexpectedly became pregnant.

Carnelley and Rowe (2010) examined how individuals experience security priming and how its effects differ from those produced by other positive-affect-related or relationship-related primes. Specifically, they analyzed the written protocols produced by participants in different priming conditions and found that security primes, as compared to other positive primes, led to more thoughts related to felt security, positive care, a sense of merging with another, positive emotion, and communion. In a further examination of the effects of security priming, Canterberry and Gillath (2013) scanned the brains of participants during rapid exposures to security-related words. Compared to a neutral prime, security priming was associated with widespread activation in the medial frontal and prefrontal cortical areas, which are associated with cognitive control and self-regulation. Additionally, security priming was uniquely associated with activation in the striatum (e.g., the putamen, globus pallidus, caudate), insula, and anterior cingulate cortex (ACC)—areas associated with positive affect and approach motivation.

There is also accumulating evidence that exposing people to security-related symbolic stimuli in the laboratory allows them to engage confidently in attachment-unrelated activities, such as exploring the environment, considering possible goals for the future, or caring for a needy other. For example, we (Mikulincer, Shaver, & Rom, 2011) examined the effects of security priming on exploration and learning. In two experiments, participants were primed with security-related or neutral stimuli, and their creative problem solving was assessed with the Remote Associates Test. In the first experiment, implicit security priming (subliminal presentation of attachment figures' names) led to more creative problem solving (compared with control conditions), regardless of participants' dispositional attachment anxiety and avoidance. In the second study, the effects of explicit security priming (recalling experiences of being cared for) were moderated by dispositional attachment anxiety and avoidance. That is, explicit priming of attachment security led to better performance on the Remote Associates Test only among those who scored lower on measures of dispositional attachment insecurity.

Security priming also facilitates effective provision of care and support to needy others. In two experiments, Mikulincer, Gillath, et al. (2001) and Mikulincer et al. (2003) found that subliminal priming with names of security providers, as compared with neutral priming, increased empathic concern for a suffering stranger and endorsement of prosocial values (concern for close others and for all of humanity). In another experimental study, we (Mikulincer, Shaver, Gillath, & Nitzberg, 2005, Study 1) examined the effects of security priming on the decision to help or not help a person in distress. Participants watched a confederate while she performed a series of aversive tasks. As the study progressed, the confederate became increasingly distressed, and the participant was given an opportunity to take her place, in effect sacrificing self for the welfare of another. Shortly before being exposed to the person's distress, participants were subliminally primed with either the name of a security provider (security priming) or a neutral name (neutral priming). We found that security priming, as compared with neutral priming, increased participants' compassion and willingness to take the distressed person's place. This effect occurred in both Israel and the United States, and occurred not only with subliminal primes but also when the priming was done supraliminally by asking participants to think of a familiar security provider (Mikulincer et al., 2005, Study 2).

In two additional studies, we (Mikulincer et al., 2005, Studies 3–4) tested whether contextual activation of mental representations of attachment security override egoistic motives for helping, such as mood enhancement (Schaller & Cialdini, 1988) and empathic joy (Smith, Keating, & Stotland, 1989). Study participants were randomly assigned to one of two priming conditions (security priming, neutral priming); read a true newspaper article about a woman in dire personal and financial distress; and then rated their emotional reactions to the article in terms of compassion and personal distress. In one study, half of the participants anticipated mood enhancement by means other than helping (e.g., expecting, immediately after this part of the experiment, to watch a comedy film). In the other study, half of the participants were told that the needy woman was chronically depressed and that her mood might be beyond their ability to improve it (the "no empathic joy" condition). Schaller and Cialdini (1988) and Smith et al. (1989) have previously found that these two conditions reduce egoistic motivations for helping, because a person gains no special mood-related benefit from helping the needy person. In our studies, however, these conditions failed to inhibit security-induced altruistic motives for helping, which were expressed even when the manipulated egoistic motives were absent (Batson, 1991).

The findings indicated that expecting to improve one's mood by means other than helping, or expecting not to be able to share a needy person's joy following the provision of help, reduced compassion and willingness to help in the neutral priming condition, but not in the security priming condition. Instead, security priming led to greater compassion and willingness to help even when there was no egoistic reason for helping (i.e., no empathic joy or no mood relief).

In sum, the combined evidence from our experimental studies indicates that attachment security makes compassion and altruism more likely. Although there are other reasons for helping, the prosocial effects of attachment security do not depend on alternative egoistic motives, such as a person's desire to improve his or her mood or the desire to share a suffering person's relief. We infer that a sense of attachment security reduces one's need for defensive self-protection and allows one to direct attention to others' needs, feel compassion toward a suffering other, and engage in altruistic behavior with the primary goal of benefiting others.

This reasoning received further support in a recent experiment in which we (Mikulincer, Shaver, Sahdra, & Bar-On, 2013) tested two hypotheses: (1) Contextually augmented attachment security would foster effective care provision toward a romantic partner who disclosed a personal problem; and (2) increased security would overcome barriers to responsive caregiving induced by mental depletion. Dating couples came to the laboratory and provided names of people (other than their dating partners) who acted as security providers for them. Each couple was then informed that the partners would be video-recorded during an interaction in which one of them ("the care seeker") disclosed a personal problem to the other ("the caregiver"). One partner was randomly preassigned to the care seeker's role, and the other to the caregiver's role. Care seekers chose and wrote about a personal problem they were willing to discuss (except ones that involved conflict with the partner). While this was happening, caregivers were taken to another room, where they performed a Stroop color-naming task in which we manipulated mental depletion and subliminally exposed them to either the names of security providers or names of unfamiliar persons. Following these manipulations, the members of each couple were video-recorded while they talked for 10 minutes about the problem the care seeker wanted to discuss. Independent judges then viewed the video recordings and coded participants' degree of responsiveness and supportiveness to their disclosing partners.

We found that security priming was associated with greater responsiveness and supportiveness toward a dating partner who was sharing a personal problem. Moreover, security priming overrode the detrimental effects of mental depletion on responsiveness and supportiveness. These effects were remarkably consistent across Israeli and American samples, and were unexplained by relationship satisfaction. Overall, these findings indicate that attachment security facilitates effective caregiving, and that experimental enhancement of security can counteract dispositional and situational barriers to compassion and helping.

Evidence Regarding the Effects of Security-Enhancing Interpersonal Contexts

Beyond examining the effects of security-enhancing mental representations, adult attachment researchers have examined whether the same broaden-and-build effects occur within interpersonal contexts in which an actual relationship partner's responsiveness and supportive behaviors augment one's sense of security. Such behavior on the part of a relationship partner, therapist, or leader may enhance a person's confidence in the availability and responsiveness of his or her social interaction partners, setting in motion the broaden-and-build cycle of attachment security. In other words, a relationship partner who acts as a reliable security provider can reactivate the secure-base script and help a person function more securely.

There is extensive evidence showing that proximity to a romantic partner can alleviate distress and contribute to emotional stability. In a naturalistic study of cohabiting and married couples, Gump, Polk, Kamarck, and Shiffman (2001) asked participants' partners to wear ambulatory blood pressure monitors for a week, report what they were doing and feeling, and indicate whether anyone was with them each time their blood pressure was recorded. Blood pressure was lower when participants were interacting with their romantic partners than when they were interacting with other people or were alone. Additionally, in an observational study of dating couples who were each video-recorded while one partner disclosed a personal concern to the other, Collins and Feeney (2000) found that observed supportiveness from partners reduced the distress reported by the support recipients. That is, people whose romantic partners provided more responsive support (as judged by independent coders) felt better after disclosing a personal problem than they did before doing so. In another observational study of dating couples who were video-recorded while trying to resolve their most important relationship problem, Simpson, Winterheld, Rholes, and Oriña (2007) found that participants were rated as calmer during peak distress points in the discussion if their partners were coded as more supportive. Interestingly, whereas securely attached individuals were rated as calmer when their partners provided more emotional care, avoidant individuals were rated as calmer when their partners provided more instrumental support.

In addition to these correlational studies, several experimental studies have shown that a romantic partner can be a source of distress regulation and emotional equanimity. For example, Coan, Schaefer, and Davidson

(2006) examined brain responses (via fMRI) of married women who underwent a laboratory stressor (the threat of electric shock) while each one was holding her husband's hand, holding the hand of an unfamiliar male experimenter, or holding no hand at all. Holding a spouse's hand reduced activation in brain regions associated with stress and distress (i.e., the right anterior insula, superior frontal gyrus, and hypothalamus). The stress-reducing effects of hand holding were greater for women who were more satisfied with their marriages, probably because of the stronger sense of security induced by physical contact with a responsive and supportive husband. In another study, Master et al. (2009) found that holding the hand of a romantic partner reduced perceptions of pain in response to heat stimuli.

Following this line of research, Kane, McCall, Collins, and Blascovich (2012) asked young adults to complete a threatening cliff-walking task in an immersive virtual environment. In this virtual world, each participant's romantic partner was, in three different experimental conditions, absent from the virtual world; present in the world and attentive to the participant during the task (waving, clapping at successes, head nodding, and actively orienting his or her body toward the participant); or present but inattentive (looking away from the participant). Participants in the attentive-partner condition experienced the task as less stressful than those who were alone; they also reported feeling more secure during the task and were less vigilant of their partners' behavior, compared to those in the inattentive-partner condition. These findings suggest that a romantic partner can alleviate distress, particularly if he or she acts in an attentive and responsive manner—that is, as a security-enhancing attachment figure.

Conceptually similar findings were reported by Guichard and Collins (2008), who manipulated the quality of a romantic partner's support by having the partner send messages (actually written by the researchers) before and after the focal person participated in a stressful speech-delivering task. Participants who received highly supportive messages were in a better mood after their speech, had higher state self-esteem, and felt more satisfied with their relationships, compared to those who received low-support messages or no message from their partners. In a similar study, Collins, Jaremka, and Kane (2009) found that experimentally manipulated supportive messages from a romantic partner during a stressful speech task (as compared to low-support messages) yielded lower cortisol levels and more rapid emotional recovery from the stressful task.

There is also evidence that a responsive and supportive romantic partner can enhance a person's autonomous exploration and goal pursuit, which is a component of the broaden-and-build cycle of attachment security. According to Bowlby (1988), an important function of an attachment figure is to provide a secure base from which another person can "make sorties into the outside world" (p. 11), with confidence that he or she can return for assistance and comfort if obstacles arise. Indeed, Feeney (2007) found that participants' perceptions of their romantic partners' availability and assistance in removing obstacles to goal pursuit were associated with a stronger sense of independence, greater self-efficacy in goal achievement, and deeper engagement in autonomous exploration. Moreover, during couples' discussions of future personal goals, participants were more likely to engage in exploration of these goals (as coded by external judges) when their partners were coded as communicating more availability and responsiveness in relation to the exploratory efforts.

Using longitudinal data, Feeney (2007) also found that individuals whose partners were more responsive to their needs for support (as reported by the partners or coded by external judges) reported increases in autonomous exploration over a 6-month period and were more likely to have achieved at least one personal goal that they had identified 6 months earlier. In another laboratory study, Feeney and Thrush (2010) found that when spouses were coded by external judges as more available during a video-recorded exploration task, as less interfering with their partners' exploration, or as more accepting of this activity, the exploring partners persisted longer at the activity and reported heightened self-esteem and a better mood following the exploration task. Similarly, Overall, Fletcher, and Simpson (2010) found that participants whose romantic partners were more responsive to their self-improvement desires during a laboratory discussion showed more self-improvement during the following year.

These broaden-and-build effects of security-enhancing interpersonal contexts have also been found in studies examining other kinds of relationships, including leader–follower and therapist–client relationships. For example, we (Davidovitz, Mikulincer, Shaver, Ijzak, & Popper, 2007) conducted two field studies examining the extent to which a military officer's responsiveness and supportiveness contributed to his soldiers' military performance and mental health. In one study, Israeli soldiers in regular military service from 60 different military units who were participating in a leadership workshop rated their instrumental and socioemotional functioning within their units. The 60 direct officers also completed ratings describing their own attachment orientations and their efficacy in providing support to their soldiers. Soldiers' instrumental and socioemotional functioning within their units was positively associated with officers' self-reported sense of attachment security (lower scores on the avoidance and anxiety dimensions) and officers' appraisal of their efficacy in supporting soldiers' emotional needs. Moreover, these officers' effects were not moderated by soldiers' own attachment insecurities.

In a second study (Davidovitz et al., 2007), we approached Israeli military recruits and their 72 direct officers at the beginning of a 4-month period of intensive combat training and asked them to report their attachment styles. At the same time, soldiers completed a self-report scale measuring their baseline mental health. Two months later, soldiers reported their mental health again and provided appraisals of their officers as providers of security (i.e., the officers' ability and willingness to be available in times of need, and to accept and care for their soldiers rather than rejecting and criticizing them). Two months after that (i.e., 4 months after combat training began), soldiers once again evaluated their mental health. The findings indicated that appraisals of officers as security providers (by their soldiers) predicted desirable changes in soldiers' mental health during combat training. At the beginning of training, baseline mental health was exclusively associated with soldiers' own level of attachment security. However, appraisals of officers' provisions of security during combat training produced significant changes in soldiers' mental health across the training (taking the baseline assessment into account). The higher the officers were appraised by their soldiers as being more sensitive and responsive, the more the soldiers' mental health improved over 2 and 4 months of intensive combat training. These findings highlight the important effects of leaders' functioning as security providers on their followers' mental health and emotional well-being under stressful conditions.

This research has been conceptually extended from the military setting to other organizational settings. For example, Ronen and Mikulincer (2012) collected data from subordinates and their direct managers in a variety of business organizations and found that managers' responsiveness and supportiveness as caregivers (as measured by a self-report scale) predicted lower job burnout and higher job satisfaction among subordinates. Importantly, these effects were not moderated by subordinates' own attachment insecurities.

There is also evidence that a counselor's functioning as a security provider has beneficial effects on a client's outcomes during and after career counseling. In a 3-session career counseling study, Littman-Ovadia (2008) found that counselees' appraisal of their counselors as security-enhancing attachment figures (following the second session) was a significant predictor of heightened career exploration following counseling compared to baseline career exploration, even after the researcher controlled for counselees' own attachment orientations. This appraisal of the therapist as a security-enhancing attachment figure also mitigated the detrimental effects of attachment anxiety and avoidance on career exploration. In another study based on data from the National Institute of Mental Health Treatment of Depression Collaborative Research Program, Zuroff and Blatt (2006) found that a client's positive appraisals of his or her therapist's sensitivity and supportiveness significantly predicted relief from depression and maintenance of therapeutic benefits 18 months later. And these results were not attributable to patient characteristics or severity of depression.

Conclusions

In line with Bowlby's theorizing, the diverse research findings reviewed in this chapter indicate that attachment security is key to the optimal functioning not only of the attachment behavioral system, but also of other behavioral systems such as exploration and caregiving. This research also shows that a person's sense of security, which allows creative, undefensive interactions with other people and fosters accurate perception of and effective reactions to others' needs, is an important asset in both personal and organizational relationships.

Fortunately, research conducted to date suggests that a person's attachment system, along with his or her core sense of security, can be changed for the better. Moreover, the change can occur both immediately (and presumably temporarily) and more permanently, and can occur both consciously and unconsciously. The strong emphasis in the attachment research field on individual differences—including much of our own work—may have made those differences seem too deep-seated and robust to alter, even though the documented benefits of good relationships and skilled psychotherapy have always indicated that change for the better is possible. Fortunately, in both behavioral and neuroscience research, it is becoming increasingly possible to measure positive changes in systematically coded interpersonal behavior and in functional brain images. This is therefore a hopeful time for testing the efficacy of a variety of security-enhancing procedures.

One of the key remaining questions concerns how best to conceptualize the sense of security and its role in mental and social processes. Is it a "feeling," an emotion, a background mood? How is it sustained when a person is under pressure or suffering injuries or losses? How does it regulate defenses, allowing a person to be generous and supportive even when mentally depleted—a process with important implications for parents, lovers, teachers, and care providers of all kinds? More specifically, how does a subliminal security prime, presumably acting through associative networks in memory, alter a person's sense of security, reduce defenses, and counter compassion fatigue? Are its effects mainly cognitive, emotional, or neurochemical? The well-documented effects reviewed in this chapter are major discoveries, in our opinion, but their nature is still largely mysterious at several different levels of analysis.

Acknowledgment

Preparation of this chapter was facilitated by a grant from the Fetzer Institute.

References

Ainsworth, M. D. S., Blehar, M. C., Waters, E., & Wall, S. (1978). *Patterns of attachment: A psychological study of the Strange Situation.* Hillsdale, NJ: Erlbaum.

Arndt, J., Schimel, J., Greenberg, J., & Pyszczynski, T. (2002). The intrinsic self and defensiveness: Evidence that activating the intrinsic self reduces self-handicapping and conformity. *Personality and Social Psychology Bulletin, 28,* 671–683.

Baccus, J. R., Baldwin, M. W., & Packer, D. J. (2004). Increasing implicit self-esteem through classical conditioning. *Psychological Science, 15,* 498–502.

Baldwin, M. W., Fehr, B., Keedian, E., Seidel, M., & Thomson, D. W. (1993). An exploration of the relational schemata underlying attachment styles: Self-report and lexical decision approaches. *Personality and Social Psychology Bulletin, 19,* 746–754.

Batson, C. D. (1991). *The altruism question: Toward a social-psychological answer.* Hillsdale, NJ: Erlbaum.

Berant, E., Mikulincer, M., & Florian, V. (2001). The association of mothers' attachment style and their psychological reactions to the diagnosis of infants' congenital heart disease. *Journal of Social and Clinical Psychology, 20,* 208–232.

Bowlby, J. (1969/1982). *Attachment and loss: Vol. 1. Attachment.* New York: Basic Books.

Bowlby, J. (1973). *Attachment and loss: Vol. 2. Separation: Anxiety and anger.* New York: Basic Books.

Bowlby, J. (1979). *The making and breaking of affectional bonds.* London: Tavistock.

Bowlby, J. (1980). *Attachment and loss: Vol. 3. Sadness and depression.* New York: Basic Books.

Bowlby, J. (1988). *A secure base: Clinical applications of attachment theory.* London: Routledge.

Brennan, K. A., Clark, C. L., & Shaver, P. R. (1998). Self-report measurement of adult attachment: An integrative overview. In J. A. Simpson & W. S. Rholes (Eds.), *Attachment theory and close relationships* (pp. 46–76). New York: Guilford Press.

Canterberry, M., & Gillath, O. (2013). Neural evidence for a multifaceted model of attachment security. *International Journal of Psychophysiology, 88,* 232–240.

Carnelley, K. B., & Rowe, A. C. (2007). Repeated priming of attachment security influences immediate and later views of self and relationships. *Personal Relationships, 14,* 307–320.

Carnelley, K. B., & Rowe, A. C. (2010). Priming a sense of security: What goes through people's minds. *Journal of Social and Personal Relationships, 27,* 253–261.

Cassidy, J., & Kobak, R. R. (1988). Avoidance and its relationship with other defensive processes. In J. Belsky & T. Nezworski (Eds.), *Clinical implications of attachment* (pp. 300–323). Hillsdale, NJ: Erlbaum.

Cassidy, J., & Shaver, P. R. (Eds.). (2008). *Handbook of attachment: Theory, research, and clinical applications* (2nd ed.). New York: Guilford Press.

Coan, J. A., Schaefer, H. S., & Davidson, R. J. (2006). Lending a hand: Social regulation of the neural response to threat. *Psychological Science, 17,* 1–8.

Collins, N. L. (1996). Working models of attachment: Implications for explanation, emotion, and behavior. *Journal of Personality and Social Psychology, 71,* 810–832.

Collins, N. L., & Feeney, B. C. (2000). A safe haven: An attachment theory perspective on support-seeking and caregiving in intimate relationships. *Journal of Personality and Social Psychology, 78,* 1053–1073.

Collins, N. L., Jaremka, L. M., & Kane, H. (2009). *Social support buffers stress, promotes emotional recovery, and enhances relationship security.* Unpublished manuscript, University of California, Santa Barbara.

Collins, N. L., & Read, S. J. (1990). Adult attachment, working models, and relationship quality in dating couples. *Journal of Personality and Social Psychology, 58,* 644–663.

Cooper, M. L., Shaver, P. R., & Collins, N. L. (1998). Attachment styles, emotion regulation, and adjustment in adolescence. *Journal of Personality and Social Psychology, 74,* 1380–1397.

Davidovitz, R., Mikulincer, M., Shaver, P. R., Ijzak, R., & Popper, M. (2007). Leaders as attachment figures: Their attachment orientations predict leadership-related mental representations and followers' performance and mental health. *Journal of Personality and Social Psychology, 93,* 632–650.

Eisenberger, N. I., Master, S. L., Inagaki, T. K., Taylor, S. E., Shirinyan, D., Lieberman, M. D., et al. (2011). Attachment figures activate a safety signal-related neural region and reduce pain experience. *Proceedings of the National Academy of Sciences USA, 108,* 11721–11726.

Emilien, G., Penasse, C., Charles, G., Martin, D., Lasseaux, L., & Waltregny, A. (2000). Post-traumatic stress disorder: Hypotheses from clinical neuropsychology and psychopharmacology research. *International Journal of Psychiatry in Clinical Practice, 4,* 3–18.

Feeney, B. C. (2007). The dependency paradox in close relationships: Accepting dependence promotes independence. *Journal of Personality and Social Psychology, 92,* 268–285.

Feeney, B. C., & Thrush, R. L. (2010). Relationship influences on exploration in adulthood: The characteristics and function of a secure base. *Journal of Personality and Social Psychology, 98,* 57–76.

Fraley, R. C., & Waller, N. G. (1998). Adult attachment patterns: A test of the typological model. In J. A. Simpson & W. S. Rholes (Eds.), *Attachment theory and close relationships* (pp. 77–114). New York: Guilford Press.

Fredrickson, B. L. (2001). The role of positive emotions in positive psychology: The broaden-and-build theory of positive emotions. *American Psychologist, 56,* 218–226.

Guichard, A., & Collins, N. (2008, February). *The influence of social support and attachment style on performance, self-evaluations, and interpersonal behaviors.* Poster presented at the meeting of the Society for Personality and Social Psychology, Albuquerque, NM.

Gump, B. B., Polk, D. E., Kamarck, T. W., & Shiffman, S. M. (2001). Partner interactions are associated with reduced blood pressure in the natural environment: Ambulatory monitoring evidence from a healthy, multiethnic adult sample. *Psychosomatic Medicine, 63,* 423–433.

Kane, H., McCall, C., Collins, N., & Blascovich, J. B. (2012). Mere presence is not enough: Responsive support in a virtual world. *Journal of Experimental Social Psychology, 48,* 37–44.

Littman-Ovadia, H. (2008). The effect of client attachment style and counselor functioning on career exploration. *Journal of Vocational Behavior, 73,* 434–439.

Master, S. L., Eisenberger, N. I., Taylor, S. E., Naliboff, B. D., Shirinyan, D., & Lieberman, M. D. (2009). A picture's worth: Partner photographs reduce experimentally induced pain. *Psychological Science, 20*, 1316–1318.

Mickelson, K. D., Kessler, R. C., & Shaver, P. R. (1997). Adult attachment in a nationally representative sample. *Journal of Personality and Social Psychology, 73*, 1092–1106.

Mikulincer, M. (1995). Attachment style and the mental representation of the self. *Journal of Personality and Social Psychology, 69*, 1203–1215.

Mikulincer, M., & Florian, V. (1995). Appraisal of and coping with a real-life stressful situation: The contribution of attachment styles. *Personality and Social Psychology Bulletin, 21*, 406–414.

Mikulincer, M., Gillath, O., Halevy, V., Avihou, N., Avidan, S., & Eshkoli, N. (2001). Attachment theory and reactions to others' needs: Evidence that activation of the sense of attachment security promotes empathic responses. *Journal of Personality and Social Psychology, 81*, 1205–1224.

Mikulincer, M., Gillath, O., Sapir-Lavid, Y., Yaakobi, E., Arias, K., Tal-Aloni, L., et al. (2003). Attachment theory and concern for others' welfare: Evidence that activation of the sense of secure base promotes endorsement of self-transcendence values. *Basic and Applied Social Psychology, 25*, 299–312.

Mikulincer, M., Hirschberger, G., Nachmias, O., & Gillath, O. (2001). The affective component of the secure base schema: Affective priming with representations of attachment security. *Journal of Personality and Social Psychology, 81*, 305–321.

Mikulincer, M., & Shaver, P. R. (2001). Attachment theory and intergroup bias: Evidence that priming the secure base schema attenuates negative reactions to out-groups. *Journal of Personality and Social Psychology, 81*, 97–115.

Mikulincer, M., & Shaver, P. R. (2003). The attachment behavioral system in adulthood: Activation, psychodynamics, and interpersonal processes. In M. P. Zanna (Ed.), *Advances in experimental social psychology* (Vol. 35, pp. 53–152). San Diego, CA: Academic Press.

Mikulincer, M., & Shaver, P. R. (2007a). *Attachment in adulthood: Structure, dynamics, and change.* New York: Guilford Press.

Mikulincer, M., & Shaver, P. R. (2007b). Boosting attachment security to promote mental health, prosocial values, and inter-group tolerance. *Psychological Inquiry, 18*, 139–156.

Mikulincer, M., Shaver, P. R., Gillath, O., & Nitzberg, R. A. (2005). Attachment, caregiving, and altruism: Boosting attachment security increases compassion and helping. *Journal of Personality and Social Psychology, 89*, 817–839.

Mikulincer, M., Shaver, P. R., & Horesh, N. (2006). Attachment bases of emotion regulation and posttraumatic adjustment. In D. K. Snyder, J. A. Simpson, & J. N. Hughes (Eds.), *Emotion regulation in families: Pathways to dysfunction and health* (pp. 77–99). Washington, DC: American Psychological Association.

Mikulincer, M., Shaver, P. R., & Rom, E. (2011). The effects of implicit and explicit security priming on creative problem solving. *Cognition and Emotion, 25*, 519–531.

Mikulincer, M., Shaver, P. R., Sahdra, B. K., & Bar-On, N. (2013). Can

security-enhancing interventions overcome psychological barriers to responsiveness in couple relationships? *Attachment and Human Development, 15,*
246–260.

Mikulincer, M., Shaver, P. R., Sapir-Lavid, Y., & Avihou-Kanza, N. (2009). What's
inside the minds of securely and insecurely attached people?: The secure-base
script and its associations with attachment-style dimensions. *Journal of Personality and Social Psychology, 97,* 615–633.

Overall, N. C., Fletcher, G. J. O., & Simpson, J. A. (2010). Helping each other
grow: Romantic partner support, self-improvement, and relationship quality.
Personality and Social Psychology Bulletin, 36, 1496–1513.

Pierce, T., & Lydon, J. (1998). Priming relational schemas: Effects of contextually
activated and chronically accessible interpersonal expectations on responses
to a stressful event. *Journal of Personality and Social Psychology, 75,* 1441–
1448.

Radecki-Bush, C., Farrell, A. D., & Bush, J. P. (1993). Predicting jealous responses:
The influence of adult attachment and depression on threat appraisal. *Journal
of Social and Personal Relationships, 10,* 569–588.

Ronen, S., & Mikulincer, M. (2012). Predicting employees' satisfaction and burnout from managers' attachment and caregiving orientations. *European Journal of Work and Organizational Psychology, 21,* 828–849.

Rowe, A., & Carnelley, K. B. (2003). Attachment style differences in the processing
of attachment-relevant information: Primed-style effects on recall, interpersonal expectations, and affect. *Personal Relationships, 10,* 59–75.

Schaller, M., & Cialdini, R. B. (1988). The economics of empathic helping: Support for a mood management motive. *Journal of Experimental Social Psychology, 24,* 163–181.

Schimel, J., Arndt, J., Pyszczynski, T., & Greenberg, J. (2001). Being accepted for
who we are: Evidence that social validation of the intrinsic self reduces general
defensiveness. *Journal of Personality and Social Psychology, 80,* 35–52.

Selcuk, E., Zayas, V., Günaydin, G., Hazan, C., & Kross, E. (2012). Mental representations of attachment figures facilitate recovery following upsetting autobiographical memory recall. *Journal of Personality and Social Psychology,
103,* 362–378.

Shaver, P. R., & Mikulincer, M. (2002). Attachment-related psychodynamics.
Attachment and Human Development, 4, 133–161.

Simpson, J. A. (1990). Influence of attachment styles on romantic relationships.
Journal of Personality and Social Psychology, 59, 971–980.

Simpson, J. A., Winterheld, H. A., Rholes, W. S., & Oriña, M. M. (2007). Working models of attachment and reactions to different forms of caregiving from
romantic partners. *Journal of Personality and Social Psychology, 93,* 466–
477.

Smith, K. D., Keating, J. P., & Stotland, E. (1989). Altruism revisited: The effect
of denying feedback on a victim's status to an empathic witness. *Journal of
Personality and Social Psychology, 57,* 641–650.

Sroufe, L. A., & Waters, E. (1977). Attachment as an organizational construct.
Child Development, 48, 1184–1199.

Waters, H. S., & Waters, E. (2006). The attachment working models concept:

Among other things, we build script-like representations of secure base experiences. *Attachment and Human Development, 8*, 185–198.

Younger, J., Aron, A., Parke, S., Chatterjee, N., & Mackey, S. (2010). Viewing pictures of a romantic partner reduces experimental pain: Involvement of neural reward systems. *PLoS ONE, 5*, e13309.

Zuroff, D. C., & Blatt, S. J. (2006). The therapeutic relationship in the brief treatment of depression: Contributions to clinical improvement and enhanced adaptive capacities. *Journal of Consulting and Clinical Psychology, 74*, 199–206.

6

Attachment and Dyadic Regulation Processes

Nickola C. Overall
Edward P. Lemay, Jr.

Annette loves her partner, David, but worries about whether David truly loves her. Annette's fears are particularly acute when David appears to be unhappy with her in some way, such as when they disagree. During these times, Annette's distress can be overwhelming, and she can't stop thinking about what David's reactions mean in terms of his feelings toward her. She becomes propelled to ensure that David still loves her, and often expresses to David how much she is hurting and how much she needs him. David typically responds by comforting and reassuring Annette, which helps her feel better and more secure. Over the course of their relationship, David learns that he needs to be careful not to trigger Annette's fears, and so he sometimes hides his negative feelings and makes a special effort to be affectionate and loving. This helps Annette feel happier and more confident in David's commitment to her.

Annette is high in attachment anxiety. Research investigating the effects of attachment anxiety suggests that the difficulties Annette has in regulating her emotions will cause problems in her relationship. However, Annette and David's responses to each other also involve *dyadic regulation*. Annette's efforts to draw David closer and gain reassurance involve Annette trying to influence or regulate how David is feeling, thinking, and behaving. Similarly, David's efforts to soothe Annette's concerns and help her feel loved involve David trying to regulate Annette's thoughts, feelings, and behavior.

In this chapter, we outline why dyadic regulation processes are so important, present recent research examining how insecure individuals and their partners regulate one another, and show how dyadic regulation is central to understanding how attachment insecurity is manifested in and affects adult relationships.

Attachment and Regulation Processes

Regulation processes are at the core of attachment dynamics. When individuals are threatened or challenged, the attachment system becomes activated and triggers efforts to alleviate distress and restore felt-security (Mikulincer & Shaver, 2003; Simpson & Rholes, 2012). The particular ways this goal is managed depend on people's expectations regarding whether close others will be a reliable source of support. Attachment security arises when proximity-seeking efforts have typically been successful in gaining responsive care. Knowing that they can trust their partners, secure people seek physical and psychological proximity to their partners when threatened (Collins & Feeney, 2000; Simpson, Rholes, & Nelligan, 1992) and use constructive, problem-focused modes of emotion regulation (Shaver & Mikulincer, 2007).

Attachment anxiety arises when attachment figures have sometimes responded to bids for support with love and care, but at other times responded with anger or rejection (Bowlby, 1969/1982, 1973, 1980). These experiences create intense fears of abandonment, a profound hunger for closeness, and a hyperactived attachment system reflected by chronic attempts to secure the closeness highly anxious individuals crave (Mikulincer & Shaver, 2003). Hyperactivation is characterized by excessive proximity seeking (Shaver, Schachner, & Mikulincer, 2005) and intense, ruminative reactions to distressing situations (Shaver & Mikulincer, 2007).

Attachment avoidance occurs when people have encountered persistent rejection from past attachment figures (Bowlby, 1969/1982, 1973, 1980), which produces a deep-seated distrust of others and entrenched beliefs that partners cannot be relied on to be loving caregivers. To prevent the pain of expected rejection, avoidant individuals defensively avoid dependence and suppress their attachment needs. When threatened, avoidant individuals manage negative emotions by suppressing their feelings, disengaging from their partners, and rejecting offers of support (Diamond, Hicks, & Otter-Henderson, 2006; Collins & Feeney, 2000; Simpson et al., 1992).

These different regulation patterns are most often conceptualized and studied as individual-based *internal* strategies, such as excessively seeking reassurance or suppressing emotions. But relationships involve two people, as does the set goal of the attachment system. In fact, a primary way an individual regulates felt-security involves manipulating closeness with the partner, which is a dyadic state. Pursuing proximity or creating distance inherently involves attempts to regulate the *partner's* thoughts, emotions, and behaviors, such as trying to get the partner to express love and provide reassurance (as Annette does in the chapter-opening example) or trying to get the partner to provide space and accept less intimacy. The way the *partner* reacts to these regulation attempts should determine the success and costs of insecure reactions to threat. Moreover, to manage and sustain the relationship, the *partner* needs to engage in counterregulation strategies of his or her own to down-regulate the insecure reactions enacted by the highly anxious or avoidant individual (just as David tries to soothe Annette's anxieties). If successful, the *partner's* regulation efforts could offset the destructive outcomes typically associated with attachment insecurity.

In the next sections, we describe and evaluate these dyadic regulation processes, using the examples summarized in Table 6.1. We first consider how highly anxious individuals regulate closeness and felt-security by trying to influence their partners' cognitions, emotions, and behaviors, and the consequences of these regulation attempts (see top left of Table 6.1). We then examine what the *partners* of anxious individuals might do to help anxious individuals feel more secure and behave more constructively (see top right of Table 6.1). The remaining sections consider the same dyadic regulation processes in relation to attachment avoidance, including exploring the ways highly avoidant individuals might cope with dependence by regulating their partners' power (see bottom left of Table 6.1) and how partners can overcome these defensive strategies (see bottom right of Table 6.1). In each section, we show that a dyadic regulation perspective reconciles inconsistencies in the literature, expands our understanding of how attachment insecurity shapes relationships, and pushes research in new directions.

TABLE 6.1. Examples of the Regulation Strategies Enacted by Insecurely Attached Individuals and Their Partners

	Regulation *of* the partner			Regulation *by* the partner		
	Regulation strategies	Potential benefits	Potential costs	Regulation strategies	Potential benefits	Potential costs
Anxiety	Guilt induction	Reassurance of partner's love and commitment	Partner dissatisfaction and rejection	Exaggerated affection	Reassurance of partner's love and commitment	Partner dissatisfaction and rejection
Avoidance	Disengagement and withdrawal	Restoration of power and control	Partner dependence and dissatisfaction	Softening influence	Reduced disengagement and withdrawal	Less change and partner dissatisfaction

Attachment Anxiety and Regulation *of* the Partner

People high in attachment anxiety intensely desire closeness and intimacy, but fear that their partners may reject or abandon them (Mikulincer & Shaver, 2003). This combination produces an acute sensitivity to rejection. For example, anxious individuals experience more pronounced feelings of rejection, stress, and hurt during relationship-threatening interactions such as conflict (Campbell, Simpson, Boldry, & Kashy, 2005; Overall & Sibley, 2009; Simpson, Rholes, & Phillips, 1996; Tran & Simpson, 2009). Prior studies also suggest that this affective reactivity often leads to more hostile, punishing responses toward their partners (e.g., Creasy, 2002; Overall & Sibley, 2009; Simpson et al., 1996). However, hostile reactions to conflict also tend to incite rejection and dissatisfaction in partners (Lemay, Overall, & Clark, 2012)—reactions that are incongruent with the principal goal of anxious individuals to secure intimacy and sustain closeness. Moreover, several studies have found no associations between attachment anxiety and observer-rated hostility during conflict (e.g., Bouthillier, Julien, Dube, Belanger, & Hamelin, 2002; Campbell et al., 2005; Roisman et al., 2007; Simpson et al., 1996). We think that this is because anxious reactions are not as hostile as often assumed, and because the behaviors measured in prior research may not capture the specific proximity-seeking strategies used by highly anxious individuals.

Regulating the Partner by Inducing Guilt

The yearning for proximity at the core of attachment anxiety should produce behaviors specifically designed to obtain care and attention from the partner, which involve attempts to regulate the *partner's* emotions and behaviors. For example, the emotionally charged responses displayed during conflict by many highly anxious individuals most likely represent forms of "protest" at the potential loss of the relationship bond and subsequent attempts to ensure that partners attend to the self and modify hurtful behaviors (Bowlby, 1973; Cassidy & Berlin, 1994; Rholes, Simpson, & Oriña, 1999). One proximity-maintaining strategy that should achieve these goals, and has been theorized to operate in infancy (Cassidy & Berlin, 1994), adolescence (Kobak, Cole, Ferenz-Gillies, Fleming, & Gamble, 1993) and adulthood (Shaver & Mikulincer, 2007), involves exaggerated emotional displays that emphasize dependence and vulnerability. When individuals express hurt feelings, they convey commitment and dependence to their partners, and in turn elicit guilt and caring responses (Lemay et al., 2012). Given that these partner reactions are exactly what highly anxious individuals desire, they may exaggerate expressions of hurt to extract guilt and care from their partners.

Guilt induction strategies are commonly employed in close relationships to influence others (Baumeister, Stillwell, & Heatherton, 1994; Vangelisti, Daly, & Rudnick, 1991). These strategies involve conveying or amplifying emotional expressions of hurt (e.g., tears, sulking, making a sad face, pouting); emphasizing the negative impact a partner's behavior or the situation is having on the self ("how much it hurts me"); or appealing to a partner's love, concern, and relationship obligations (Overall, Fletcher, Simpson, & Sibley, 2009). All of these tactics involve emphasizing hurt, dependence, and vulnerability to induce guilt and motivate the partner to take responsibility and soothe the individual's hurt feelings. Moreover, because guilt powerfully motivates people to make amends, guilt induction tactics tend to be successful in getting close others to apologize, cease hurtful behavior, and express commitment, empathy and concern (e.g., Baumeister et al., 1994; Tangney, Wagner, Hill-Barlow, Marschall, & Gramzow, 1996; Vangelisti et al., 1991).

In a recent set of studies, we (Overall, Girme, Lemay, & Hammond, 2014) tested whether highly anxious individuals engage in guilt induction strategies in response to conflict. The first study involved couples' recording their daily experiences for 3 weeks. Highly anxious participants reported more pronounced hurt feelings on days they reported conflict or their partners reported behaving in a critical or hurtful manner. On those "hurt-felt" days, the *partners* of anxious individuals also overestimated the intensity of anxious individuals' hurt feelings. These biased perceptions indicate that anxious individuals were exaggerating how hurt they were, which led the partners to perceive more hurt than anxious individuals were actually feeling.

In a second study (Overall et al., 2014), we directly measured the degree to which guilt induction tactics were exhibited during couples' video-recorded conflict discussions. Trained coders independently rated the extent to which individuals exhibited guilt induction tactics, such as using or exaggerating emotional expressions of hurt (e.g., sulking, making a sad face); appealing to their partners' love, concern, or relationship obligations; or portraying themselves as needing help or being less capable or powerful than their partners. Coders also rated the degree to which participants exhibited hostile communication, such as derogating their partners or expressing threats or anger. As predicted, individuals higher in anxiety engaged in more observer-rated guilt induction strategies, but they did *not* exhibit greater hostile behavior. These results provide evidence that highly anxious individuals are not lashing out with hostility, but instead engage their hurt feelings as a tool to influence their partners and restore proximity.

The Benefits and Costs of Guilt Induction Strategies

Guilt induction tactics are an effective way of altering a partner's emotions and motivations while limiting the risk of immediate partner reactance and rejection. Illustrating this point, in both studies, we (Overall et al., 2014) gathered ratings of partners' feelings of guilt. As predicted, anxious individuals' guilt induction attempts successfully produced higher levels of partner guilt. As outlined above, guilt typically triggers empathy, apologies, and other amends-making efforts. Moreover, because guilt induction tactics work only if a partner cares about and is committed to the relationship, guilt also provides evidence of the partner's caring (Baumeister et al., 1994). Accordingly, partner guilt, even in the absence of reparative actions, can improve the hurt person's emotional state because guilt conveys concern and commitment.

Intriguingly, given that the principal goal of anxious individuals is to obtain love and acceptance, successfully inducing guilt may provide them the evidence they need to feel somewhat secure and satisfied in their relationships. We tested this possibility (Overall et al., 2014) by examining whether guilt experienced by a partner during a couple's daily life (Study 1) and conflict-related discussions (Study 2) predicted longitudinal changes in perceptions of the partner's commitment and satisfaction. When their partners reported higher levels of guilt, highly anxious individuals reported more positive evaluations of the partners' commitment and relationship quality across time. In contrast, anxious individuals experienced significant declines in perceived commitment and relationship quality across time when their partners reported lower levels of guilt, consistent with the detrimental outcomes typically associated with attachment insecurity. These novel results demonstrate that the partner regulation strategies engaged by highly anxious individuals actually do produce the reassurance they crave, and in turn bolster their feelings of security and relationship satisfaction.

Unfortunately, our research (Overall et al., 2014) also demonstrated that the benefits of partner guilt for anxious individuals had a substantial drawback. In both studies, the greater guilt felt by partners of highly anxious individuals was associated with declines in partners' satisfaction across time. We think that this detrimental outcome occurs because the guilt experienced by the partners of anxious individuals is "pulled" from them rather than intrinsically generated, and any resulting pro-relationship behavior is thus designed to minimize and prevent conflict rather than to create intimacy and closeness. Indeed, even positive behaviors motivated by these types of avoidance goals are associated with lower relationship satisfaction (Impett et al., 2010). Feeling guilty also leads people to prioritize making amends and reassuring insecure individuals instead of pursuing their own personal needs (Baumeister et al., 1994). This shift in partners' goal pursuit often involves partners' suppressing negative emotions and desires, which impedes closeness and satisfaction (Gross & John, 2003; Lemay & Dudley, 2011), generates resentment and distress, and impairs satisfaction (Clark, Graham, Williams, & Lemay, 2008; Jones & Kugler, 1993).

Implications and Future Research Directions

The results of our research demonstrate that understanding how attachment anxiety influences relationship functioning involves identifying the specific ways individuals regulate their *partners'* emotions and behaviors in desired ways, and thereby successfully forge feelings of closeness (at least in the minds of anxious individuals). Rather than simply identifying "negative" reactions to threat and classifying them as destructive, it is necessary to explore how anxious individuals' threat regulation strategies pay off by creating a sense of being loved and cared for. Anxious individuals may garner evidence of their partners' commitment and love when their partners feel hurt, experience jealousy or engage in mate guarding, seek reassurance, or feel insecure in other ways, and thus they may purposely try to elicit these states in their partners or be less discouraging of them when they occur. As with guilt induction tactics, these regulation attempts may bolster security but undermine the partner's satisfaction.

Other partner regulation strategies that anxious individuals enact to achieve closeness may yield a different distribution of benefits and costs. Murray and colleagues (2009) found that people with low self-worth, who underestimate the extent to which they are valued by their partners, try to be invaluable in their relationships to increase their partners' commitment and dependence. Thus highly anxious individuals may try to emphasize the rewards (e.g., being a good support provider) or novel experiences (e.g., great sex, fun activities) that they can offer to their partners. These regulation strategies may produce benefits for partners, although some tactics may be costly for anxious individuals (e.g., focusing too much on the partners' sexual needs rather than their own). Other proximity-seeking strategies may sustain both individuals' own and their partners' levels of satisfaction. For example, anxious individuals display greater relationship-oriented disclosure during conversations with their partners, which enhances relationship quality over time (Tan, Overall, & Taylor, 2012). Such relationship-strengthening behaviors may help counteract the damage of the reactions enacted by highly anxious individuals in threatening contexts that tend to harm partner satisfaction.

Our analysis has important therapeutic implications. The relative benefits of partner guilt highlight that attempting to alter what might be considered dysfunctional behavior could have unexpected and potentially damaging consequences if the underlying needs associated with that behavior are not addressed. Trying to reduce the use of guilt induction strategies may produce more constructive problem solving and bolster the satisfaction of the partners, but it also removes a central route by which anxious individuals can draw reassurance and security from their relationship. Similarly, fostering potentially positive behavior in the partners, such as by quelling the hyperactivating strategies of anxious individuals, could have unintended consequences. For example, we found that partners of anxious individuals who did not feel guilty maintained stable levels of satisfaction, but that this undermined anxious individuals' feelings of relationship-specific security and satisfaction (Overall et al., 2014). Consequently, any intervention aimed at altering the experience and use of guilt induction strategies (or other potentially maladaptive regulation strategies) needs to devise alternative, ultimately more constructive methods of gaining and providing reassurance to ensure that concerns about the partners' commitment are not left unabated.

Attachment Anxiety and Regulation *by* the Partner

The security benefits of guilt induction strategies highlight an important point: Attachment anxiety does not have blanket destructive effects. Indeed, there is growing evidence that when partners clearly demonstrate they are available and supportive, anxious individuals' typically negative expectations and evaluations are neutralized. When partners are more supportive, for example, highly anxious people tend to be more optimistic about their relationships (Campbell et al., 2005; Rholes, Simpson, Campbell, & Grich, 2001). Satisfying sex also attenuates the lower marital satisfaction typically associated with attachment anxiety, in part because sex bolsters the perceived availability of the partner (Little, McNulty, & Russell, 2010). These reassuring partner behaviors may not simply be happenstance; just as anxious individuals try to purposely pull reassurance from their partners, their *partners* may also learn to approach anxious individuals in ways that ease their insecurities and compensate for their heightened reactions to threat. This involves *partners'* regulating the insecurities and reactivity of anxiously attached individuals (see top right of Table 6.1).

    This central idea is laid out by Lemay and Dudley (2011) in their model of *interpersonal insecurity compensation*. Lemay and Dudley (2011) have proposed that partners learn quickly about the insecurities of their mates because of the strong affective and behavioral reactivity to threat that is displayed by highly anxious individuals. Experiencing the difficulties that attachment anxiety can generate in relationships should lead partners to become vigilant to signs of anxious individuals' distress and insecurity, and thus enact behaviors intended to avoid or alleviate their distress and insecurity. Lemay and Dudley (2011) have described this process as partners' "walking on eggshells," such as exaggerating their affection and concealing their negative feelings in order to prevent activating the insecurities of highly anxious individuals and help them feel more secure. In three studies, Lemay and Dudley (2011) found evidence for this process across various indices of interpersonal insecurity, including high attachment anxiety, low self-esteem, and high proneness to hurt feelings. We focus here on the analyses examining attachment anxiety.

In their first study, Lemay and Dudley (2011) asked friends and romantic partners to privately rate each other's attachment anxiety and sentiments toward each other. Consistent with their prediction that partners can and do detect insecure individuals' high anxiety, there was a significant link between the partners' perceptions of individuals' attachment anxiety and individuals' reports of their own attachment anxiety. To test whether perceiving individuals' anxiety led partners to conceal their negative feelings about those individuals, toward the end of the experimental session participants were unexpectedly asked to report their feelings toward each other again. This time, however, half of the participants were assigned to a "public" condition in which they were told that they would see each other's responses. As expected, partners who believed their responses would be public and perceived they were in relationships with highly anxious individuals concealed their negative evaluations by providing more positive ratings than they had first provided. In contrast, partners who perceived they were in relationships with individuals low in anxiety exhibited very few differences between their private and public responses, illustrating that they did not attempt to conceal negative feelings.

A follow-up diary study with romantic couples provided further support that partners detect and regulate anxious individuals' insecurity during their daily interactions (Lemay & Dudley, 2011, Study 3). Replicating their first study, partners accurately detected when they were involved in relationships with anxious individuals. This detection of anxiety in turn predicted efforts to regulate the insecurity of highly anxious individuals. Across their daily interactions, partners who detected individuals' attachment anxiety reported more vigilance about upsetting anxious individuals and greater motivations to up-regulate their feelings of relationship security. Self-reports of vigilance were also corroborated by partners demonstrating greater accuracy in anxious individuals' daily sentiments. In particular, partners who reported greater vigilance about upsetting their mates were more accurate at detecting and remembering anxious individuals' feelings about their relationships. Thus partners' vigilance appeared to optimize detection of anxious individuals' feelings of insecurity.

Lemay and Dudley (2011) also found that individuals who perceived their partners to be more anxious reported a series of behaviors intended to regulate their partners' feelings of security, including concealing negative sentiments about anxious partners, exaggerating affection and positive sentiments, and providing unmitigated forms of caregiving that involved attending to the needs of anxious individuals at the expense of their own needs. These regulation strategies were also effective; highly anxious individuals felt more secure in their partners' care and regard when their partners enacted these daily regulation behaviors. Combined, the results reported by Lemay and Dudley (2011) provide strong evidence that (1) partners try to avoid triggering anxious individuals' insecurities by cautiously camouflaging discontent and accentuating how positive they feel in their relationships, and (2) these regulation strategies are effective at helping insecure individuals feel more valued and regarded.

The novel results reported by Lemay and Dudley (2011) highlight that the impact of attachment insecurity on relationships depends on whether and how successfully partners regulate the insecurity of anxious individuals. Their findings also show that partners' regulation efforts appear to be intentional and calibrated to the assessed need for regulation. In particular, partners attempted to conceal negative feelings and reassure anxious individuals *when* they detected feelings of insecurity and *when* they encountered situations that were likely to exacerbate those anxieties, such as exposure to negative evaluations. Simpson and Overall (2014) also highlight that partners may be most likely to enact regulation behaviors in stressful contexts that activate the attachment system, and in turn the rejection sensitivity and emotion-focused strategies arising from attachment anxiety. For example, confronting the pronounced distress and guilt induction strategies that highly anxious individuals exhibit during conflict should initiate counterattempts by their partners to down-regulate these potentially damaging emotions and behaviors.

A study by Tran and Simpson (2009) provides further support for the role partners play in down-regulating insecurities in conflict situations. Tran and Simpson (2009) video-recorded couples discussing areas of relationship conflict, gathered measures of emotional reactions during the discussion, and objectively coded the presence of accommodation behaviors. *Accommodation* involves resisting hurtful impulses and instead trying to resolve a problem in a calm, forgiving, and supportive manner (Rusbult, Verette, Whitney, Slovik, & Lipkus, 1991). Accommodation is good for relationships, but it is hard to do; it requires self-control and high levels of commitment (Arriaga & Rusbult, 1998; Finkel & Campbell, 2001). Because of this, accommodation also conveys the qualities that highly anxious individuals desire—love, commitment, and trustworthiness (Wieselquist, Rusbult, Foster, & Agnew, 1999)—all of which should soothe anxious reactivity.

As expected, Tran and Simpson (2009) found that highly anxious individuals felt less accepted, reported more negative emotions, and in turn behaved in less accommodating ways during the discussion. The partners of highly anxious individuals also tended to respond with greater negative emotions and less accommodation. However, when partners were highly committed, they were able to prevent the reactivity of their highly anxious mates from infecting their own responses and displayed more accommodation. Additional dyadic analyses reported by Tran and Simpson (2011) indicated that partners' accommodation helped to counteract the effects of attachment anxiety. For example, when partners were highly committed, highly anxious individuals felt greater acceptance and behaved as positively as less anxious or more secure individuals. Moreover, across the sample, greater accommodation repaired feelings of rejection and elicited more positive emotions. This overall pattern indicates that partners who are committed to their relationships and try to accommodate the destructive reactions of their anxious mates may help anxious individuals respond more constructively during conflict.

The Benefits and Costs of Regulating Insecurities

By allaying rejection concerns and reducing threat-based reactions, the regulation by partners of highly anxious individuals should have important benefits. First, anxious individuals should feel more accepted and valued, which may help them develop a stronger sense of trust and more secure beliefs across the course of their relationships (Lemay & Dudley, 2011; Tran & Simpson, 2011; Simpson & Overall, 2014). Second, through this down-regulating of potentially damaging reactions within threatening contexts, a couple should negotiate challenging dilemmas more effectively. This should not only build greater commitment and satisfaction in both partners, but protect the relationship from the toll that poor conflict management takes on relationships. In short, attachment insecurity does not destine relationships to failure; partners' security regulation can contain the reactivity of highly anxious individuals and prevent such difficulties from spreading through their relationships.

Regulating the insecurities of anxious individuals, however, may not always be easy and may have unintentional detrimental effects if it is not done skillfully. Lemay and Clark (2008a, 2008b) have found that insecure people are more likely to perceive that their partners sometimes deliver inauthentic and exaggerated expressions of regard, in part because of biases related to insecurity and in part because people tend to detect their partners' deceptive communications. Instead of perceiving the partners' regulation efforts as a sign of care, detecting these efforts can problematically fuel doubts about the authenticity of their expressions of regard. Doubting the veracity of the partners' expressions can in turn increase feelings of rejection and diminish trust (Lemay & Clark, 2008a). One way partners' positive evaluations may be perceived as more authentic is if partners also show a willingness to express dissatisfaction about relatively trivial or nonthreatening domains, thereby revealing their honesty without the risk of eliciting distress and feelings of rejection in insecure individuals (Lemay & O'Leary, 2012). Thus regulation by the partners may need to strike a balance between positivity and credibility.

Partners of insecure individuals may also tire of having to continually regulate the insecurity of their mates. Censoring complaints, exaggerating affection, and accommodating hurt reactions take a great deal of effort, and regulating anxious individuals' reactivity may run the risk of damaging the partners' relationship evaluations. Lemay and Dudley (2011) provide mixed support for this possibility: Partners viewed their relationships more negatively on days they reported engaging in more exaggerated affection, but they did *not* report more negative evaluations the following day. We think this pattern indicates that insecurity regulation by partners can produce dissatisfaction and resentment, but it can also yield benefits that offset these costs, including having happier and more secure mates. Such benefits may also be more acutely appreciated by committed partners who are invested, prioritize relationship maintenance, and value the salubrious effects of their regulation efforts. In fact, people whose self-concept is intricately tied to their relationships report greater satisfaction when they suppress their emotions while sacrificing for their partners, whereas people who do not strongly identify with their relationships report the reverse (Le & Impett, 2013).

Implications and Future Research Directions

The way in which highly anxious individuals manage threat (regulation *of* the partner) and the ways in which partners try to manage the insecure reactions of these individuals (regulation *by* the partner) emphasize the dyadic nature of attachment dynamics (see also Overall & Simpson, 2013). The manifestation, impact, and stability of attachment anxiety depend on whether and how well anxious individuals successfully evoke signs of commitment from their partners, as well as how effectively partners behave in ways that contain anxious fears and bolster felt security. Indeed, these co-occurring processes probably work in unison (see top row of Table 6.1). For example, the exaggerated expressions of hurt that anxious individuals use to induce guilt probably constitute a key way in which their partners learn about anxious individuals' insecurity, which should in turn trigger regulation efforts by the partners to soothe expressed hurt and insecurity. Moreover, as partners acquire knowledge of anxious individuals' insecurities and feel responsible for compensating for them, partners may be more vigilant, preemptively try to avoid triggering insecurities, and become more responsive to anxious individuals' reassurance-seeking efforts. Thus what we have considered regulation *by* partners is intricately linked to, and may even arise from, anxious individuals' regulation *of* partners.

The coordinated regulation of highly anxious individuals and their partners also implies that regulation by partners does not simply occur because highly anxious individuals happen to stumble into partners and relationships that adequately regulate them. Instead, partners appear to be trying to provide anxious individuals exactly what they want and need (e.g., reassurance of love and commitment) exactly when they need it (e.g., when anxious individuals feel insecure, encounter threatening contexts, or try to pull reassurance from their partners). Nonetheless, some partners may be better able than others to respond to the needs of their anxious mates, such as those who are secure, are strongly invested, have high self-control, or believe that people can grow and change. Moreover, we have only just begun to identify the regulation processes that are effective in bolstering security. For example, partners may more effectively foster security if insecurity management behaviors are enacted only when they are truly needed and are complemented by other, less reactive security-building behaviors, such as facilitating anxious individuals' personal achievements and thriving outside the relationship (Arriaga, Kumashiro, Finkel, VanderDrift, & Luchies, 2014). Identifying the different ways partners can counteract the insecurity of highly anxious individuals, and in turn foster security and relationship stability over time, is an important goal for future research.

Finally, the ways in which anxious individuals' regulation *of* their partners intersects with the regulation *by* their partners imply a form of collaboration in building more secure, happy, and well-functioning relationships. However, the research we have presented indicates that the subsequent benefits and costs are distributed unevenly, in that these dyadic regulation processes primarily help anxious individuals feel more secure in their relationships, but they often breed dissatisfaction in their partners. Future longitudinal research, however, may reveal other patterns. Anxious people may, for instance, perceive the toll it takes on their partners and try to balance or repair these costs. And if partners' regulation efforts are successful and anxious individuals do become more secure, this should both modify how anxious individuals manage threat and allow partners to discontinue the more costly behaviors they need to enact in order to sustain their relationships. In sum, the manner in which regulation cycles across a dyad (and the consequences that ensue) are critical to understanding how attachment anxiety shapes, and is shaped by, relationships. These dyadic processes should be central to future investigations.

Attachment Avoidance and Regulation *of* the Partner

Dyadic regulation processes should also be central to understanding the reactions and relationship consequences associated with attachment avoidance. Highly avoidant individuals believe they cannot trust and depend on others, so they defensively avoid closeness and strive to maintain independence (Mikulincer & Shaver, 2003). To achieve these goals, highly avoidant individuals simply ignore threatening relationship information (Dykas & Cassidy, 2011; Simpson et al., 2011) and deactivate the attachment system by disengaging from intimacy and support (e.g., Tan et al., 2012; Collins & Feeney, 2000; Simpson et al., 1992). However, these preemptive strategies are difficult to maintain during the interdependent context of relationship exchanges, when avoidant individuals have to confront their partners' needs, emotions, and desires. In these "interdependent" situations, such as when their partners need support or are trying to influence them during conflict, highly avoidant individuals exhibit greater anger, hostility, and withdrawal (e.g., Rholes et al., 1999; Simpson, Rholes, Oriña, & Grich, 2002; Overall & Sibley, 2009; Simpson et al., 1996); these reactions create emotional distance, reduce how much partners can encroach on and hurt the highly avoidant individuals, and thus down-regulate negative affect and reestablish a sense of personal control.

Importantly, applying our dyadic regulation perspective highlights that the ways these distancing strategies influence or regulate their partners is crucial to whether highly avoidant people achieve their goals. Defensive distancing is enacted in the service of restoring the "security" that avoidant individuals feel when they are safe from the vulnerability of being too close to, dependent on, and susceptible to influence by others. This sense of safety and independence is most effectively achieved by regulating their partner in ways that encourage emotional distance and minimize their partners' influence, such as getting their partners to back off, cease seeking support or change, or accept less intimacy. We can therefore consider deactivating strategies to be *dyadic*, as they involve avoidant individuals trying to regulate their own sense of autonomy and safety by affecting their partner's emotions and behaviors (see bottom left of Table 6.1).

Regulating the Partner by Reducing Power

There is solid evidence that highly avoidant individuals engage in distancing behaviors (e.g., Fraley & Shaver, 1998; Simpson et al., 1992; Simpson, Winterheld, Rholes, & Oriña, 2007), but whether these halt the partner's influence has received little attention. In a recent study, Overall, Simpson, and Struthers (2013) assessed the degree to which highly avoidant individuals enacted withdrawal and disengagement during video-recorded discussions in which relationship partners (couples) were trying to produce desired changes in each other's thoughts or behaviors. Independent coders rated the degree to which individuals attempted to deactivate attachment concerns and maintain independence by avoiding or dismissing the problem, disengaging from their partners, and/or withdrawing from the conversation. To test whether these strategies were effective in thwarting the partner's influence, Overall et al. (2013) asked both members of each couple to report how successful the partner was in producing the changes he or she desired. Highly avoidant individuals displayed greater withdrawal and disengagement when their partners were trying to influence them, which reduced the degree to which partners generated desired change.

Disengagement and withdrawal display to the partner that avoidant individuals cannot be influenced, do not need their partners' love, and are not wholly invested in their relationships. For these reasons, distancing strategies are likely to have far-reaching effects beyond undercutting their partners' influence in specific interactions. In particular, such tactics should create wider asymmetries in power and dependence by parading avoidant individuals' lower levels of commitment. According to the principle of least interest (Kelley & Thibaut, 1978; Waller & Hill, 1951), the partner who is less committed, and thus less affected if a relationship ends, has relatively greater power in the relationship. In contrast, the partner who is more committed, and whose happiness and goals are more dependent on the relationship, possesses less power. By conveying relative disparities in commitment and diluting the partner's influence, an avoidant individual's distancing may engineer larger power imbalances within the relationship—making the partner feel less powerful, lowering his or her expectations, or resigning the partner to what the avoidant mate wants.

Reducing their partners' perception of power should be satisfying for avoidant individuals because it minimizes the degree to which avoidant individuals must adjust their autonomous desires and goals to coincide with those of their partners. People who have (or perceive they have) less power expend more effort in trying to understand their partners' perspective (Gordon & Chen, 2013), which often leads to greater accommodation of negative and hurtful behavior (Arriaga & Rusbult, 1998). People higher in dependence (or lower in power) may also be more willing to sacrifice their own goals and desires, conform to the wishes of their partners, and avoid causing friction in their relationships (Simpson, Farrell, Oriña, & Rothman, 2014). Thus, expecting that influence attempts will be futile, partners may be forced to concede during conflict and also more generally succumb to what they believe their avoidant mates want.

The Benefits and Costs of Power-Reducing Strategies

Strategies that minimize their partners' power may appear ideal for highly avoidant people to use, but they have important disadvantages. Inequities in power are unlikely to remain stable because partners will try to redress their lack of control in the relationship. Withdrawal from conflict is often met with greater demanding behavior (Christensen & Heavey, 1990), and feeling less power in relationship interactions tends to trigger anger and hostility (Overall & Sibley, 2009). Even if partners learn that more direct attempts to restore power exacerbate the distancing of avoidant individuals, they are unlikely to cease efforts to equalize power. Instead, partners may engage more indirect strategies, such as trying to be valuable and desirable partners. Feeling unable to control potential rejection should also spark reassurance seeking, which conveys desired support and can make avoidant individuals feel uncomfortable. Ultimately, therefore, avoidant individuals' attempts to protect their own autonomy by trying to attain interpersonal power may exacerbate their partners' dependence needs and generate power-balancing strategies by their partners that will be very aversive to highly avoidant individuals.

The difficulties produced by avoidant distancing may also undermine their partners' satisfaction. People who possess lower power are less happy in their relationships (Sprecher, Schmeeckle, & Felmlee, 2006), and even if partners manage to regain a sense of control, the lack of responsiveness communicated by avoidant tactics is likely to erode feelings of regard, trust, commitment, and satisfaction (Reis, Clark, & Holmes, 2004). These consequences might account for why greater avoidance is associated with reductions in partners' satisfaction (Tan et al., 2012) and higher rates of relationship dissolution (Kirkpatrick & Davis, 1994).

Finally, by reducing the satisfaction and commitment of their partners, avoidant individuals are ironically eroding an important source of their relative power—their partners' dependence on them. Avoidant individuals' potential power is derived from conveying less commitment than their partners do. However, this also means that behaving in ways that reduce the partners' commitment could ultimately transfer some power from avoidant individuals *to* their partners, leaving avoidant individuals in the predicament of having to express ever-decreasing levels of commitment in order to maintain power over partners who are always just one step behind. Such a process, if left unfettered, should contribute to relationship decline and dissolution.

Implications and Future Research Directions

Applying a dyadic regulation perspective to understanding the way avoidant individuals manage relationships enhances our understanding of how avoidance shapes relationships. First, this perspective outlines interpersonal mechanisms that explain the development and maintenance of avoidance strategies; these strategies should weaken a partner's power and sustain an individual's own desired autonomy, and thus these tactics will be reinforced across time. Second, distancing strategies may paradoxically elicit insecurity and dependence-balancing reactions in a partner, which heighten an avoidant individual's need to create distance. Although these partner responses have not been investigated, they are likely to create self-perpetuating cycles that exacerbate the dependence-based challenges faced by avoidant individuals and their partners in their relationships. Third, these dynamics undoubtedly contribute to poorer relationship outcomes. By undermining their partners' satisfaction and commitment, distancing strategies will reduce avoidant individuals' power-regulating capabilities, destabilize their relationships, and confirm their expectations that people cannot be trusted to remain loving partners.

We have conceptualized avoidant distancing strategies as dyadic because highly avoidant individuals need to modify their partners' behavior, desires, and influence in order to comfortably attain the autonomy and distance they desire. Regulating the partner's power may arise from purposeful attempts to change the partner's behavior and influence, or it may simply by a by-product of the deactivation strategies that highly avoidant individuals engage in to manage their own negative emotions. We suspect that both are true, because the inevitable interdependence of relationship interactions means that avoidant individuals must manage both their own emotions and their partners' emotions and behaviors, particularly if they want to protect themselves from being susceptible to influence and hurt by their partners. Nonetheless, even when avoidant individuals are trying to alter their partners' behavior and motivations, it is unlikely to be the concept of "power" that these individuals are trying to manipulate; rather, they are probably trying to alter the behaviors, emotions, and dyadic dynamics arising from the power that intimates have over one another.

Many of these propositions require further testing, but they do highlight a much-needed approach to investigating attachment dynamics in relationships. In particular, future research should consider how the regulation strategies associated with avoidance—often conceptualized as "internal"—involve dyadic processes. Highly avoidant individuals need to manage the desires, dependence, and influence of their partners, not just their own reactions to threat and dependence. And the partners' responses ultimately shape the use, effectiveness, and consequences of distancing strategies. Although we have focused on the detrimental outcomes for partners on the "receiving end" of avoidant distancing, certain partners may be able to respond in ways that curtail the destructive cycles we have hypothesized. Indeed, because avoidant individuals defensively disengage and may lack motivation to maintain relationships, their partners probably need to play a significant role in regulating their reactivity in order to sustain their relationships. We turn to this topic next (see bottom right of Table 6.1).

Attachment Avoidance and Regulation *by* the Partner

Partners' attempts to regulate the defenses of highly avoidant individuals must be responsive to the underlying concerns and vulnerabilities that trigger the avoidant individuals' distance-based coping strategies (Overall & Simpson, 2013; Simpson & Overall, 2014). Overall et al. (2013) identified two main ingredients of partner behavior that should down-regulate avoidant individuals' defenses: (1) behaviors that are sensitive to the autonomy needs of avoidant targets, and (2) behaviors that contradict the negative expectations avoidant individuals hold of their partners (cf. Bowlby, 1973). When avoidant individuals are targets of their partners' influence, for example, partners may be able to curtail the anger and withdrawal that highly avoidant individuals typically display by "softening" their communication through (1) reducing direct influence attempts that challenge avoidant targets (by downplaying problem severity, acknowledging progress made, and validating targets' point of view); and (2) offering clear evidence that avoidant targets are valued (by reducing friction, inhibiting negativity, and expressing positive regard). In the study described above, Overall et al. (2013) measured these types of softening behaviors. Avoidant targets whose partners displayed more softening communication exhibited less anger and withdrawal, which in turn generated more success in resolving the relationship problems couples discussed.

These types of softening behaviors should be particularly effective at alleviating avoidant defenses because they are less autonomy-threatening and they contradict the hostile intentions that avoidant individuals often anticipate from their partners. Other research also shows that behaviors sidestepping the emotional dependence that highly avoidant individuals find disconcerting help in down-regulating avoidant reactivity. Simpson et al. (2007) assessed the degree to which individuals were visibly calmed by different types of caregiving at moments during conflict discussions when individuals were most visibly upset. Individuals low in avoidance (i.e., those who were more securely attached as assessed by the Adult Attachment Interview) were rated as more calmed when their partners gave them more emotional care, such as encouraging them to talk about their emotions/experiences; by contrast, individuals high in avoidance were more calmed when their partners delivered instrumental caregiving, such as giving specific advice and concrete solutions to problems (see also Mikulincer & Florian, 1997). Although high levels of emotional caregiving may counteract avoidant individuals' negative expectations, the emotionally laden and intimacy-inducing nature of this type of caregiving requires too much vulnerability and intimacy for highly avoidant people to lower their self-protective defenses. Thus partners of avoidant individuals need to convey their trustworthiness and availability, while simultaneously being sensitive to the avoidant individuals' needs to maintain emotional independence and autonomy.

Salvatore, Kuo, Steele, Simpson, and Collins (2011) also demonstrated that recovery following couples' conflict interactions is important in minimizing the damage that insecure attachment can cause to relationships. Salvatore et al. (2011) examined conflict recovery during a 4-minute "cool-down" task that immediately followed adult couples' discussions of a major relationship problem. Better conflict recovery was evident when partners focused on the positive aspects of their relationships and were responsive to each other's repair attempts. Attachment insecurity (primarily avoidance) during infancy as assessed in the Strange Situation approximately 20 years earlier predicted poorer conflict recovery, and insecure individuals whose *partners* could not "move beyond the conflict" were less likely to be together 2 years later. In contrast, insecure participants involved with partners who exhibited better conflict recovery were more likely to be together 2 years later. As with softening and instrumental caregiving behaviors, recovering from conflict should signal that their partners can be trusted to let go of negativity, which should provide avoidant individuals with the room they need to restore comfortable levels of autonomy. These critical ingredients are what may have helped couples maintain their relationships.

Implications and Future Research Directions

The defensiveness of highly avoidant individuals is likely to escalate relationship problems and, in turn, increase dissatisfaction and instability in most relationships over time. Thus finding a way around avoidant defenses is crucial for partners involved with avoidant intimates if they want to develop and maintain successful relationships. By bypassing reactance and being responsive to the broader needs and goals associated with avoidance, partner softening may help to build greater trust and commitment in avoidant people (Simpson & Overall, 2014). However, as with regulating anxious insecurities, softening avoidant defenses may incur costs for a partner. Soft, loyal responses during conflict can downplay the need for change in a relationship and be less effective in generating improvement in it across time (Overall et al., 2009; Overall, Sibley, & Travaglia, 2010). The effort and motivation required to deliver influence and support attempts in ways that bypass avoidant reactivity may also generate resentment if desired changes are not made or if avoidant individuals' reactions do not improve. In addition, softening involves inhibiting or suppressing negativity, which, as described earlier, can be a source of dissatisfaction. On the other hand, experiencing success in down-regulating avoidant defenses during important interactions may be enough to maintain satisfaction in partners, particularly if avoidant intimates show positive change. Again, future longitudinal research is needed to track the ways in which dyadic regulation shapes the manifestation and consequences of attachment insecurity.

Some partners will be better at regulating avoidant defenses, and skillful regulation may be particularly crucial with avoidant individuals. Avoidant individuals' deep-rooted distrust of others often causes them to perceive their partners' actions as intentionally controlling or undermining (Mikulincer, 1998; Rholes et al., 1999). Their goal to resist dependence and maintain control may also make highly avoidant individuals more vigilant to their partners' regulation efforts. These concerns and this "myopic focus" could result in highly avoidant individuals' interpreting their partners' regulation attempts as manipulative, only exacerbating their defenses. If their partners' softening and other regulation efforts contradict avoidant expectations, however, avoidant individuals' focus on their partners' motives may enhance the effectiveness of their partners' regulation attempts (Overall et al., 2013). Identifying the characteristics of fluid and persuasive partner regulation is an important aim for future research.

Finally, the regulation attempts of avoidant individuals and the regulation attempts of their partners target the same underlying needs and concerns (see the bottom row of Table 6.1), most likely operate in unison, and probably reciprocally influence each other. In particular, the ways in which an avoidant individual tries to sustain power and control (regulation *of* the partner) are balanced by the partner being sensitive to the individual's autonomy needs and contradicting the individual's underlying fears that trigger distancing (regulation *by* the partner). And effective regulation by the partner probably develops across time as the partner encounters avoidant reactions in threatening contexts and learns how to bypass such defenses or soothe them when they arise. Some partners may be less able to adjust to avoidant reactivity, such as those who are highly anxious or experience acute rejection and felt dependence in response to avoidant distancing tactics. In contrast, partners who are secure or highly invested may develop successful regulation repertoires more quickly. Moreover, once partners learn to be sensitive to the autonomy needs of their avoidant mates and repeatedly demonstrate that they are trustworthy, this should provide the safety avoidant individuals need to commit and invest in their relationships fully, reduce avoidant distancing, and in turn reduce the need for their partners to regulate them. Thus, to reiterate a central point, understanding how members of dyads regulate and influence one another provides a clearer picture of how avoidance *affects* and is *affected by* intimate relationships.

Themes and Conclusions

The aim of this chapter has been to illustrate how a dyadic regulation perspective enhances our understanding of the ways in which attachment insecurity shapes and is shaped by intimate relationships. We close by briefly reiterating three important themes that illustrate the importance of a dyadic regulation approach. First, the threat management strategies arising from attachment anxiety and avoidance involve influencing or regulating partners' emotions and behavior, such as trying to induce guilt and obtain reassurance (anxiety) or reduce the partner's power and restore independence (avoidance). Importantly, the ways these strategies influence the partner, and in turn fulfill the specific needs and motives of anxious and avoidant individuals, highlight why these regulation strategies emerge and are subsequently reinforced. The partner regulation strategies enacted by highly anxious individuals elicit the reassurance they need to feel more secure and satisfied in their relationships. Similarly, distancing strategies protect highly avoidant individuals by minimizing their partners' power to hurt or influence them.

Second, regulation *of* the partner by an insecure individual operates within a dyadic system involving regulation *by* the partner (see Table 6.1). Most prior research has focused on how anxiety and avoidance can damage relationships. Not only can insecure individuals' own regulation strategies produce reinforcing benefits, but their partners can also recognize and regulate the concerns and defenses of highly anxious and avoidant people in ways that match and satisfy their specific needs. As highly anxious individuals try to elicit reassurance from their partners, their partners vigilantly try to avoid triggering anxious worries and soothe rejection-sensitive reactions. Successful regulation *by* the partners circumvents the destructive interaction cycles that can be produced by anxiety and can promote greater security. Similarly, by minimizing the threat of dependence, partners who soften their influence can reduce avoidant distancing, foster more effective emotion regulation in highly avoidant people, and thus help sustain close relationships.

Third, these dyadic regulation processes highlight that attachment insecurity does not destine relationships to failure and dissatisfaction. Instead, couples may often collaborate to manage, contain, and perhaps even alter levels of attachment insecurity. Nonetheless, we do not think that regulating insecurity is easy, and it may not be sustainable if the burden of caring for insecure individuals outweighs the security-enhancing benefits. We need to know more about the dyadic processes that reinforce and perpetuate the regulation strategies enacted by insecure individuals, and we need to identify the factors that optimize partners' attempts to downregulate and buffer these responses. Indeed, understanding the benefits and costs of the regulation strategies enacted by insecure individuals and their partners is essential for a full understanding of attachment dynamics. We hope this chapter motivates attachment researchers to consider dyadic regulation processes more seriously in the future.

References

Arriaga, X. B., Kumashiro, M., Finkel, E. J., VanderDrift, L. E., & Luchies, L. B. (2014). Filling the void: Bolstering attachment security in committed relationships. *Social Psychological and Personal Science, 5*(4), 398–406.

Arriaga, X. B., & Rusbult, C. E. (1998). Standing in my partner's shoes: Partner perspective taking and reactions to accommodative dilemmas. *Personality and Social Psychology Bulletin, 24,* 927–948.

Baumeister, R. F., Stillwell, A. M., & Heatherton, T. F. (1994). Guilt: An interpersonal approach. *Psychological Bulletin, 115,* 243–267.

Bouthillier, D., Julien, D., Dube, M., Belanger, I., & Hamelin, M. (2002). Predictive validity of adult attachment measures in relation to emotion regulation behaviors in marital interactions. *Journal of Adult Development, 9,* 291–305.

Bowlby, J. (1969/1982). *Attachment and loss: Vol. 1. Attachment.* New York: Basic Books.

Bowlby, J. (1973). *Attachment and loss: Vol. 2. Separation.* New York: Basic Books.

Bowlby, J. (1980). *Attachment and loss: Vol. 3. Loss.* New York: Basic Books.

Campbell, L., Simpson, J. A., Boldry, J., & Kashy, D. A. (2005). Perceptions of conflict and support in romantic relationships: The role of attachment anxiety. *Journal of Personality and Social Psychology, 88,* 510–531.

Cassidy, J., & Berlin, L. J. (1994). The insecure/ambivalent pattern of attachment: Theory and research. *Child Development, 65,* 971–981.

Christensen, A., & Heavey, C. L. (1990). Gender and social structure in the demand/withdraw pattern of marital conflict. *Journal of Personality and Social Psychology, 59,* 73–81.

Clark, M. S., Graham, S. M., Williams, E., & Lemay, E. P. (2008). Understanding relational focus of attention may help us understand relational phenomena. In J. P. Forgas & J. Fitness (Eds.), *Social relationships: Cognitive, affective, and motivational processes* (pp. 131–146). New York: Psychology Press.

Collins, N. L., & Feeney, B. C. (2000). A safe haven: An attachment theory perspective on support seeking and caregiving in intimate relationships. *Journal of Personality and Social Psychology, 78,* 1053–1073.

Creasey, G. (2002). Associations between working models of attachment and conflict management behavior in romantic couples. *Journal of Counseling Psychology, 49,* 365–375.

Diamond, L. M., Hicks, A. M., & Otter-Henderson, K. (2006). Physiological evidence for repressive coping among avoidantly attached adults. *Journal of Social and Personal Relationships, 23,* 205–229.

Dykas, M. J., & Cassidy, J. (2011). Attachment and the processing of social information across the life span: Theory and evidence. *Psychological Bulletin, 137,* 19–46.

Finkel, E. J., & Campbell, W. K. (2001). Self-control and accommodation in close relationships: An interdependence analysis. *Journal of Personality and Social Psychology, 81,* 263–277.

Fraley, R. C., & Shaver, P. R. (1998). Airport separations: A naturalistic study of adult attachment dynamics in separating couples. *Journal of Personality and Social Psychology, 75,* 1198–1212.

Gordon, A. M., & Chen, S. (2013). Does power help or hurt?: The moderating role of self–other focus on power and perspective-taking in romantic relationships. *Personality and Social Psychology, 39,* 1097–1110.

Gross, J. J., & John, O. P. (2003). Individual differences in two emotion regulation processes: Implications for affect, relationships, and well-being. *Journal of Personality and Social Psychology, 85,* 348–362.

Impett, E. A., Gordon, A. M., Kogan, A., Oveis, C., Gable, S. L., & Keltner, D. (2010). Moving toward more perfect unions: Daily and long-term consequences of approach and avoidance goals in romantic relationships. *Journal of Personality and Social Psychology, 99,* 948–963.

Jones, W. H., & Kugler, K. (1993). Interpersonal correlates of the guilt inventory. *Journal of Personality Assessment, 61,* 246–258.

Kelley, H. H., & Thibaut, J. W. (1978). *Interpersonal relations: A theory of interdependence.* New York: Wiley.

Kirkpatrick, L. A., & Davis, K. E. (1994). Attachment style, gender, and relationship stability: A longitudinal analysis. *Journal of Personality and Social Psychology, 66,* 502–512.

Kobak, R. R., Cole, H. E., Ferenz-Gillies, R., Fleming, W. S., & Gamble, W. (1993). Attachment and emotion regulation during mother–teen problem solving: A control theory analysis. *Child Development, 64,* 231–245.

Le, B. M., & Impett, E. A. (2013). When holding back helps: Suppressing negative emotions during sacrifice feels authentic and is beneficial for highly interdependent people. *Psychological Science, 24,* 1809–1815.

Lemay, E. P., Jr., & Clark, M. S. (2008a). "Walking on eggshells": How expressing relationship insecurities perpetuates them. *Journal of Personality and Social Psychology, 95,* 420–441.

Lemay, E. P., Jr., & Clark, M. S. (2008b). "You're just saying that": Contingencies of self-worth, suspicion, and authenticity in the interpersonal affirmation process. *Journal of Experimental Social Psychology, 44,* 1376–1382.

Lemay, E. P., Jr., & Dudley, K. L. (2011). Caution: Fragile! Regulating the interpersonal security of chronically insecure partners. *Journal of Personality and Social Psychology, 100,* 681–702.

Lemay, E. P., Jr., & O'Leary, K. (2012). Alleviating interpersonal suspicions of low self-esteem individuals: Negativity as honesty credentials. *Journal of Social and Clinical Psychology, 31,* 251–288.

Lemay, E. P., Jr., Overall, N. C., & Clark, M. S. (2012). Experiences and interpersonal consequences of hurt feelings and anger. *Journal of Personality and Social Psychology, 103,* 982–1006.

Little, K. C., McNulty, J. K., & Russell, M. (2010). Sex buffers intimates against the negative implications of attachment insecurity. *Personality and Social Psychology Bulletin, 36,* 484–498.

Mikulincer, M. (1998). Adult attachment style and individual differences in functional versus dysfunctional experiences of anger. *Journal of Personality and Social Psychology, 74,* 513–524.

Mikulincer, M., & Florian, V. (1997). Are emotional and instrumental supportive interactions beneficial in times of stress?: The impact of attachment style. *Anxiety, Stress and Coping, 10,* 109–127.

Mikulincer, M., & Shaver, P. R. (2003). The attachment behavioral system in adulthood: Activation, psychodynamics, and interpersonal processes. In M. P. Zanna (Ed.), *Advances in experimental social psychology* (Vol. 35, pp. 53–152). San Diego, CA: Academic Press.

Murray, S. L., Aloni, M., Holmes, J. G., Derrick, J. L., Stinson, D. A., & Leder, S. (2009). Fostering partner dependence as trust insurance: The implicit contingencies of the exchange script in close relationships. *Journal of Personality and Social Psychology, 96,* 324–348.

Overall, N. C., Fletcher, G. J. O., Simpson, J. A., & Sibley, C. G. (2009). Regulating partners in intimate relationships: The costs and benefits of different communication strategies. *Journal of Personality and Social Psychology, 96,* 620–639.

Overall, N. C., Girme, Y. U., Lemay, E. P., Jr., & Hammond, M. T. (2014). Attachment anxiety and reactions to relationship threat: The benefits and costs of inducing guilt in romantic partners. *Journal of Personality and Social Psychology, 106*, 235–256.

Overall, N. C., & Sibley, C. G. (2009). Attachment and dependence regulation within daily interactions with romantic partners. *Personal Relationships, 16*, 239–261.

Overall, N. C., Sibley, C. G., & Travaglia, L. K. (2010). Loyal but ignored: The benefits and costs of constructive communication behavior. *Personal Relationships, 17*, 127–148.

Overall, N. C., & Simpson, J. A. (2013). Regulation processes in close relationships. In J. A. Simpson & L. Campbell (Eds.), *The Oxford handbook of close relationships* (pp. 427–451). New York: Oxford University Press.

Overall, N. C., Simpson, J. A., & Struthers, H. (2013). Buffering attachment avoidance: Softening emotional and behavioral defenses during conflict discussions. *Journal of Personality and Social Psychology, 104*, 854–871.

Reis, H. T., Clark, M. S., & Holmes, J. (2004). Perceived partner responsiveness as an organizing construct in the study of intimacy and closeness. In D. J. Mashek & A. Aron (Eds.), *Handbook of closeness and intimacy* (pp. 201–225). Mahwah, NJ: Erlbaum.

Rholes, W. S., Simpson, J. A., Campbell, L., & Grich, J. (2001). Adult attachment and the transition to parenthood. *Journal of Personality and Social Psychology, 81*, 421–435.

Rholes, W. S., Simpson, J. A., & Oriña, M. M. (1999). Attachment and anger in an anxiety-provoking situation. *Journal of Personality and Social Psychology, 76*, 940–957.

Roisman, G. I., Holland, A., Fortuna, K., Fraley, R. C., Clausell, E., & Clarke, A. (2007). The Adult Attachment Interview and self-reports of attachment style: An empirical rapprochement. *Journal of Personality and Social Psychology, 92*, 678–697.

Rusbult, C. E., Verette, J., Whitney, G. A., Slovik, L. F., & Lipkus, I. (1991). Accommodation processes in close relationships: Theory and preliminary empirical evidence. *Journal of Personality and Social Psychology, 60*, 53–78.

Salvatore, J. E., Kuo, S. I., Steele, R. D., Simpson, J. A., & Collins, W. A. (2011). Recovering from conflict in romantic relationships: A developmental perspective. *Psychological Science, 22*, 376–383.

Shaver, P. R., & Mikulincer, M. (2007). Adult attachment strategies and the regulation of emotion. In J. J. Gross (Ed.), *Handbook of emotion regulation* (pp. 446–465). New York: Guilford Press.

Shaver, P. R., Schachner, D. A., & Mikulincer, M. (2005). Attachment style, excessive reassurance seeking, relationship processes, and depression. *Personality and Social Psychology Bulletin, 31*, 343–359.

Simpson, J. A., Farrell, A., Oriña, M. M., & Rothman, A. J. (2015). Power and social influence in relationships. In M. Mikulincer, P. R. Shaver, J. A. Simpson, & J. F. Dovidio (Eds.), *APA handbook of personality and social psychology: Vol. 3. Interpersonal relations* (pp. 393–420). Washington, DC: American Psychological Association.

Simpson, J. A., Kim, J. S., Fillo, J., Ickes, W., Rholes, W. S., Oriña, M. M., et al. (2011). Attachment and the management of empathic accuracy in relationship-threatening situations. *Personality and Social Psychology Bulletin, 37*, 242–254.

Simpson, J. A., & Overall, N. C. (2014). Partner buffering of attachment insecurity. *Current Directions in Psychological Science, 23,* 54–59.

Simpson, J. A., & Rholes, W. S. (2012). Adult attachment orientations, stress, and romantic relationships. In T. Devine & A. Plante (Eds.), *Advances in experimental social psychology* (Vol. 45, pp. 279–328). New York: Elsevier.

Simpson, J. A., Rholes, W. S., & Nelligan, J. S. (1992). Support-seeking and support-giving within couples in an anxiety-provoking situation: The role of attachment styles. *Journal of Personality and Social Psychology, 62,* 434–446.

Simpson, J. A., Rholes, W. S., Oriña, M. M., & Grich, J. (2002). Working models of attachment, support giving, and support seeking in a stressful situation. *Personality and Social Psychology Bulletin, 28,* 598–608.

Simpson, J. A., Rholes, W. S., & Phillips, D. (1996). Conflict in close relationships: An attachment perspective. *Journal of Personality and Social Psychology, 71,* 899–914.

Simpson, J. A., Winterheld, H. A., Rholes, S., & Oriña, M. (2007). Working models of attachment and reactions to different forms of caregiving from romantic partners. *Journal of Personality and Social Psychology, 93,* 466–477.

Sprecher, S., Schmeeckle, M., & Felmlee, D. (2006). The principle of least interest: Inequality in emotional involvement in romantic relationships. *Journal of Family Issues, 27,* 1255–1280.

Tan, R., Overall, N. C., & Taylor, J. K. (2012). Let's talk about us: Attachment, relationship-focused disclosure, and relationship quality. *Personal Relationships, 19,* 521–534.

Tangney, J. P., Wagner, P., Hill-Barlow, D., Marschall, D. E., & Gramzow, R. (1996). Relation of shame and guilt to constructive versus destructive responses to anger across the life-span. *Journal of Personality and Social Psychology, 70,* 797–809.

Tran, S., & Simpson, J. A. (2009). Pro-relationship maintenance behavior: The joint roles of attachment and commitment. *Journal of Personality and Social Psychology, 97,* 685–698.

Tran, S., & Simpson, J. A. (2011). Attachment, commitment and relationship maintenance: When partners really matter. In L. Campbell, J. La Guardia, J. Olson, & M. Zanna (Eds.), *The Ontario Symposium: Vol. 10. The science of the couple* (pp. 95–117). New York: Psychology Press.

Vangelisti, A. L., Daly, J. A., & Rudnick, J. R. (1991). Making people feel guilty in conversations: Techniques and correlates. *Human Communication Research, 18,* 3–39.

Waller, W. W., & Hill, R. (1951). *The family: A dynamic interpretation.* New York: Dryden Press.

Wieselquist, J., Rusbult, C. E., Foster, C. A., & Agnew, C. R. (1999). Commitment, pro-relationship behavior, and trust in close relationships. *Journal of Personality and Social Psychology, 77,* 942–966.

7

On the Convergence of Sexual Urges and Emotional Bonds

The Interplay of the Sexual and Attachment Systems during Relationship Development

Gurit E. Birnbaum

Sex is typically perceived as an integral aspect of romantic love and adult attachment relationships (e.g., Regan & Berscheid, 1999; Shaver, Hazan, & Bradshaw, 1988). Sexual urges and emotional attachments, however, are not necessarily interrelated. A person can feel emotionally attached to someone without being sexually attracted to him or her, and vice versa; sexual partners may have sex without being emotionally attached to each other, such as in the case of one-night stands. Indeed, attachment and sexual mating are distinct behavioral systems that evolved to serve different goals (maintaining proximity to a caregiver and gene reproduction, respectively); as such, their behavioral manifestation may occur in isolation (Bowlby, 1969/1982; Diamond, 2003). Still, sex does not generally occur in a "relational vacuum," and romantic partners are usually both attracted to and attached to each other. Thus, when it comes to romantic relationships, the attachment and sexual systems mutually influence one another and operate jointly to affect relationship quality (Birnbaum, 2010; Hazan & Zeifman, 1994).

The attachment system is the earliest-developing social behavioral system in humans. As such, it shapes the regulatory functioning of the later-developing sexual system (Bowlby, 1969/1982; Shaver et al., 1988).

Specifically, attachment processes may influence the way in which adolescents and adults construe their sexual interactions (e.g., Birnbaum, 2010; Mikulincer & Shaver, 2012). Nevertheless, the sexual behavioral system may also influence attachment by serving as a powerful motivational force across different stages of relationship development (Birnbaum, 2014; Hazan & Zeifman, 1994). Sexual attraction is often what brings potential partners together initially, and it helps determine whether subsequent interactions will occur. In later stages, as relationships progress from initial encounters to serious dating, sex may foster emotional bonding between sexual partners and strengthen their emerging relationship (Hazan & Zeifman, 1994, 1999). Yet, toward the end of a weakening relationship, sexual desire—or, more specifically, the lack of it—may be what makes partners grow apart.

In this chapter, I review research that points to a reciprocal relation between the attachment and sexual systems. The chapter begins with an overview of the literature on the contribution of attachment orientations to the appraisal of sexual interactions. In doing so, I discuss the role of attachment processes in linking sexuality with relationship quality and in shaping sexual responses to relationship-threatening events. I then focus on the role of sex as a promoter of emotional bonds, and review research indicating that sexual desire may be a mechanism that keeps sexual partners attached to each other. I also introduce a model of the functional significance of sex at different stages of relationship development, and present initial findings that support this model. I conclude by discussing the need for more research exploring the dual role of sex as a relationship maintenance mechanism and as a force motivating people to pursue alternative partners in a world of changing societal trends.

Contribution of Attachment Processes to the Construal of Sexual Interactions

According to Bowlby's (1969/1982, 1973) attachment theory, the attachment behavioral system evolved to increase the infant's survival chances and future reproductive success by maintaining proximity to supportive figures. Over the course of development, the quality of repeated interactions with these attachment figures gradually shapes chronic patterns of relational cognitions and goals. Interactions with attachment figures who are responsive to one's bids for proximity facilitate optimal functioning of the attachment system and promote a sense of attachment security. This sense of felt security provides confidence that one is worthy of others' love and that significant others will be supportive when needed, thereby leading to the consolidation of interpersonal goals aimed at forming nurturing intimate relationships. Recurrent failure to attain the primary goal of felt security results in the adoption of alternative regulatory strategies for dealing with the ensuing insecurity: hyperactivation and deactivation of the attachment system (Mikulincer & Shaver, 2007b). Hyperactivation strategies, which characterize anxious attachment, are intended to motivate attachment figures, who are perceived as insufficiently responsive, to pay attention and provide relief from stress. Deactivation strategies, which characterize avoidant attachment, are intended to maintain emotional distance and self-reliance in close relationships (Main, 1990; Mikulincer & Shaver, 2007b).

Early-developing attachment strategies are theorized to play a central role in molding a person's cognitive models of social life. These mental models guide interpersonal interactions over the entire lifespan by shaping relationship goals and affecting desired levels of intimacy and independence with adult romantic partners. Accordingly, they may influence the sexual system, which matures later in life (Shaver et al., 1988). Indeed, empirical evidence has supported the view that these different interpersonal goals and strategies explain variations in the functioning of the sexual system in romantic relationships (see Birnbaum, 2010; Mikulincer & Shaver, 2007a). In particular, people who are secure with respect to attachment tend to pursue committed intimate relationships and are thus likely to seek fulfillment of their sexual needs within such relationships (Mikulincer & Shaver, 2007a). In line with their intimacy goals, they engage in sex mainly to promote emotional bonding (e.g., to express love for their partners; Tracy, Shaver, Albino, & Cooper, 2003) and are less likely than less secure individuals to engage in casual sex (e.g., Brennan & Shaver, 1995; Paul, McManus, & Hayes, 2000; Stephan & Bachman, 1999).

Beyond encouraging the channeling of sexual desires into a committed intimate relationship, smooth functioning of the attachment system promotes a secure state of mind that facilitates relaxed engagement in sexual activities. Securely attached people, as compared to their less secure counterparts, are less likely to be preoccupied with attachment concerns and with worries about their sexual performance, and are generally more comfortable with their sexuality (Mikulincer & Shaver, 2007a). Specifically, they have more positive sexual self-schemas (Cyranowski & Andersen, 1998); they are less erotophobic (i.e., they experience fewer negative affective–evaluative responses to sexual cues); and they experience fewer negative emotions and more positive, passionate emotions during sexual activity (e.g., Birnbaum, Reis, Mikulincer, Gillath, & Orpaz, 2006; Tracy et al., 2003). This relaxed and confident approach to sexuality allows securely attached people to respond to partners' sexual preferences without compromising their own needs, and to enjoy affectionate and exploratory sexual activities that foster mutual sexual satisfaction (Mikulincer & Shaver, 2007a; Shaver et al., 1988). Overall, securely attached individuals' sense of sexual confidence, comfort with sexual intimacy, and enjoyment of sexual interactions with their long-term partners contribute to maintaining satis-fying romantic relationships (Birnbaum et al., 2006).

Chronic dysfunctions of the attachment system may distort the acti-vation of the sexual system and interfere with sexual activities (Bowlby, 1969/1982). In other words, to the extent that a person feels chronically insecure about being loved, whether this is manifested in relational worries or in being uncomfortable with intimacy, it is unlikely that this person's sexual system will function optimally. Consistent with this contention, research has shown that even though anxious and avoidant attachment are associated with different approaches to sex, they both bias the functioning of the sexual system (see reviews by Birnbaum, 2010; Stefanou & McCabe, 2012).

Anxiously attached people are preoccupied with rejection fears (Bar-tholomew & Horowitz, 1991; Mikulincer & Shaver, 2007b). These fears may motivate them to use sex, which is a prominent route for seeking prox-imity, to serve their unmet attachment needs for love and security (e.g., Davis, Shaver, & Vernon, 2004). The resulting subordination of sexual activity to the attachment system may account for diverse sexual motives, thoughts, and behaviors. For example, anxiously attached people tend to engage in sex for attachment-related reasons (e.g., achieving intimacy, approval, and reassurance; Birnbaum, Mikulincer, & Austerlitz, 2013; Impett, Gordon, & Strachman, 2008; Schachner & Shaver, 2004) and to be attracted to partners who seem willing to provide the sense of reassur-ance that they crave (Birnbaum & Reis, 2012; Holmes & Johnson, 2009; Wei, Mallinckrodt, Larson, & Zakalik, 2005). Along with this motivation, they prefer the affectionate aspects of sex (e.g., holding, cuddling, kissing) rather than sex per se (Hazan, Zeifman, & Middleton, 1994), and they fan-tasize about giving and receiving affection during sexual activity. It is inter-esting that their sexual fantasies also involve submission themes that may serve the need for experiencing the power of their partners and eliciting caregiving (Birnbaum, 2007b; Birnbaum, Mikulincer, & Gillath, 2011).

Ironically, anxiously attached individuals channel not only their rela-tional expectations into the sexual realm, but also excessive relational worries (Birnbaum et al., 2006). In particular, anxiously attached people fear disappointing their partners and engage in sex to avoid abandonment (Davis et al., 2004; Schachner & Shaver, 2004). Accordingly, they tend to please their partners during sexual intercourse, to inhibit the expres-sion of their own sexual needs (e.g., Davis et al., 2006), and to succumb to unwanted sexual advances (Feeney, Peterson, Gallois, & Terry, 2000; Gentzler & Kerns, 2004; Impett & Peplau, 2002).

The overall construal of highly anxiously attached people's sexuality is therefore quite ambivalent. On the one hand, the erotophilic tendencies that lead them to channel relational goals into the sexual route (Bogaert & Sadava, 2002) may intensify the pleasurable aspects of sex (Birnbaum et al., 2006). On the other hand, attachment-related worries may lead simultaneously to aversive feelings during sexual intercourse (Birnbaum, 2007a). Indeed, when describing their experiences of sexual intercourse, anxiously attached people report relatively high levels of a "letting go" state of mind and desire for emotional involvement, warmth, and attention from their partners. At the same time, they also report negative emotions and doubts about being loved (Birnbaum et al., 2006). Unsurprisingly, this pattern of sexual experiences often fail to meet their unrealistic relationship expectations, resulting in frustrated attachment needs and sexual disappointment (Birnbaum, 2007a; Birnbaum et al., 2006).

More avoidant individuals, in contrast, feel uncomfortable being close to others (Mikulincer & Shaver, 2007b) and may thus be threatened by the demand for personal disclosure implied by sexual interactions. These intimacy fears may motivate them either to abstain from sexual activity altogether (or at least delay its onset; Gentzler & Kerns, 2004; Kalichman et al., 1993; Tracy et al., 2003) or to approach sex in various distancing ways. Avoidant people typically downplay sexual motives associated with the promotion of emotional closeness and instead pursue self-serving goals, such as having sex to feel good about oneself (see Cooper et al., 2006; Mikulincer & Shaver, 2007a, for reviews). Consequently, they are less likely than less avoidant people to be sexually interested in potential partners who want to be close, and are more likely to be attracted to partners with similar needs for independence (Birnbaum & Reis, 2012; Holmes & Johnson, 2009).

Avoidant people are also more likely than less avoidant people to be promiscuous and nonexclusive in intimate relationships. They hold more permissive attitudes about casual sex and are more likely to engage in uncommitted sex with different partners (Brennan & Shaver, 1995; Feeney, Noller, & Patty, 1993; Gentzler & Kerns, 2004). Consistent with this pattern, they tend to respond favorably to mate-poaching attempts (i.e., attempts to lure them away from their current partners) in a short-term context, but not when the poaching is for a long-term relationship (Schachner & Shaver, 2002). As might be expected, avoidant people's tendency to have sex outside their relationships is explained by low levels of commitment to their relationship partners (DeWall et al., 2011) and is reinforced by their primary partners' desire for intimacy (Beaulieu-Pelletier, Philippe, Lecours, & Couture, 2011).

Avoidant people distance themselves from their partners not only by engaging in extradyadic sex, but also by relying on the solitary sexual activity of masturbation (Bogaert & Sadava, 2002) and by having less frequent sex with their partners (Brassard, Shaver, & Lussier, 2007). When avoidant people do have sex with their partners, they display relatively low levels of physical affection and experience difficulties in attending to their partners' needs. In addition, they experience relatively strong feelings of estrangement and alienation (Birnbaum & Reis, 2006; Birnbaum et al., 2006), which may impair their sexual functioning (e.g., Birnbaum, 2007a; Cohen & Belsky, 2008). These aversive experiences migrate into their sexual fantasy lives in the form of interpersonal distance and hostility themes, which may serve the goal of self-reliance and control in close relationships (Birnbaum, 2007b; Birnbaum, Mikulincer, et al., 2011). Viewed together, avoidant individuals' detached stance may impede the experience of genuine intimate interactions, often resulting in sex lives that are devoid of affectional bonding, even within the context of their ongoing romantic relationships.

Gender Differences in the Sexual Manifestations of Attachment Insecurities

Attachment dynamics in the sexual arena may differ for men and women, as they experience sexual activity somewhat differently (e.g., Birnbaum & Laser-Brandt, 2002). These differences are congruent with both evolutionary models (e.g., Buss & Schmitt, 1993; Ellis & Symons, 1990) and social approaches (DeLamater, 1987; Gagnon & Simon, 1973) to gender differences in human sexuality. Both perspectives agree, though for different reasons (evolutionary vs. cultural socialization processes), that women develop a more emotional/interpersonal orientation toward sexuality than do men. For example, women are more concerned with their romantic relationships during sexual intercourse and tend to be more affectionate and nurturing. Men, by comparison, tend to adopt a more individualistic/recreational orientation. For example, men are more likely to be active, to take the initiator role, and to focus on satisfying their partners during sexual activity (Birnbaum & Laser-Brandt, 2002; Byers & Heinlein, 1989; Carroll, Volk, & Hyde, 1985; O'Sullivan & Byers, 1992).

Given that men and women diverge in their approach to sex, it is hardly surprising that they also express attachment insecurities differently in the sexual domain. Specifically, both avoidant men and women tend to restrict expressions of intimacy in sexual interactions (e.g., Birnbaum et al., 2006; Cooper et al., 2006). However, the avoidant effect is more marked in men's sexuality than in women's. For example, avoidant men, but not avoidant women, are less likely to experience sexual fantasies that involve romantic themes (Birnbaum, 2007b). Avoidant men are also more inclined to engage in extrapair sex and to use sex for relationship-irrelevant reasons (e.g., coping with upset feelings) as compared to avoidant women (e.g., Birnbaum, Hirschberger, & Goldenberg, 2011; Cooper et al. 2006). It is possible that male sex-role norms, which emphasize the quest for sexual conquering and restrict the expression of vulnerability, exacerbate the destructive effects of avoidance on expressions of intimacy, whereas women's habitual nurturing tendencies mitigate these effects.

Gender differences in the sexual manifestations of attachment anxiety are more salient. Among men, attachment anxiety is associated with relatively restricted sexual expression. For example, anxiously attached men are less likely than less anxiously attached men to have sex to bolster their self-esteem or to cheat on their partners (Cooper et al., 2006), and they have fewer sex partners overall (Gentzler & Kerns, 2004). At the same time, they are particularly likely to exert pressure on their current partners to have sex (Brassard et al., 2007). Among women, attachment anxiety is associated with unrestricted and risky sexual behaviors. For example, anxiously attached women are inclined to engage in extrapair sex (Bogaert & Sadava, 2002; Gangestad & Thornhill, 1997), as well as in unprotected and consensual unwanted sex (e.g., Feeney & Noller, 2004; Impett & Peplau, 2002). Expectedly, they also report higher rates of unplanned pregnancy than less anxiously attached women do (Cooper, Shapiro, & Powers, 1998).

These findings suggest that the same relational worries that inhibit initiating sex with new partners among men and lead them to invest more in current relationships also lead men to use coercive sex as a means for regaining proximity to partners who are perceived as unresponsive. Similar relational worries appear to create difficulty in negotiating sexual encounters among women and lead them to secure alternatives to their current partners, both in the real and in the virtual worlds. Indeed, a corresponding pattern emerges in the content of sexual fantasies: More anxiously attached women are more likely than less anxiously attached women to experience fantasies that involve unrestricted sex and are less likely to fantasize about their current partners. More anxiously attached men, by comparison, are more likely than less anxiously attached men to experience sexual fantasies that involve romantic themes and to express the desire to satisfy their partners (Birnbaum, 2007b). The content of these fantasies seems to reflect the typical defense mechanisms employed by anxiously attached men and women, further supporting the notion that sexual expressions constitute a route by which men and women uniquely cope with their attachment insecurities.

The Contribution of Attachment and Sex to Relationship Well-Being

Both attachment anxiety and avoidance are positively associated with aversive sexual experiences among men and women, regardless of whether or not gender-specific construal of sex buffers the adverse effects of attachment insecurities on sexual expressions. Nevertheless, attachment anxiety and avoidance represent two extremes relevant to the potential effects of sex on relationship well-being: Attachment anxiety may intensify the association between sexual experiences and the quality of relationship interactions, whereas attachment avoidance may inhibit this association. In particular, anxiously attached individuals tend to conflate sex and intimacy, such that their perception of relationship quality relies heavily on their sexual experiences. Hence they are likely to equate gratifying sexual experiences with a sense of being loved, and to perceive negative sexual experiences as an indicator of their partners' rejection or of overarching relational difficulties. Conversely, avoidant people tend to isolate sexuality from psychological intimacy, and are thus prone to experience a sense of disconnection between sexual activity and relationship quality. Within this conceptualization is embedded the assertion that optimal functioning of the attachment system—such as in the case of securely attached partners—involves intermediate levels of interdependence between sexual and emotional aspects of a relationship, rather than high or low levels of dependence between these two aspects (Birnbaum, 2010, 2014; Birnbaum et al., 2006).

Several dyadic studies support this conceptualization. We (Birnbaum et al., 2006), for example, had both members of heterosexual cohabiting couples reported on their attachment orientations and provide daily diary measures of relationship quality and sexual activity for 42 consecutive days. In addition, each time they had sex, participants reported their feelings and cognitions during that sexual episode (e.g., "During or after sexual intercourse, I felt some frustration and disappointment," "During sexual intercourse, I felt passionately attracted to my partner"). The findings showed that attachment anxiety amplified the effects of positive and negative sexual experiences on relationship quality, implying that sex is most beneficial, but also most detrimental, to the relationships of couples with an anxiously attached partner. Attachment avoidance, in contrast, inhibited both the detrimental relational effects of negative sexual interactions and the positive relational effect of having sex. Hence couples with an avoidant partner neither suffer the adverse effects of bad experiences nor enjoy the beneficial effects of positive sexual experiences.

The latter conclusion is qualified by a more recent diary study of newlywed couples (Little, McNulty, & Russell, 2010). The surprising results of this study revealed that under nonthreatening circumstances, frequent and satisfying sex may benefit not only the relationships of anxiously attached spouses, but those of avoidant spouses as well. In particular, engaging in highly frequent and satisfying sexual activity may lead to positive expectancies for partner availability, thereby attenuating the adverse relational effects of attachment insecurities. Gratifying sex can therefore make both anxiously and avoidantly attached partners feel more satisfied in their relationships, as long as it helps them perceive their partners as more available and responsive.

The Coordination of Attachment and Sex during Relationship-Distressing Events

Of course, the sexual expressions of attachment dynamics and their relational outcomes may change in relationship-threatening circumstances (e.g., insecurity regarding the love of one's partner, possible mate poaching, prospective separation). Such threatening conditions are likely to activate attachment concerns that call for distress regulation (e.g., Davis, Shaver, & Vernon, 2003; Mikulincer, Gillath, & Shaver, 2002; Simpson, Rholes, & Phillips, 1996) and may therefore elicit attachment defensive strategies in insecurely attached individuals (e.g., Mikulincer & Shaver, 2007b; Simpson & Rholes, 1994). Given that behaviors characteristic of the sexual system may serve the goals of deactivation and hyperactivation strategies (e.g., maintaining distance by engaging in emotionless sex, and avoiding abandonment by deferring to partners' sexual needs, respectively; Birnbaum, 2010; Davis et al., 2006), it is reasonable to expect that under relationship-threatening conditions, the sexual manifestations of these defensive strategies may be particularly pronounced.

This reasoning has received support from studies that examined sexual responses to a variety of relationship-threatening conditions (e.g., hypothetical relationship threat scenarios, actual troubled interactions). For example, in two series of experiments, participants imagined relationship-threatening scenes (e.g., a partner's considering breaking up, a partner's infidelity), non-relationship-threatening scenes (failure on an exam), or nonthreatening scenarios (e.g., a partner going to a grocery store). Following this procedure, participants rated or described their desire to have sex, reasons for engaging in sex (Birnbaum, Weisberg, & Simpson, 2011), and what sexual activities they would like to engage in (i.e., their sexual fantasies) (Birnbaum, Svitelman, Bar-Shalom, & Porat, 2008). The results indicated that relationship threat generated mixed emotions in anxiously attached people. Specifically, it decreased their pursuit of sexual pleasure (Birnbaum, Weisberg, et al., 2011) and increased their habitual negative self-representations, such that highly anxious people represented themselves as more alienated and hostile in their fantasies (Birnbaum et al., 2008). This negative reaction, which may reflect the intensification of anger toward the threatening partners and self-relevant thoughts typical of relationship-threatening events (e.g., Campbell & Marshall, 2011; Mikulincer & Shaver, 2007b), was accompanied by a heightened desire to satisfy others sexually (Birnbaum et al., 2008).

The findings of these studies suggest that anxiously attached people have trouble enjoying sex when being flooded with the relationship worries imposed by threat. Threats to their relationships exacerbate their habitual insecurity, motivating them to respond to threats with relationship-maintaining behaviors (e.g., using sex to please their partners) while denying their own sexual needs. The ensuing frustration may pose additional obstacles to their erotic pleasure. Tragically, the ambivalent reaction that relationship threat invokes in anxiously attached people may lead them to display relationship-destructive behaviors (e.g., recurring bouts of uncontrollable anger, partner surveillance; Guerrero, 1998; Mikulincer & Shaver,

2005). Such behaviors may eventually sabotage their attempts to repair the threatened relationship and lead them to realize their worst fear—relationship loss (e.g., Campbell & Marshall, 2011; Campbell, Simpson, Boldry, & Kashy, 2005; Simpson et al., 1996).

The studies on sexual reactions to threats also indicate that, as expected, avoidant people use distancing strategies when being threatened. Specifically, relationship threat lessened avoidant people's desire to have sex with their partners (Birnbaum, Weisberg, et al., 2011). In addition, reminders of death—the final separation and possibly the ultimate threat—increased the likelihood that avoidant people have sex for self-serving reasons (e.g., affirming their self-worth) as well as the likelihood that avoidant men engage in casual sex (Birnbaum, Hirschberger, et al., 2011). These findings show that unlike anxiously attached people, who use sex to repair threatened relationships, avoidant people react to threat by withdrawing sexually from their partners and by using sex as a means to feel better about themselves. That is, avoidant people attempt to protect themselves against anticipated rejection by engaging in compensatory self-enhancement and defensive distancing from their potentially rejecting partners.

A similar pattern was observed in a dyadic study conducted in a more natural context (Birnbaum, Mikulincer, et al., 2011). In this study, members of heterosexual cohabiting couples reported their attachment orientations and then provided daily diary measures of their relationship interactions for 21 consecutive days. In addition, immediately after every occasion in which they experienced a sexual fantasy during the 21-day study period, participants described it in narrative form. The results revealed that negative couple interactions increased habitual attachment-related wishes and self-representations. Specifically, distressful relationship events led anxiously attached people to shift from fantasizing about mutually nurturing themes to fantasizing about submission themes that emphasize their neediness (e.g., representations of the self as weak and helpless), which could serve the goal of eliciting caregiving from a powerful partner (Birnbaum, 2007b; Davis et al., 2004). Avoidant people, in contrast, reacted to troubled interactions with distancing themes and enhancement fantasies. They expressed more avoidant wishes (escaping reality) and represented themselves as less weak and helpless.

Considered together, these findings demonstrate the involvement of sexual mental imagery in handling attachment-related stressful events and imply that such negative events amplify habitual defensive tendencies. These events elicit compensatory self-enhancement (i.e., protective responses in which the self is represented as sexually potent) among avoidant people, and compensatory relational restoration strategies (i.e., protective responses designed to improve the relationship) among anxiously attached people.

This conclusion is tempered, however, by results from a recent series of studies indicating that subliminally activated attachment insecurity exerts a uniformly avoidant effect on the content of sexual fantasies. In these studies (Birnbaum, Simpson, Weisberg, Barnea, & Assulin-Simhon, 2012, Studies 2 and 3), participants were subliminally exposed to either a security or an insecurity picture prime (pictorial representations of either maternal caring or maternal rejection), after which they described a sexual fantasy narratively or completed a fantasy checklist. The results showed that, regardless of dispositional attachment orientations, subliminally activated attachment insecurity inhibited relationship-promoting themes and produced fantasies that involved interpersonal distance and hostility themes. These presumably self-protective fantasy responses (i.e., distancing oneself from the potential source of distress) resemble the typical thematic content of avoidant people's sexual fantasies (Birnbaum, 2007b; Birnbaum, Mikulincer, et al., 2011). The finding that this effect was independent of dispositional attachment orientations suggests the involvement of unconscious processes in which rejection concerns automatically activate self-protection goals while inhibiting relationship-promoting ones.

The discrepancies between the results of this research and those of earlier studies are likely due to differences in methodology. For example, the finding that activated attachment insecurity inhibited, rather than prompted, relationship-promoting themes may be related to the type of threat studied and to the goals that are more likely to be challenged by this specific threat. A situation in which a partner considers to end the relationship is likely to challenge interpersonal goals aimed at maintaining nurturing intimate relationships. As such, it may elicit reactions that focus on fighting for the specific threatened relationship, at least among those who are motivated by intimacy needs (e.g., Davis et al., 2003). Conversely, consistent exposure to a rejecting mother image fits with the conceptualization of an avoidant prime and should therefore produce general rejection concerns. These general concerns are likely to challenge self-image goals (i.e., maintaining a positive self-image) and thus to activate avoidance motivation geared toward protecting the self from the pain of rejection (Andersen & Chen, 2002; Bartz & Lydon, 2004).

The Contribution of the Partner's Attachment Characteristics to Sexual Dynamics

Obviously, people are motivated by a variety of purely personal goals in the sexual domain (e.g., enhancement, stress reduction, hedonism) under both threatening and nonthreatening conditions, and often engage in sex that involves a solitary act of pleasure. Nevertheless, given that sexual experiences are generally integrated into some sort of relational context that guides their construal, sexual responses should be determined not only by each individual's characteristics, but also by the partner's characteristics. In the case of relationship threat, for example, people may be less likely to turn to their partners for sexual consolation if they realize that their partners are not likely to respond positively to such advances. Corroborating this view, a study examining the effects of relational conflict on sexual motivation showed that major conflict inhibited self-serving sexual motives (e.g., having sex to obtain relief from stress) among people with avoidant partners (Birnbaum et al., 2013). These findings imply that people are unlikely to use avoidant partners as a source of comfort while engaging in so-called "make-up" sex, because they do not view them as responsive figures that can alleviate their distress, either inside or outside the bedroom. Indeed, avoidant people habitually distance themselves from emotional partners, dismiss their signals of sexual and nonsexual needs, and provide them with less support (Birnbaum et al., 2006; Mikulincer & Shaver, 2007b; Reis, 2007).

Other studies have demonstrated the value of adopting a dyadic perspective for understanding the manifestations of attachment dynamics in everyday sexual experience. These studies show, for example, that partners of anxiously attached people do not report greater levels of sexual dissatisfaction than partners of less anxiously attached people do, at least in nonclinical samples (Butzer & Campbell, 2008; Impett & Peplau, 2002; but see Brassard, Péloquin, Dupuy, Wright, & Shaver, 2012, for different results in couples seeking marital therapy). This is probably because anxiously attached people tend to please their partners and defer to their sexual needs (e.g., Davis et al., 2006). Still, partners of anxiously attached women do experience relational distress following negative sexual interactions—a finding that may reflect their negative reaction to the destructive behavior that anxiously attached women exhibit after having experienced negative feelings during sex (Birnbaum et al., 2006). In contrast, and as expected, partners of avoidant people report greater levels of sexual dissatisfaction than do partners of less avoidant people (e.g., Butzer & Campbell, 2008). Furthermore, partners of avoidant men, compared to partners of less avoidant men, show fewer reductions in relationship-damaging behaviors following sexual interactions, possibly because sex with an avoidant male may contribute minimally to women's intimacy goals in close relationships (Birnbaum et al., 2006).

Taking into consideration the unique configuration of both partners' attachment orientations extends these studies by unraveling the interactive nature of couples' sexuality. The predictive power of this approach has been demonstrated in a study in which members of established couples reported their attachment orientations and sexual experiences (Brassard et al., 2007). This study revealed dyadic interaction patterns in which two anxiously attached partners have a relatively high rate of sexual intercourse. However, anxiously attached men have sex less often if their female partners are less anxiously attached. This pattern suggests that anxiously attached men's intense efforts to have sex are well received by partners with similar intimacy needs, but deter less anxiously attached partners, who may perceive such excessive demands as irritating. Somewhat similarly, anxiously attached women have sex less often if their male partners are avoidantly attached, probably because anxiously attached women's needs for reassurance clash with their avoidant partners' intimacy fears. Avoidant men are also more likely to avoid sexual activities in their current relationships, to experience sexual difficulties, and to have sex less often if their female partners are avoidantly attached. It seems that fears of intimacy that burden both partners in a couple may be particularly detrimental to their sexuality, because neither of them is motivated to resolve their relationship difficulties.

Contribution of Sex to Attachment Processes

The studies reviewed above illustrate how attachment processes may affect the construal of sexual interactions in close relationships. Other studies suggest that influences in the reverse direction, from sexual to attachment processes, are also possible. There is no doubt that sex has the potential to be an intensely meaningful experience—one that can be a powerful motivational force during relationship development. Indeed, although the sexual behavioral system evolved to facilitate reproduction (via pregnancy or impregnation; Buss & Kenrick, 1998), impregnation is generally not sufficient for the survival of human offspring, who have a long period of development and vulnerability. Sexual partners therefore need to remain together long enough to enable their offspring to survive the most vulnerable period of infancy, to increase chances of future reproductive success (Fisher, 1998; Hazan & Zeifman, 1994; Mellen, 1981). Accordingly, mechanisms that keep sexual partners attached to each other for an extended period and motivate them to care jointly for their offspring should have arisen in the course of human evolution (Birnbaum & Gillath, 2006; Birnbaum & Reis, 2006).

Several characteristics of human sexuality insinuate that sexual needs may act as such a mechanism because they encourage extended intimate contact, which is likely to contribute to the formation and maintenance of attachment bonds (e.g., Birnbaum, 2014; Hazan & Zeifman, 1994). For example, humans tend to prefer the ventro-ventral sexual position, which allows belly-to-belly contact and mutual gaze. Humans also tend to have sex in private and to sleep together after intercourse (Ford & Beach, 1951). These tendencies are likely to enhance intimacy and emotional bonding between sexual partners. In addition, oxytocin and vasopressin, the neuropeptides involved in mediating the rewarding aspects of attachment (e.g., Carter et al., 2005; Young, Gobrogge, Liu, & Wang, 2011), are secreted in humans during foreplay, during sexual intercourse, and in the moments preceding orgasm (e.g., Carmichael et al., 1987; Carter, 1992; Filippi et al., 2003; Murphy, Seckl, Burton, Checkley, & Lightman, 1987). Moreover, in contrast to most mammalian species, humans have sex on every day of the menstrual cycle; they may therefore experience an extended release of oxytocin and vasopressin that further reinforces sexual bonding, which over time promotes enduring attachment bonds between sexual partners (Young & Wang, 2004).

Research assessing mental representations of the sexual aspect of romantic relationships provides additional support for the theorized link between sex and attachment. Specifically, studies exploring people's accounts of their motives for having sex show that some of the most frequently endorsed reasons for having sex involve relationship-related motives, such as the desire for emotional closeness and the desire to intensify the relationship (e.g., Meston & Buss, 2007). Similarly, research examining the functional meaning of sex has indicated that prevalent meanings attached to sex reflect the beliefs that sexual activity promotes intimacy between partners and enhances their emotional bond (e.g., Birnbaum, 2003; Birnbaum & Gillath, 2006; Birnbaum & Reis, 2006). Subsequent research has extended these studies by providing evidence for the hypothesized causal pathway from activation of the sexual system to attachment formation and maintenance (Gillath, Mikulincer, Birnbaum, & Shaver, 2008). In this series of experiments, participants were subliminally exposed to erotic stimuli (vs. neutral stimuli). The results revealed that subliminal exposure to sexually arousing stimuli increased the willingness to self-disclose intimate information to a potential new partner, as well as the willingness to engage in relationship-promoting behaviors with existing partners. These findings imply that sexual arousal leads people to employ strategies that allow them to get closer to potential new partners or to strengthen relationships with existing ones.

A Model of the Functional Significance of Sex within Romantic Relationships

Although research suggests that activation of the sexual system facilitates both relationship initiation and relationship maintenance strategies (e.g., Gillath et al., 2008), as yet there is still no compelling theoretical framework for understanding changes in the functional significance of sex across major relationship phases. The underlying function of sex is likely to change as the relationship develops, due to corresponding changes in the emotional bonding process (e.g., the transformation from preattachment to a full-blown attachment relationship, and then on to potential detachment and dissolution; Birnbaum, 2014). A model depicting these changes may thus include, but is not limited to, relationship initiation and maintenance. Furthermore, to the extent that the meaning of sex varies in individuals (e.g., Birnbaum, 2003, 2014) and across contexts (e.g., relationship threat;

Birnbaum et al., 2008; Birnbaum, Weisberg, et al., 2011), such a model should clarify under which circumstances and for whom sex is most likely to promote the bonding process and benefit the relationship.

The model presented here offers such an initial person × context interactive framework. In particular, the proposed model identifies six roles that sex may play in attachment processes, which roughly correspond to major relationship phases (see Figure 7.1). Initially, the desire for sex may motivate a person to look for either short-term or long-term mating opportunities with potential sexual partners (Fisher, Aron, Mashek, Li, & Brown, 2002). Once a potential partner is identified, sexual responses to this new acquaintance may serve as a diagnostic test of his or her suitability and compatibility (Birnbaum & Reis, 2006), determining whether future interactions will occur (Berscheid & Reis, 1998). Increased sexual desire for this potential partner may signify suitability and therefore motivate the individual to pursue this desirable partner. In contrast, a lack of sexual desire may signal relationship incompatibility and therefore motivate withdrawal from

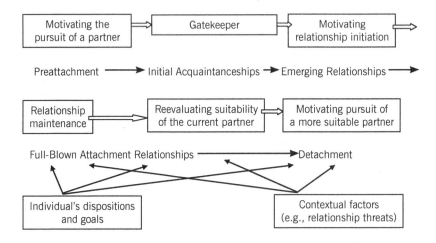

FIGURE 7.1. A model of the functional significance of sex at different relationship phases: (1) motivating an individual's pursuit of either short-term or long-term mating opportunities with potential sexual partners; (2) serving as a means of evaluating the suitability and compatibility of a newly met potential partner, and as a gatekeeper ensuring that only suitable partners will be pursued; (3) motivating relationship initiation with a suitable potential partner; (4) promoting intimacy, trust, and commitment; (5) serving as a means of reevaluating the suitability and compatibility of a current long-term partner; (6) motivating the individual to solve relational problems or pursue an alternative, more suitable partner.

future interactions with this person (Birnbaum & Reis, 2006, 2012). Once a suitable partner is found, sexual desire for this partner may motivate the individual to form a relationship that extends beyond a single sexual episode (Birnbaum & Gillath, 2006).

As a relationship progresses from initial encounters to casual dating to steady dating, sex may serve as a binding force that fosters emotional bonding between sexual partners and strengthens their emerging relationship. A recent longitudinal study has supported this theorizing (Mizrahi, Birnbaum, Hirschberger, Mikulincer, & Szepsenwol, 2015). In this study, members of couples who had been dating for less than 4 months completed measures of sexual desire, frequency of sexual intercourse, and relationship-specific attachment avoidance and anxiety three times over an 8-month period. The results indicated that relationship-specific attachment insecurities declined over time, but only among participants who reported relatively high levels of sexual desire and high frequency of sexual intercourse. These findings suggest that sexual activity reduces attachment defenses in the early stages of dating, thereby fostering the formation of genuine intimacy (see also Rubin & Campbell, 2012).

In later phases of relationship development, sex may still help maintain a relationship (e.g., Bell, Daly, & Gonzalez, 1987; Birnbaum et al., 2006), but may become less important to its quality and stability than other aspects of the relationship, such as the provision of mutual support, warmth, and interdependence (Kotler, 1985; Reedy, Birren, & Schaie, 1981; Sternberg, 1986). Nevertheless, sex may turn out to be especially beneficial to the relationship of most people in relationship-threatening situations, which provoke anxiety and elicit proximity seeking. In these situations, people may use sex to repair their threatened relationships (e.g., Birnbaum, 2014; Birnbaum et al., 2008). Frequent sexual activity can also buffer against the detrimental relational implications of potentially destructive personality traits of romantic partners (e.g., neuroticism; Russell & McNulty, 2011) or deficits in nonsexual relational dimensions (e.g., poor communication; Litzinger & Gordon, 2005). It is possible that the intimacy inherent in sexual contact provides an alternative, compensatory route for satisfying the otherwise unmet attachment needs for security and love.

Yet relationship restoration is not always feasible, such as in the case of major and insoluble relational conflict. Hence sex may eventually tear partners apart. For example, prolonged major conflict may lead to a decline in the desire for sex with one's partner (e.g., Birnbaum et al., 2013), which in turn may contribute to reevaluation of his or her suitability. When loss of sexual interest signals incompatibility with the partner's relationship goals, it may motivate the individual to seek resolution of these interpersonal problems, either with the current partner or by looking for a more suitable one (Birnbaum & Reis, 2006).

Concluding Comments and Directions for Future Work

Sex has the potential to motivate intensely meaningful experiences whose nature and quality may vary in individuals, across contexts, and during relationship development. Attachment processes may explain some of the individual differences in sexual experiences. As indicated in this chapter, early attachment experiences seem to shape what people want out of sexual encounters, how they get their needs met, and what role(s) sex plays in their close relationships. Still, little is known about how current attachment experiences intersect with earlier experiences to affect the construal of sex across different stages of relationship development. For example, the effects of a partner's attachment behavior (e.g., provision of responsiveness, safe haven caregiving) on the desire to have sex with the partner may vary across relationship phases. In the initial relationship stages, partners often experience relatively strong and spontaneous sexual urges. At later relationship stages, when couples are more likely to experience habituation, sexual urges may reflect general interpersonal circumstances rather than a spontaneous event (Basson, 2000; Baumeister & Bratslavsky, 1999). In these later stages, a partner's attachment behavior may have the greatest potential to affect sexual response (particularly that of an anxiously attached person), as it is more likely to be influenced by the relational atmosphere (Birnbaum, 2010). Future studies should address this possibility by examining the interactive contribution of early and current attachment experiences to sexual responses over the course of relationship development.

Another promising direction for future research is to identify the mechanisms through which sex promotes emotional bonding. The model presented in this chapter embodies three components that could modify the functional significance of sexuality for relationship quality: person, context, and time. A closer consideration of these components leads to the conclusion that sex is more likely to affect attachment processes when the attachment relationship is more vulnerable, such as in couples with partners who have negative characteristics, during conflicts that endanger a relationship, or in the early stages of emerging relationships. Although the model indicates for whom, under which circumstances, and when sex is more likely to influence the quality of a relationship, it does not include the component that specifies the processes by which such effects occur in each stage of relationship development. For example, positive sexual experiences may be more likely to reduce attachment insecurities during the uncertainty stage of dating than in later relationship stages, when certainty about partners' commitment intentions is relatively high.

The current line of theorizing suggests that just as optimal sexual functioning can foster the development of attachment relationships, so can disruptions in the sexual system's functioning lead to corresponding disruptions of attachment processes. These possibilities raise questions about how and why the sexual system develops either optimally or nonoptimally. Individual differences in the functioning of any behavioral system were theorized to result from a history of positive and negative outcomes of system activation in various contexts across the lifespan (Bowlby, 1969/1982, 1973). Behavioral genetic studies have challenged this view by revealing that, at least in the case of the attachment system, heritable factors may account for some of these individual differences (e.g., Crawford et al., 2007; see also Fraley & Roisman, Chapter 1, this volume). It is possible, of course, that genetic factors interact with early life experiences (e.g., parental attitudes toward sex, early sexual experiences) and current changes in the social context (e.g., partners' responses, social norms of sexuality) to shape the functioning of the sexual system. Future studies should identify the origins of individual differences in the sexual system's functioning, and should clarify the extent to which these differences are heritable and the extent to which they are produced by historical and contemporary contextual factors.

Future work should also more fully explore the dual role of sex: on the one hand, as a potent relationship maintenance mechanism, and on the other hand, as a force motivating people to pursue alternative sexual partners. Several studies have delineated some of the conditions that encourage the pursuit of these seemingly conflicting goals. For example, a recent study has indicated that women who are strongly attached to their partners are more likely to desire sexual intimacy with the partners when they themselves are fertile than when nonfertile, whereas women who are not strongly attached to their long-term partners show the opposite pattern (Eastwick & Finkel, 2012). Another study revealed that men's investment in their spouses is associated with lower testosterone levels (Gray, Kahlenberg, Barrett, Lipson, & Ellison, 2002). These findings suggest that activation of attachment processes can inhibit relationship-threatening tendencies (i.e., extradyadic mating efforts near ovulation, extrapair desires that are enhanced by higher testosterone levels).

Studies that pursue this line of investigation should take into account the new challenges for traditional committed romantic relationships presented by the increase in social acceptability of alternative lifestyles (e.g., swinging, open relationships, polyamory; Conley, Ziegler, Moors, Matsick, & Valentine, 2013) and the rise of Internet technology and social media (e.g., greater availability of alternative partners, engaging in online sexual activities without a partner). Clearly, these changing societal trends may also create new opportunities for sexual expression in existing relationships. For example, sexting and engaging in partnered online sexual activities may connect romantic partners across geographical distance, enabling them to interact more intimately than at any time in the past. Future studies should examine whether the new patterns of sexual communication promote the quality of previously challenged relationships, whether virtual sexual expressions have similar beneficial effects on attachment processes as actual ones, and whether the effects of sex on relationship development vary in different relationship arrangements.

References

Andersen, S. M., & Chen, S. (2002). The relational self: An interpersonal social-cognitive theory. *Psychological Review, 109,* 619–645.

Bartholomew, K., & Horowitz, L. M. (1991). Attachment styles among young adults: A test of a four-category model. *Journal of Personality and Social Psychology, 61,* 226–244.

Bartz, J. A., & Lydon, J. E. (2004). Close relationships and the working self-concept: Implicit and explicit effects of priming attachment on agency and communion. *Personality and Social Psychology Bulletin, 30,* 1389–1401.

Basson, R. (2000). The female sexual response: A different model. *Journal of Sex and Marital Therapy, 26,* 51–65.

Baumeister, R. F., & Bratslavsky, E. (1999). Passion, intimacy, and time: Passionate love as a function of change in intimacy. *Personality and Social Psychology Review, 3,* 49–67.

Beaulieu-Pelletier, G., Philippe, F., Lecours, S., & Couture, S. (2011). The role of attachment avoidance in extradyadic sex. *Attachment and Human Development, 13,* 293–313.

Bell, R. A., Daly, J. A., & Gonzalez, C. (1987). Affinity-maintenance in marriage and its relationship to women's marital satisfaction. *Journal of Marriage and the Family, 49,* 445–454.

Berscheid, E., & Reis, H. T. (1998). Attraction and close relationships. In D. T. Gilbert, S. T. Fiske, & G. Lindzey (Eds.), *The handbook of social psychology* (3rd ed., Vol. 2, pp. 193–281). New York: McGraw-Hill.

Birnbaum, G. E. (2003). The meaning of heterosexual intercourse among women with female orgasmic disorder. *Archives of Sexual Behavior, 32,* 61–71.

Birnbaum, G. E. (2007a). Attachment orientations, sexual functioning, and relationship satisfaction in a community sample of women. *Journal of Social and Personal Relationships, 24,* 21–35.

Birnbaum, G. E. (2007b). Beyond the borders of reality: Attachment orientations and sexual fantasies. *Personal Relationships, 14,* 321–342.

Birnbaum, G. E. (2010). Bound to interact: The divergent goals and complex interplay of attachment and sex within romantic relationships. *Journal of Social and Personal Relationships, 27,* 245–252.

Birnbaum, G. E. (2014). Sexy building blocks: The contribution of the sexual system to attachment formation and maintenance. In M. Mikulincer & P. R. Shaver (Eds.), *Mechanisms of social connection: From brain to group* (pp. 315–332). Washington, DC: American Psychological Association.

Birnbaum, G. E., & Gillath, O. (2006). Measuring subgoals of the sexual behavioral system: What is sex good for? *Journal of Social and Personal Relationships, 23,* 675–701.

Birnbaum, G. E., Hirschberger, G., & Goldenberg, J. L. (2011). Desire in the face of death: Terror management, attachment, and sexual motivation. *Personal Relationships, 18,* 1–19.

Birnbaum, G. E., & Laser-Brandt, D. (2002). Gender differences in the experience of heterosexual intercourse. *Canadian Journal of Human Sexuality, 11,* 143–158.

Birnbaum, G. E., Mikulincer, M., & Austerlitz, M. (2013). A fiery conflict: Attachment orientations and the effects of relational conflict on sexual motivation. *Personal Relationships, 20,* 294–310.

Birnbaum, G. E., Mikulincer, M., & Gillath, O. (2011). In and out of a daydream: Attachment orientations, daily relationship quality, and sexual fantasies. *Personality and Social Psychology Bulletin, 37,* 1398–1410.

Birnbaum, G. E., & Reis, H. T. (2006). Women's sexual working models: An evolutionary-attachment perspective. *Journal of Sex Research, 43,* 328–342.

Birnbaum, G. E., & Reis, H. T. (2012). When does responsiveness pique sexual interest?: Attachment and sexual desire in initial acquaintanceships. *Personality and Social Psychology Bulletin, 38,* 946–958.

Birnbaum, G. E., Reis, H. T., Mikulincer, M., Gillath, O., & Orpaz, A. (2006). When sex is more than just sex: Attachment orientations, sexual experience, and relationship quality. *Journal of Personality and Social Psychology, 91,* 929–943.

Birnbaum, G. E., Simpson, J. A., Weisberg, Y. J., Barnea, E., & Assulin-Simhon, Z. (2012). Is it my overactive imagination?: The effects of contextually activated attachment insecurity on sexual fantasies. *Journal of Social and Personal Relationships, 29,* 1131–1152.

Birnbaum, G. E., Svitelman, N., Bar-Shalom, A., & Porat, O. (2008). The thin line between reality and imagination: Attachment orientations and the effects of relationship threats on sexual fantasies. *Personality and Social Psychology Bulletin, 34,* 1185–1199.

Birnbaum, G. E., Weisberg, Y. J., & Simpson, J. A. (2011). Desire under attack: Attachment orientations and the effects of relationship threat on sexual motivations. *Journal of Social and Personal Relationships, 28,* 448–468.

Bogaert, A. F., & Sadava, S. (2002). Adult attachment and sexual behavior. *Personal Relationships, 9,* 191–204.

Bowlby, J. (1969/1982). *Attachment and loss: Vol. 1. Attachment.* New York: Basic Books.

Bowlby, J. (1973). *Attachment and loss: Vol. 2. Separation: Anxiety and anger.* New York: Basic Books.

Brassard, A., Péloquin, K., Dupuy, E., Wright, J., & Shaver, P. R. (2012). Romantic attachment predicting sexual satisfaction in couples seeking marital therapy. *Journal of Sex and Marital Therapy, 38,* 245–262.

Brassard, A., Shaver, P. R., & Lussier, Y. (2007). Attachment, sexual experience, and sexual pressure in romantic relationships: A dyadic approach. *Personal Relationships, 14,* 475–494.

Brennan, K. A., & Shaver, P. R. (1995). Dimensions of adult attachment, affect regulation, and romantic relationship functioning. *Personality and Social Psychology Bulletin, 21,* 267–283.

Buss, D. M., & Kenrick, D. T. (1998). Evolutionary social psychology. In D. T. Gilbert, S. T. Fiske, & G. Lindzey (Eds.), *The handbook of social psychology* (3rd ed., Vol. 2, pp. 982–1026). New York: McGraw-Hill.

Buss, D. M., & Schmitt, D. P. (1993). Sexual strategies theory: An evolutionary perspective on human mating. *Psychological Review, 100,* 204–232.

Butzer, B., & Campbell, L. (2008). Adult attachment, sexual satisfaction, and relationship satisfaction: A study of married couples. *Personal Relationships, 15*, 141–154.

Byers, E. S., & Heinlein, L. (1989). Predicting initiations and refusals of sexual activities in married and cohabiting heterosexual couples. *Journal of Sex Research, 26*, 210–231.

Campbell, L., & Marshall, T. (2011). Anxious attachment and relationship processes: An interactionist perspective. *Journal of Personality, 79*, 917–947.

Campbell, L., Simpson, J. A., Boldry, J. G., & Kashy, D. (2005). Perceptions of conflict and support in romantic relationships: The role of attachment anxiety. *Journal of Personality and Social Psychology, 88*, 510–531.

Carmichael, M. S., Humbert, R., Dixen, J., Palmisano, G., Greenleaf, W., & Davidson, J. M. (1987). Plasma oxytocin increases in the human sexual response. *Journal of Clinical Endocrinology and Metabolism, 64*, 27–31.

Carroll, J. L., Volk, K. D., & Hyde, J. S. (1985). Differences between males and females in motives for engaging in sexual intercourse. *Archives of Sexual Behavior, 14*, 131–139.

Carter, C. S. (1992). Oxytocin and sexual behavior. *Neuroscience and Biobehavioral Reviews, 16*, 131–144.

Carter, C. S., Ahnert, L., Grossmann, K. E., Hrdy, S. B., Lamb, M. E., Porges, S. W., et al. (Eds.). (2005). *Attachment and bonding: A new synthesis.* Cambridge, MA: MIT Press.

Cohen, D., & Belsky, J. (2008). Avoidant romantic attachment and female orgasm: Testing an emotion-regulation hypothesis. *Attachment and Human Development, 10*, 1–11.

Conley, T. D., Ziegler, A., Moors, A. C., Matsick, J. L., & Valentine, B. (2013). A critical examination of popular assumptions about the benefits and outcomes of monogamous relationships. *Personality and Social Psychology Review, 17*, 124–141.

Cooper, M. L., Pioli, M., Levitt, A., Talley, A., Micheas, L., & Collins, N. L. (2006). Attachment styles, sex motives, and sexual behavior: Evidence for gender-specific expressions of attachment dynamics. In M. Mikulincer & G. S. Goodman (Eds.), *Dynamics of romantic love: Attachment, caregiving, and sex* (pp. 243–274). New York: Guilford Press.

Cooper, M. L., Shapiro, C. M., & Powers, A. M. (1998). Motivations for sex and risky sexual behavior among adolescents and young adults: A functional perspective. *Journal of Personality and Social Psychology, 75*, 1528–1558.

Crawford, T. N., Livesley, W. J., Jang, K. L., Shaver, P. R., Cohen, P., & Ganiban, J. (2007). Insecure attachment and personality disorder: A twin study of adults. *European Journal of Personality, 21*, 191–208.

Cyranowski, J. M., & Andersen, B. L. (1998). Schemas, sexuality, and romantic attachment. *Journal of Personality and Social Psychology, 74*, 1364–1379.

Davis, D., Shaver, P. R., & Vernon, M. L. (2003). Physical, emotional, and behavioral reactions to breaking up. *Personality and Social Psychology Bulletin, 29*, 871–884.

Davis, D., Shaver, P. R., & Vernon, M. L. (2004). Attachment style and subjective motivations for sex. *Personality and Social Psychology Bulletin, 30*, 1076–1090.

Davis, D., Shaver, P. R., Widaman, K. F., Vernon, M. L., Follette, W. C., & Beitz, K. (2006). "I can't get no satisfaction": Insecure attachment, inhibited sexual communication, and sexual dissatisfaction. *Personal Relationships, 13,* 465–483.

DeLamater, J. D. (1987). Gender differences in sexual scenarios. In K. Kelley (Ed.), *Females, males, and sexuality* (pp. 127–140). Albany: State University of New York Press.

DeWall, C., Lambert, N., Slotter, E., Pond, R., Deckman, T., Finkel, E., et al. (2011). So far away from one's partner, yet so close to romantic alternatives: Avoidant attachment, interest in alternatives, and infidelity. *Journal of Personality and Social Psychology, 101,* 1302–1316.

Diamond, L. M. (2003). What does sexual orientation orient?: A biobehavioral model distinguishing romantic love and sexual desire. *Psychological Review, 110,* 173–192.

Eastwick, P. W., & Finkel, E. J. (2012). The evolutionary armistice: Attachment bonds moderate the function of ovulatory cycle adaptations. *Personality and Social Psychology Bulletin, 38,* 174–184.

Ellis, B. J., & Symons, D. (1990). Sexual differences in sexual fantasy: An evolutionary psychological approach. *Journal of Sex Research, 27,* 527–555.

Feeney, J. A., & Noller, P. (2004). Attachment and sexuality in close relationships. In J. H. Harvey, A. Wenzel, & S. Sprecher (Eds.), *The handbook of sexuality in close relationships* (pp. 183–201). Mahwah, NJ: Erlbaum.

Feeney, J. A., Noller, P., & Patty, J. (1993). Adolescents' interactions with the opposite sex: Influence of attachment style and gender. *Journal of Adolescence, 16,* 169–186.

Feeney, J. A., Peterson, C., Gallois, C., & Terry, D. J. (2000). Attachment style as a predictor of sexual attitudes and behavior in late adolescence. *Psychology and Health, 14,* 1105–1122.

Filippi, S., Vignozzi, L., Vannelli, G. B., Ledda, F., Forti, G., & Maggi, M. (2003). Role of oxytocin in the ejaculatory process. *Journal of Endocrinological Investigation, 26,* 82–86.

Fisher, H. E. (1998). Lust, attraction, and attachment in mammalian reproduction. *Human Nature, 9,* 23–52.

Fisher, H. E., Aron, A., Mashek, D., Li, H., & Brown, L. L. (2002). Defining the brain systems of lust, romantic attraction, and attachment. *Archives of Sexual Behavior, 31,* 413–419.

Ford, C. S., & Beach, F. A. (1951). *Patterns of sexual behavior.* New York: Harper & Row.

Gagnon, J. H., & Simon, W. (1973). *Sexual conduct: The social sources of human sexuality.* Chicago: Aldine.

Gangestad, S. W., & Thornhill, R. (1997). The evolutionary psychology of extrapair sex: The role of fluctuating asymmetry. *Evolution and Human Behavior, 18,* 69–88.

Gentzler, A. L., & Kerns, K. A. (2004). Associations between insecure attachment and sexual experiences. *Personal Relationships, 11,* 249–265.

Gillath, O., Mikulincer, M., Birnbaum, G. E., & Shaver, P. R. (2008). When sex primes love: Subliminal sexual priming motivates relational goal pursuit. *Personality and Social Psychology Bulletin, 34,* 1057–1069.

Gray, P. B., Kahlenberg, S. M., Barrett, E. S., Lipson, S. F., & Ellison, P. T. (2002). Marriage and fatherhood are associated with lower testosterone in males. *Evolution and Human Behavior, 23,* 193–201.

Guerrero, L. K. (1998). Attachment-style differences in the experience and expression of romantic jealousy. *Personal Relationships, 5,* 273–291.

Hazan, C., & Zeifman, D. (1994). Sex and the psychological tether. In K. Bartholomew & D. Perlman (Eds.), *Advances in personal relationships: Vol. 5. Attachment processes in adulthood* (pp. 151–177). London: Jessica Kingsley.

Hazan, C., & Zeifman, D. (1999). Pair bonds as attachments: Evaluating the evidence. In J. Cassidy & P. R. Shaver (Eds.), *Handbook of attachment: Theory, research, and clinical applications* (pp. 336–354). New York: Guilford Press.

Hazan, C., Zeifman, D., & Middleton, K. (1994, July). *Adult romantic attachment, affection, and sex.* Paper presented at the 7th International Conference on Personal Relationships, Groningen, The Netherlands.

Holmes, B. M., & Johnson, K. R. (2009). Adult attachment and romantic partner preference: A review. *Journal of Social and Personal Relationships, 26,* 33–52.

Impett, E. A., Gordon, A. M., & Strachman, A. (2008). Attachment and daily sexual goals: A study of dating couples. *Personal Relationships, 15,* 375–390.

Impett, E. A., & Peplau, L. A. (2002). Why some women consent to unwanted sex with a dating partner: Insights from attachment theory. *Psychology of Women Quarterly, 26,* 359–369.

Kalichman, S. C., Sarwer, D. B., Johnson, J. R., Ali, S. A., Early, J., & Tuten, J. T. (1993). Sexually coercive behavior and love styles: A replication and extension. *Journal of Psychology and Human Sexuality, 6,* 93–106.

Kotler, T. (1985). Security and autonomy within marriage. *Human Relations, 38,* 299–321.

Little, K. C., McNulty, J. K., & Russell, V. M. (2010). Sex buffers intimates against the negative implications of attachment insecurity. *Personality and Social Psychology Bulletin, 36,* 484–498.

Litzinger, S., & Gordon, K. C. (2005). Exploring relationships among communication, sexual satisfaction, and marital satisfaction. *Journal of Sex and Marital Therapy, 31,* 409–424.

Main, M. (1990). Cross-cultural studies of attachment organization: Recent studies, changing methodologies, and the concept of conditional strategies. *Human Development, 33,* 48–61.

Mellen, S. L. W. (1981). *The evolution of love.* Oxford, UK: Freeman.

Meston, C. M., & Buss, D. M. (2007). Why humans have sex. *Archives of Sexual Behavior, 36,* 477–507.

Mikulincer, M., Gillath, O., & Shaver, P. R. (2002). Activation of the attachment system in adulthood: Threat-related primes increase the accessibility of mental representations of attachment figures. *Journal of Personality and Social Psychology, 83,* 881–895.

Mikulincer, M., & Shaver, P. R. (2005). Attachment theory and emotions in close relationships: Exploring the attachment-related dynamics of emotional reactions to relational events. *Personal Relationships, 12,* 149–168.

Mikulincer, M., & Shaver, P. R. (2007a). A behavioral systems perspective on the psychodynamics of attachment and sexuality. In D. Diamond, S. J. Blatt, & J. D. Lichtenberg (Eds.), *Attachment and sexuality* (pp. 51–78). New York: Analytic Press.

Mikulincer, M., & Shaver, P. R. (2007b). *Attachment in adulthood: Structure, dynamics, and change.* New York: Guilford Press.

Mikulincer, M., & Shaver, P. R. (2012). Attachment theory expanded: A behavioral systems approach to personality. In K. Deaux & M. Snyder (Eds.), *The Oxford handbook of personality and social psychology* (pp. 467–492). New York: Oxford University Press.

Mizrahi, M., Birnbaum, G. E., Hirschberger, G., Mikulincer, M., & Szepsenwol, O. (2015). *Reassuring sex: Can sex repair attachment insecurities?* Manuscript submitted for publication.

Murphy, M. R., Seckl, J. R., Burton, S., Checkley, S. A., & Lightman, S. L. (1987). Changes in oxytocin and vasopressin secretion during sexual activity in men. *Journal of Clinical Endocrinology and Metabolism, 65,* 738–742.

O'Sullivan, L. F., & Byers, E. S. (1992). College students' incorporation of initiator and restrictor roles in sexual dating interactions. *Journal of Sex Research, 29,* 435–446.

Paul, E. L., McManus, B., & Hayes, A. (2000). "Hookups": Characteristics and correlates of college students' spontaneous and anonymous sexual experiences. *Journal of Sex Research, 37,* 76–88.

Reedy, M. N., Birren, J. E., & Schaie, K. W. (1981). Age and sex differences in satisfying love relationships across the adult lifespan. *Human Development, 24,* 52–66.

Regan, P. C., & Berscheid, E. (1999). *Lust: What we know about human sexual desire.* Thousand Oaks, CA: Sage.

Reis, H. T. (2007). Steps toward the ripening of relationship science. *Personal Relationships, 14,* 1–23.

Rubin, H., & Campbell, L. (2012). Day-to-day changes in intimacy predict heightened relationship passion, sexual occurrence, and sexual satisfaction: A dyadic diary analysis. *Social Psychological and Personality Science, 3,* 224–231.

Russell, V. M., & McNulty, J. K. (2011). Frequent sex protects intimates from the negative implications of neuroticism. *Social Psychological and Personality Science, 2,* 220–227.

Schachner, D. A., & Shaver, P. R. (2002). Attachment style and human mate poaching. *New Review of Social Psychology, 1,* 122–129.

Schachner, D. A., & Shaver, P. R. (2004). Attachment dimensions and motives for sex. *Personal Relationships, 11,* 179–195.

Shaver, P. R., Hazan, C., & Bradshaw, D. (1988). Love as attachment: The integration of three behavioral systems. In R. J. Sternberg & M. Barnes (Eds.), *The psychology of love* (pp. 68–99). New Haven, CT: Yale University Press.

Simpson, J. A., & Rholes, W. S. (1994). Stress and secure base relationships in adulthood. In K. Bartholomew & D. Perlman (Eds.), *Advances in personal relationships: Vol. 5. Attachment processes in adulthood* (pp. 181–204). London: Jessica Kingsley.

Simpson, J. A., Rholes, W. S., & Phillips, D. (1996). Conflict in close relationships: An attachment perspective. *Journal of Personality and Social Psychology, 71,* 899–914.

Stefanou, C., & McCabe, M. P. (2012). Adult attachment and sexual functioning: A review of past research. *Journal of Sexual Medicine, 9*, 2499–2507.

Stephan, C. W., & Bachman, G. F. (1999). What's sex got to do with it?: Attachment, love schemas, and sexuality. *Personal Relationships, 6*, 111–123.

Sternberg, R. J. (1986). A triangular theory of love. *Psychological Review, 93*, 119–135.

Tracy, J. L., Shaver, P. R., Albino, A. W., & Cooper, M. L. (2003). Attachment styles and adolescent sexuality. In P. Florsheim (Ed.), *Adolescent romance and sexual behavior: Theory, research, and practical implications* (pp. 137–159). Mahwah, NJ: Erlbaum.

Wei, M., Mallinckrodt, B., Larson, L. A., & Zakalik, R. A. (2005). Attachment, depressive symptoms, and validation from self versus others. *Journal of Counseling Psychology, 52*, 368–377.

Young, K. A., Gobrogge K. L., Liu, Y., & Wang, Z. X. (2011). The neurobiology of pair bonding: Insights from a socially monogamous rodent. *Frontiers in Neuroendocrinology, 32*, 53–69.

Young, L. J., & Wang, Z. (2004). The neurobiology of pair-bonding. *Nature Neuroscience, 7*, 1048–1054.

8

An Attachment-Theoretical Perspective on Optimal Dependence in Close Relationships

Brooke C. Feeney
Meredith Van Vleet
Brittany K. Jakubiak

All individuals in close relationships encounter issues of dependence—regardless of how conscious–unconscious, deliberate–accidental, or explicit–implicit these occurrences are. Important questions regarding dependence in relationships include these: (1) Is dependence good or bad for partners and relationships? (2) Is there an optimal level of dependence that one should strive for in close relationships, and if so, what influences the attainment of optimal dependence? In this chapter, we address these questions from an attachment-theoretical perspective, and we point to important avenues for future research.

Is Dependence Good or Bad for Individuals and Relationships?

Attachment theory provides a core perspective on dependence on others, because it emphasizes the importance of forming and maintaining close emotional bonds with particular individuals across the lifespan. An important aspect of attachment theory that we have emphasized in recent work (Feeney, 2007) is that dependence on close others is a normative and important part of human development throughout the lifespan, and that true independence and self-sufficiency emerges only *because* of an individual's ability to depend on close relationship partners in times of need. Attachment theory emphasizes the critical importance of relationships across the lifespan—throughout infancy, adolescence, and adulthood—and asserts that a healthy dependence on a reliably sensitive and responsive *attachment figure* is important for optimal functioning and well-being "from the cradle to the grave" (Bowlby, 1988, p. 62; see also Bowlby, 1969/1982, 1973, 1980). According to this perspective, attachment behavior (e.g., reliance on significant others) in certain circumstances should not be discouraged and looked down upon, but instead should be accepted as an intrinsic part of human nature and acknowledged for the important role it plays in promoting optimal human functioning. Bowlby (1969/1982, 1988) emphasized the important function of attachment figures in this regard: An attachment figure promotes healthy functioning by providing a *safe haven* to which a relationship partner can retreat for comfort, support, reassurance, assistance, and protection, and by providing a *secure base* from which a relationship partner can explore the world and strive to meet his or her full potential.

In the most healthy, stable partnerships, this can be viewed as a cyclical process in which individuals move out from their attachment figures to learn, explore, and discover when feeling secure and content, and in which they move toward the attachment figures to derive comfort and security when feeling threatened (Bowlby, 1988; Feeney, 2004; Feeney & Collins, 2004; Marvin, Cooper, Hoffman, & Powell, 2002). Bowlby stated that "this concept of the secure personal base, from which a child, an adolescent, or an adult goes out to explore and to which he returns from time to time, is one [that is] crucial for an understanding of how an emotionally stable person develops and functions *all through his life*" (1988, p. 60; emphasis in original).

Evidence for this process has been shown particularly with regard to parent–child relationships (Ainsworth, 1982; Ainsworth, Blehar, Waters, & Wall, 1978; Bowlby, 1988). Children who are brought up in affectionate homes and have attachment figures who are responsive to their needs (e.g., interpret the children's signals correctly, respond promptly and appropriately, and are cooperative and accepting in dealing with the children) are confident and clear about whom to seek out in times of need. This type of attachment figure is usually able, by his or her presence or ready accessibility, to create the conditions that enable a child to feel secure and to resume exploration in a confident way (Bowlby, 1988). Thus children raised in this type of environment typically make a series of excursions away from their attachment figures, often returning to "check in" and engage in mutually enjoyable contact before making the next excursion. When any type of threat arises (e.g., when the children become frightened, tired, ill, injured, or worried about separation), the children's top priority is to regain the presence of their attachment figures, and until that occurs, the children's explorations and organized excursions cease. In contrast, children who are raised in homes where attachment figures are less sensitive and responsive to their needs (e.g., fail to notice or misinterpret the children's signals, and respond tardily, inappropriately, or not at all; ignore or reject the children; interfere with the children's activities in an arbitrary way) are less confident about receiving care in times of need (Ainsworth et al., 1978; Bowlby, 1988). The conditions created by such unresponsive attachment figures disallow dependence and restrict the children's ability to explore the world in a confident way.

Thus, according to attachment theory, independent exploration behavior is facilitated by relationship partners who allow dependence and provide a secure base from which this behavior can occur. Bowlby (1988) described the concept of a secure base as one in which support providers create the conditions that enable their relationship partners to confidently explore the world. He described it as "a role similar to that of the officer commanding a military base from which an expeditionary force sets out and to which it can retreat, should it meet with a setback. Much of the time the role of the base is a waiting one but it is none the less vital for that. For it is only when the officer commanding the expeditionary force is confident his base is secure that he dare press forward and take risks" (p. 11). The theory states that as an individual grows older, his or her life continues to be organized as a series of excursions away from a close relationship partner. However, the excursions become steadily longer in time and space, and the threshold for activation of attachment behavior is raised because adolescents and adults have more complex representational models of themselves, the environment, and the people who are important to them (Bowlby, 1969/1982, 1973, 1988).

Thus a major proposition of attachment theory relevant to having a healthy dependence on others is that throughout adult life, the availability of a responsive attachment figure is the source of a person's feeling secure, and only when a person feels secure will he or she be able to explore most effectively, confidently, and autonomously. Important propositions of attachment theory related to dependence can be summarized as follows:

First, individuals come into the world predisposed to form strong emotional bonds with particular individuals who care for them (attachment figures). During childhood, bonds are typically with parents, who are looked to for protection, comfort, and support; during adolescence and adulthood, important bonds persist, but are supplemented by new ones (e.g., romantic partners).

Second, these bonds exist and are important because they reduce the risk of individuals' experiencing harm. In times of adversity, individuals seek proximity to known and trusted others, and they derive a sense of protection, safety, and security from doing so.

Third, the way in which an attachment figure responds to the individual's need for close contact in times of adversity has an important influence on the individual's personal functioning. If an individual's attachment figure is known to be accessible, available, and responsive when called upon, the individual should feel secure enough to explore and function autonomously. An attachment figure who is accepting of and responsive to dependence needs also serves a protective function with regard to any number of threats that the individual may encounter. Thus the desire for comfort and support during adversity should not be regarded as unhealthy or childish, unlike what may be implied by the word *dependence* (Bowlby, 1988).

Hence an important prediction of attachment theory regarding dependence is that an attachment figure's acceptance of an individual's dependence needs creates *less* rather than more dependence. Because dependence on close relationship partners, particularly in times of need, is an intrinsic part of human nature, relationship partners who are sensitive and responsive to this behavior actually promote independence and self-sufficiency rather than inhibit it. According to the theory, individuals who are unaccepting of dependence typically foster an unhealthy and anxious dependence in their relationship partners.

Research in the developmental literature has supported this prediction. For example, by the end of the first year, mothers who attend promptly to their crying babies have babies who cry much less than the babies of mothers who let them cry (Ainsworth et al., 1978; Belsky, Rovine, & Taylor, 1984; Bowlby, 1988). Thus mothers' sensitivity to distress cues in their children foster less fussiness or neediness in their children. Moreover, researchers examining autonomy and attachment in adolescence have found that adolescent autonomy is most easily established not at the expense of attachment relationships with parents, but against a backdrop of secure relationships with them (Allen & Land, 1999; Moore, 1987; Noom, Dekovic, & Meeus, 1999).

The postulate that an individual's responsiveness to his or her partner's dependence needs facilitates that partner's independent functioning has been supported in adult relationships as well (Feeney, 2007). Two samples of couples involved in established romantic relationships were used to test the idea that a close relationship partner's acceptance of dependence when needed (e.g., sensitive responsiveness to distress cues) is associated with less dependence, more autonomous functioning, and more self-sufficiency on the part of the supported individual. In Study 1, measures of acceptance of dependence needs and independent functioning were obtained through couple members' reports of general behaviors, through observing couple members' behaviors during a laboratory interaction, and through observing responses to experimentally manipulated partner assistance provided during a laboratory task. The results supported the predicted links between acceptance of dependence and independent functioning. First, one partner's reports of his or her acceptance of dependence were associated with reports of the other's independent functioning (as operationalized by the other's perceived independence and self-efficacy, engagement in independent exploration, and perceived ability to achieve independent goals). Second, the link between acceptance of dependence and independent functioning was observable in couple members' discussions of personal goals for the future. Third, one partner's acceptance of dependence (as reported and observed) predicted the other partner's autonomous functioning and self-sufficiency during a subsequent challenging task.

Study 2 replicated these results and extended them by providing a more rigorous, longitudinal test of the hypothesis that acceptance of a partner's dependence needs at one point in time predicts *changes* in that person's independent functioning 6 months later. The results of this study indicated that (1) partners' acceptance of dependence (as reported by both couple members and as observed) at Time 1 predicted *increases* in the recipients' independent functioning 6 months later at Time 2 (after controls for recipients' independent functioning at Time 1); and (2) partners' acceptance of dependence at Time 1 predicted the accomplishment of the specific goal 6 months later. In addition, the results did not support the reverse hypothesis that recipients' independent functioning at Time 1 would predict increases in the partners' acceptance of dependence at Time 2.

Attachment theory postulates that the hypothesized link between dependence acceptance and independent functioning should normatively apply to all individuals. Thus, all individuals should benefit from relationship partners who show acceptance of their dependence needs by being sensitive and responsive to distress cues, because this is precisely the type of behavior that fosters attachment security. Although individual-difference variables are likely to influence partners' acceptance of dependence needs and recipients' expectations of having their needs met (e.g., Feeney & Collins, 2001; Simpson, Rholes, & Nelligan, 1992), even insecure individuals, who report a low need for achievement and a high fear of failure (Elliot & Reis, 2003), are likely to fear failure less and function more autonomously with the support of relationship partners who provide a secure base by being appropriately accepting of (and sensitive/responsive to) their dependence needs.

Taken together, this research on dependence from an attachment theory perspective has a number of important implications. First, although it is paradoxical that the acceptance of dependence needs may promote autonomous functioning, this idea is consistent with other theorizing regarding the power of *positive dependence* in relationships (also referred to as *mature dependence* and *healthy dependence*), which incorporates the human need for connection with others as a component of healthy functioning (Bornstein, 2005; Bornstein & Languirand, 2003; Solomon, 1994). Consistent with attachment-theoretical propositions, these other theories also refute the widely held societal belief that dependence on others in adulthood is childish and unhealthy (see Bornstein & Languirand, 2003; Sutton, 2001; and Fine & Glendinning, 2005, for societal messages that argue against dependence as a fundamental component of the human condition; see Rasmussen, 2005, for views on the *dependent prototype*). Although too much dependence in relationships can be unhealthy, the research thus far suggests that too little dependence in relationships may be equally unhealthy and disadvantageous. It also suggests that one way to assist a relationship partner in reaching his or her full potential is to demonstrate availability and accessibility when the individual feels threatened or needs comfort and support.

A second implication of this work involves the emphasis on normative aspects of attachment theory. The existing research supports attachment theory's assertion that attachment dynamics are important and influential throughout life for *all* individuals. Since Bowlby's initial theoretical contribution, very little empirical work or theoretical elaboration has been advanced regarding the normative interworkings of the attachment, exploration, and caregiving systems in adulthood, because most research has focused on identifying individual differences in personal and relationship functioning. As emphasized by Simpson and Rholes (2010), a stronger focus on normative aspects of attachment theory (e.g., optimal dependence in relationships) will be important in future research on adult attachment.

Third, attachment theory's perspective on dependence also speaks to the importance of incorporating the function of intimate relationships into existing theories of human agency, such as self-determination theory (Ryan & Deci, 2000a, 2004), resource control theory (Hawley, 1999), and action control theory (Little, 1998; Little, Hawley, Heinrich, & Marsland, 2002). Self-determination theory highlights the importance of social-contextual conditions that facilitate or undermine self-motivational processes, and, consistent with attachment theory, it discusses both autonomy and relatedness as innate psychological needs (Deci & Ryan, 2000; Ryan & Deci, 2000a, 2000b). A detailed account of the function of intimate relationships in fostering intrinsic motivation and human agency is important for elaborating and extending attachment theory (see also Feeney & Collins, 2014).

Also important for future work will be to establish *why* depending on others is so helpful by identifying the mechanisms underlying this process. Why are individuals with close relationship partners who accept their dependence needs more self-efficacious and less needy than those with relationship partners who are less accepting of their dependence needs? Wouldn't complete self-reliance lead to the best outcomes for everyone, because it gives one more control over one's own experiences and requires nothing from others? Why should accepting dependence foster independence instead of dependence? And why shouldn't discouraging dependence foster the most successful independent functioning? It will be important to establish that individuals function best when they have attachment figures who accept dependence needs *because* such acceptance (and felt security) gives them the confidence and courage needed to make independent excursions away from their home base in order to grow and accomplish important goals. It is much easier for people to take risks, accept challenges, and try new things when they know that someone is available to comfort and assist them if things go wrong. An individual who feels confident in the availability and accessibility of his or her secure base does not have to cling to that base to the same extent as someone who lacks such confidence. Bowlby stated that "to remain within easy access of a familiar individual known to be willing and able to come to our aid in an emergency is clearly a good insurance policy— whatever our age" (1988, p. 27). Individuals who lack such an insurance policy should be less likely to take risks and forge new territory than those who are assured of their significant others' availability and accessibility. We have likened this process to driving a car without an insurance policy (Feeney, 2007): Just as an individual without a car insurance policy may be reluctant to drive long distances or take unnecessary risks because there will be a heavy price to pay if something goes wrong, so too might an individual be reluctant to take many (or any) independent excursions away from a relationship partner who does not provide good "coverage" in the case of an emergency. In this sense, the ready availability and accessibility of a relationship partner is necessary for a person to be an optimally functioning individual.

But how much dependence is ideal? Is there a critical level or range of dependence that one must maintain for optimal functioning? And if so, how does one attain this optimal level of dependence? We address these issues next and point to the need for research focused on identifying optimal levels of dependence in close relationships.

Is There an Optimal Level of Dependence? If So, What Influences Its Attainment?

After establishing that acceptance of dependence by close relationship partners (and being dependent on such partners) is part of the process of becoming an optimally functioning individual, we need to ask: *How much* dependence is healthy? This is an area that is lacking in empirical work; however, this question can be addressed by extending attachment-theoretical postulates and considering research on individual differences in caregiving experiences that predict individual and relationship outcomes.

Research and theory regarding the dependency paradox (that accepting dependence promotes independence instead of more dependence; see Feeney, 2007) view dependence as adaptive when it occurs because there is a need for it. We view dependence that occurs in the absence of need as *overdependence*, and a complete lack of dependence on others (even in times of need) as *underdependence*, which has also been referred to as *compulsive self-reliance* or *defensive self-reliance* (Feeney & Collins, 2014). Theoretically, both overdependence and underdependence result from having attachment figures (or close relationship partners) who are not accepting of dependence or who do not consistently provide sensitive/responsive support when needed.

A recent theoretical paper (Feeney & Collins, 2014) describes unresponsive and insensitive support behaviors as undermining thriving because they promote either overdependence or underdependence. Overdependence (an overreliance on a significant other to do what can be done by oneself) represents a means of clinging to a person whose availability and acceptance are perceived to be uncertain (e.g., inconsistently responsive support providers) or who provides support when it is not needed (e.g., compulsively overinvolved support providers). Underdependence (defensive self-reliance and lack of dependence on others) represents a means of coping with a support environment or relationship history in which significant others have been consistently unresponsive, insensitive to, or unaccepting of dependence needs (e.g., neglectful/disengaged or negative/demeaning support providers). Optimal dependence (a normative and healthy dependence on others that occurs in response to genuine need), optimal independence (a healthy autonomy to pursue opportunities for growth), and optimal interdependence (a relationship in which each member is mutually dependent on the other) is made possible when relationship partners provide sensitive and responsive support for both attachment needs and autonomous exploration (see Feeney & Collins, 2014).

Overdependence, underdependence, and optimal dependence may be based in one's relationship history and carried forward into new relationships where the strategy is no longer adaptive, or they may arise from new experiences in one's current relationship. We now discuss various types of support experiences that are likely to underlie each type of dependence. In doing so, we emphasize the need, with regard to attaining optimal levels of dependence in relationships, for partners to balance sensitive/responsive support for attachment needs (safehaven support) and sensitive/responsive support for autonomous exploration (secure base support). These support experiences are presumed to have the greatest impact when enacted by attachment figures with whom one has a strong emotional bond.

Behavior That Underlies Optimal Dependence: Sensitive and Responsive Support

From an attachment-theoretical perspective, support provision that promotes optimal dependence involves the sensitive and responsive provision of support for both attachment needs (a safe haven) and autonomous exploration behavior (a secure base). A balance of these two support functions is needed to promote healthy levels of dependence, which should underlie healthy and optimal human functioning. Figure 8.1 depicts a model of outcomes related to the receipt of responsive safe haven and secure base support (elaborated below) that should underlie optimal levels of dependence.

Responsive Safe Haven

Attachment theory stipulates that all individuals come into the world equipped with an attachment behavioral system, which is prone to activation when an individual is distressed. The goal of this system is to maintain a feeling of security, and one way individuals attain this sense of security is via attachment behaviors that bring close relationship partners into proximity and elicit support (Bowlby, 1969/1982, 1973, 1980, 1988). In support of this postulate, observational and daily diary studies have shown that support-seeking behavior increases in response to stressful or threatening events (Collins & Feeney, 2000, 2005; Collins, Kane, Guichard, & Ford, 2008). A support provider's response to this attachment behavior should determine the nature of a recipient's dependence on the relationship. Ideally, attachment behavior should motivate the support provider to provide sensitive and responsive safe haven support. This is consistent with attachment theory's notion of a caregiving system that, like the attachment system, functions to maintain felt security, but that becomes activated when a significant other is distressed and functions to maintain the security of a close relationship partner (Bowlby, 1969/1982, 1988). Thus, in a close, well-functioning partnership, support-seeking (attachment) and support-giving (caregiving) behaviors have the same goal, which is to restore the felt security of the distressed individual. In its optimal form, sensitive and responsive safe haven support provision should include a broad array of behaviors aimed at comforting and problem resolution that are flexibly enacted to meet the specific needs of the support receiver (Bowlby, 1988; Kunce & Shaver, 1994).

Safe haven behaviors that are sensitive and responsive to the support receiver's needs should be perceived as supportive by the recipient and should result in both immediate and long-term outcomes that promote optimal levels of dependence in relationships (Figure 8.1). Prior research has shown that supportive acts are most likely to be perceived as supportive when they are viewed as voluntary behaviors intended solely to benefit the person in need of support (Cutrona, Cohen, & Igram, 1990; Dunkel-Schetter, Folkman, & Lazarus, 1987; Fincham & Bradbury, 1990; Pierce, Baldwin, & Lydon, 1997); when they match the needs of the recipient (Cohen & Wills, 1985; Cutrona, 1990; Cutrona & Russell, 1990; Simpson, Winterheld, Rholes, & Oriña, 2007); and when they are delivered sensitively (e.g., the support provided protects the recipient's self-esteem and makes him or

Safe Haven Processes: Response in Times of Adversity

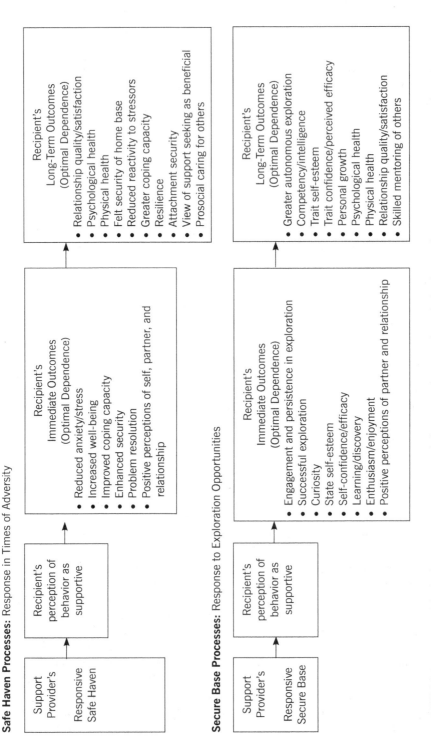

Support Provider's

Responsive Safe Haven

Recipient's perception of behavior as supportive

Recipient's
Immediate Outcomes
(Optimal Dependence)

- Reduced anxiety/stress
- Increased well-being
- Improved coping capacity
- Enhanced security
- Problem resolution
- Positive perceptions of self, partner, and relationship

Recipient's
Long-Term Outcomes
(Optimal Dependence)

- Relationship quality/satisfaction
- Psychological health
- Physical health
- Felt security of home base
- Reduced reactivity to stressors
- Greater coping capacity
- Resilience
- Attachment security
- View of support seeking as beneficial
- Prosocial caring for others

Secure Base Processes: Response to Exploration Opportunities

Support Provider's

Responsive Secure Base

Recipient's perception of behavior as supportive

Recipient's
Immediate Outcomes
(Optimal Dependence)

- Engagement and persistence in exploration
- Successful exploration
- Curiosity
- State self-esteem
- Self-confidence/efficacy
- Learning/discovery
- Enthusiasm/enjoyment
- Positive perceptions of partner and relationship

Recipient's
Long-Term Outcomes
(Optimal Dependence)

- Greater autonomous exploration
- Competency/intelligence
- Trait self-esteem
- Trait confidence/perceived efficacy
- Personal growth
- Psychological health
- Physical health
- Relationship quality/satisfaction
- Skilled mentoring of others

FIGURE 8.1. Proposed links between responsive safe haven and secure base behavior and recipient perceptions and outcomes.

her feel valued, understood, and accepted; Reis & Shaver, 1988) (see also Feeney & Collins, 2014).

Immediate consequences of receiving responsive safe haven support that have implications for a healthy dependence on others include reduced feelings of anxiety or distress; increases in the recipient's well-being (e.g., increases in positive mood, decreases in negative mood, or freeing of cognitive and emotional resources expended on ruminating about a problem); improved coping capacity; enhanced feelings of safety or security; and better problem resolution. Additional consequences of receiving responsive safe haven support include positive perceptions of one's partner and relationship (e.g., perceptions that the partner is available, and that seeking support and showing vulnerability is beneficial and will be met with compassion). Responsive safe haven support should also increase feelings of emotional closeness, trust, and satisfaction with the relationship because it provides diagnostic information about a partner's love and concern for one's welfare (Collins & Feeney, 2004), and it should also lead recipients to have positive perceptions of themselves as a result of feeling cared for (Reis & Shaver, 1988). These immediate outcomes reflect a healthy dependence on a partner, because they signify the recipient's and the relationship's positive well-being.

These outcomes are supported by studies showing that caring support from a partner in times of stress has immediate positive effects on emotional well-being and relationship functioning (e.g., Collins & Feeney, 2000, 2005; Cutrona, 1986; Jaremka, Kane, Guichard, Ford, & Collins, 2010; Kane, McCall, Collins, & Blascovich, 2012; Simpson et al., 1992; Winstead & Derlega, 1985). These studies indicate a strong link between receipt of responsive safe haven support and immediate improvements in mood, relationship satisfaction, feelings of being loved and valued, and feelings of security. Additional evidence comes from studies showing that cardiovascular reactivity is buffered in individuals who experience a stressor in the presence of a close, nonevaluative support provider, relative to individuals who experience the stressor alone, with a stranger, or with an evaluative other (e.g., Allen, Blascovich, Tomaka, & Kelsey, 1991; Edens, Larkin, & Abel, 1992; Fontana, Diegnan, Villeneuve, & Lepore, 1999; Kamarck, Manuck, & Jennings, 1990; Snydersmith & Cacioppo, 1992). Likewise, other studies show that soothing touch or close physical contact with a close partner during a stressful task decreases heart rate and blood pressure (e.g., Ditzen et al., 2007; Fishman, Turkheimer, & DeGood, 1995; Grewen, Anderson, Girdler, & Light, 2003; Lynch, Thomas, Paskewitz, Katcher, & Weir, 1977; Whitcher & Fisher, 1979), and attenuates neural activation in brain regions associated with emotional and behavioral responses to threat (Coan, Schaefer, & Davidson, 2006).

These immediate outcomes of receiving responsive safe haven support should, over many interactions, contribute to long-term tendencies toward optimal dependence on others. For example, if an individual experiences improved mood, exhibits reduced autonomic reactivity to stress, and feels supported (i.e., feels more secure) after interacting with a close partner when distressed, these positive support experiences should, over time, lead to long-term outcomes that result in a healthier dependence on the relationship partner; these include improved relationship quality/satisfaction, enhanced prospects for good health, perceptions of an effective social support network, and confidence in the security/availability of one's home base. Over time, a recipient of consistently responsive support provision should also experience reduced reactivity to stressors, higher thresholds for perceiving life events as stressful (and for needing to turn to the partner for support), greater capacity to cope with stressors, stronger feelings of security, greater resilience, and perceptions of the benefits of seeking support from others—all of which reflect, and should contribute to, the continuance of healthy dependence on others. Responsive support should contribute to healthy dependence by preventing physical and emotional withdrawal or isolation that can erode relationships; by providing a positive emotional tone in the relationship; and by engendering a sense of closeness, trust, appreciation, and goodwill that strengthens the commitment between partners, which may help a couple survive future conflicts (Cutrona, 1996; Feeney & Lemay, 2012; Kane et al., 2007). This is consistent with studies showing that the extent to which individuals are satisfied and well adjusted in their relationships depends in part on whether their partners are responsive caregivers who provide a safe haven of comfort and security (Buhrmester, Furman, Wittenberg, & Reis, 1988; Carnelley, Pietromonaco, & Jaffe, 1996; Collins & Feeney, 2000; J. A. Feeney, 1996; Feeney & Collins, 2001; Jaremka et al., 2010; Katz, Beach, & Anderson, 1996; Kotler, 1985).

Responsive support provision also should contribute to healthy dependence (and interdependence) by increasing the recipient's capacity to provide similar care to others, because (1) having his or her own needs met frees up the recipient's cognitive and emotional resources to focus on others; and (2) a responsive partner, by modeling effective support behaviors, shows the recipient how to care for others in turn. This mutual giving and receiving of support is an important indicator of healthy dependence on others that is not one-sided.

Responsive Secure Base

According to attachment theory, the urge to explore (e.g., to identify and achieve personal goals, take on new challenges, learn new skills, develop new competencies, or make new discoveries) is a basic aspect of human nature (Bowlby, 1988). Thus relationships that support this urge by providing a secure base for exploration should play a large role in promoting optimal levels of relational dependence. In previous work (Feeney & Thrush, 2010), we have shown that relationship partners function as responsive secure bases for one another by encouraging exploration, by not interfering with or intruding in one another's explorations, and by being available if needed during exploration. We showed that the three components of secure base support were significant predictors of exploration behavior. Specifically, spouse availability was associated with greater persistence at exploration, whereas spouse interference predicted less persistence, poorer performance, and less enthusiasm during exploration, and spouse encouragement predicted better performance and greater expressed enthusiasm during exploration. These results indicate that availability and encouragement facilitate exploration, whereas interference inhibits exploration. In addition, a study examining links between secure base behavior and exploration behavior in the context of discussions each couple had about one partner's personal goals showed that support providers who were coded by observers as being more supportive of and comfortable with their partners' goals had partners who discussed their goals more openly, more confidently explored avenues for achieving their goals, and were more receptive to support attempts (Feeney, 2004).

Secure base behaviors that sensitively encourage the support receiver in his or her exploratory behavior, in the attainment of goals, or in the pursuit of personally rewarding challenges, as well as behaviors that convey availability if needed and that are appropriately contingent on the needs of the recipient, should be perceived as supportive by the recipient (Feeney, 2004; Feeney & Thrush, 2010). Such behaviors should result in immediate and long-term outcomes that facilitate optimal levels of dependence in relationships (i.e., appropriately seeking support when needed, but balanced with healthy autonomy) (Figure 8.1). Because safe haven support and secure base support serve different functions, secure base support should have important immediate consequences promoting optimal dependence that are distinct from those afforded by safe haven support. For example, a secure base gives individuals the confidence and courage to explore the environment, accept challenges, and take risks (Bowlby, 1969/1982, 1988). Thus, recipients who receive responsive secure base support should be more fully engaged in exploration, experience greater curiosity, persist longer at exploration, and therefore be more productive and successful at exploration. In other words, they are likely to demonstrate healthy independence and healthy pursuit of autonomous activities. In support of these hypotheses, we found that spouse availability and encouragement predicted recipients' greater persistence and better performance on an autonomous and challenging exploration activity (Feeney & Thrush, 2010).

In addition, the greater engagement in and success at exploration should lead a recipient to experience higher state self-esteem and greater perceived competency, self-efficacy, and self-confidence immediately following an exploration activity for which a partner has provided respon-sive secure base support. These increases in self-esteem and perceived effi-cacy have implications for the recipient's ability to establish healthy levels of dependence, independence, and interdependence. Relatedly, explorations for recipients who have responsive partners should result in greater learn-ing and discovery, greater willingness to explore in the future, and greater enjoyment of exploration. This enjoyment and pursuit of exploration activi-ties are important in enabling an individual to attain a healthy balance of autonomy and relatedness. Consistent with these ideas, recipients of respon-sive secure base support report increases in state self-esteem after engaging in exploration activities (Feeney, 2004; Feeney & Thrush, 2010), as well as greater self-efficacy, self-confidence, and perceived ability to achieve their goals (Feeney, 2004, 2007). Other evidence indicates that responsive secure base support provision is linked with greater expressed enthusiasm during exploration activities and increases in positive mood after engaging in them (Feeney, 2004; Feeney & Thrush, 2010); with perceptions that explora-tion is more enjoyable and that one is smart and competent to engage in it (Feeney & Thrush, 2010); and with a greater willingness to engage in autonomous exploration (Feeney, 2007).

Another immediate outcome of receiving secure base support that has implications for healthy dependence on others involves positive percep-tions of the partner and the relationship. Recipients of secure base support are more likely to perceive that sharing their exploration experiences with their partners (i.e., capitalizing on the experience; see Gable, Gonzaga, & Strachman, 2006; Gable, Reis, Impett, & Asher, 2004) and seeking support for exploration are beneficial. Similar to immediate relationship outcomes experienced in the safe haven context, recipients of responsive secure base support are more likely to feel valued and accepted by their partners and to be satisfied with their relationships. These relational outcomes reflect an optimal dependence in which recipients are able to use their partners as a base for autonomous exploration (establishing competence and autonomy) while remaining connected to the partners.

Over many interactions, these immediate outcomes of receiving secure base support should predict indicators of healthy dependence across time. Recipients of consistently responsive secure base support should show increases in engagement in exploration, persistence in exploration, and suc-cess at exploration activities over time. Recipients should also experience greater independence during exploration because of their increased con-fidence in the security of their home base (Feeney, 2007), which may be reflected in their being more intrinsically motivated to engage in explora-tion activities (Deci & Ryan, 2000; La Guardia et al., 2000; Ryan & Deci, 2000) and feeling greater enthusiasm about engaging in them. This greater engagement in exploration should result in more learning and discovery and in the development of new competencies. Thus, recipients should experience increases in *trait* self-esteem, perceived competency/intelligence, perceived self-efficacy, and self-confidence over time—all long-term improvements in the self reflecting personal growth. This is consistent with research showing that newlyweds who receive responsive secure base support during the first year of marriage are more engaged in exploration and experience more personal growth 1 year later (Feeney & Van Vleet, 2010; Van Vleet & Feeney, 2012), and with research showing that reports of the amount of goal support received from romantic partners predict the enactment of both relationship and individual goals over time (Brunstein, Dangelmayer, & Schultheiss, 1996). This trajectory of personal growth is indicative of healthy dependence, independence, and interdependence.

Consistently responsive secure base support provision should also have beneficial effects on psychological and physical health, albeit through different mechanisms than those that explain the effects of safe haven support on health. Individuals who receive consistently responsive secure base support should actively engage in the type of exploration that makes them feel happier, more fulfilled, and more self-actualized, which in turn ought to have a beneficial impact on indicators of health. Increased exploration may lead to the development of new competencies, which may promote self-esteem, happiness, and psychological health, which may in turn have positive implications for physical health. Active engagement in exploration should contribute to physical health via increases in physical activity and mental stimulation (Blair, Cheng, & Holder, 2001; Warburton, Nicol, & Bredin, 2006). It is also likely to increase positive affect, which is linked to psychological and physical health (Cohen & Pressman, 2006; Pressman & Cohen, 2005). Moreover, it should increase an individual's social network over time, which may provide additional resources that are health-protective (e.g., Cohen, Doyle, Turner, Alper, & Skoner, 2003; Cohen & Wills, 1985). This increase in social network size (and enhanced mental and physical health) should contribute to optimal levels of dependence in relationships because it ensures that an individual does not overburden one particular source of support.

These ideas are also consistent with studies indicating that the successful pursuit of personally meaningful goals is related to indicators of well-being such as elated versus depressed mood and satisfaction with life (Brunstein, 1993; Brunstein, Schultheiss, & Grassman, 1998; Emmons, 1986; Emmons & King, 1988; Omodei & Wearing, 1990; Palys & Little, 1983; Ruehlman & Wolchik, 1988; Yetim, 1993; Zaleski, 1987). As a whole, these studies indicate that individuals high in well-being pursue goals that are important, fulfilling, challenging, fueled by optimistic expectations, and assisted by others. We propose that the interpersonal dynamics surrounding the *assistance by others* play a vital role in determining optimal levels of dependence in the pursuit of exploration opportunities.

The giving and receipt of responsive secure base support should also strengthen relationships over time by increasing relationship satisfaction, intimacy, and trust (and by reducing experiences of conflict) for both partners, which should also enable healthier levels of dependence in their relationship. This is supported by studies showing that social support for personal goals by intimate partners accounts for how satisfied people feel with their relationships (Brunstein et al., 1996; Kaplan & Maddux, 2002); by research showing that people draw closer to significant others who are instrumental in the accomplishment of their goals (Fitzsimons & Fishbach, 2010; Fitzsimons & Shah, 2008); and by research showing that responsive secure base support during the first year of marriage predicts increases in relationship quality 1 year later (Van Vleet & Feeney, 2012). These studies suggest that personal goal attainment and relationship outcomes are linked in important ways (Gore & Cross, 2006), and it highlights the importance of a healthy balance of autonomy and relatedness. Finally, individuals who feel fulfilled and successful in their own goal pursuits, and who have had responsive secure base support provision modeled for them, should become especially skilled mentors of others.

Unresponsive Safe Haven and Secure Base Behavior

Thus far, we have described outcomes reflecting a healthy dependence on others for recipients of *responsive* safe haven and secure base support. However, there are many ways in which interpersonal processes surrounding the provision of a safe haven and secure base may go awry, resulting in suboptimal levels of dependence. Although the support recipient certainly plays a role and may be unwilling to turn to a partner for support or may be unwilling to engage in exploration activities, we propose that an unhealthy balance of autonomy and relatedness is likely to result from relational histories or experiences in which an individual has not received responsive support from attachment figures for both attachment *and* exploration needs. We now consider links between various forms of unresponsive support provider behavior (in both safe haven and secure base contexts) and support recipient outcomes that indicate suboptimal levels of dependence on others. It is important to consider distinct patterns of unresponsiveness, because each pattern should lead to distinct patterns of suboptimal dependence. We discuss three patterns of unresponsiveness that present unique challenges to the establishment of optimal levels of dependence in relationships: compulsively overinvolved, negative/demeaning, and neglectful/disengaged behavior.

Compulsively Overinvolved Behavior

Compulsively overinvolved support provider behavior in safe haven and/or secure base support contexts should undermine optimal dependence by creating overdependence in the recipient. We next describe processes involving compulsively overinvolved caregiving that should have implications for unhealthy dependence on others, depicted in Figure 8.2.

Compulsively Overinvolved Support in Safe Haven Contexts

Compulsively overinvolved support provider behavior may occur either in response to a partner's support seeking (e.g., expressions of distress) or spontaneously in response to the presence of a partner's life stressor. Such behavior can include (1) giving support that is not needed (i.e., providing support regardless of the need or desire for it); (2) being responsive to actual needs while also responding to perceived needs that do not exist; (3) sacrificing oneself or one's own needs for the partner by offering or providing services that could be detrimental to the self; and (4) providing indulgent, coddling, or pampering forms of support that encourage or maintain dependence.

Recipients of this behavior should have ambivalent perceptions of it. That is, they are likely to perceive it as both supportive (in the sense that their partners are trying to provide support) and unsupportive (in the sense that the support is excessive and out of synchrony with the recipients' actual needs). These behaviors and perceptions should result in immediate outcomes indicative of a lack of healthy dependence on others. Although recipients are likely to experience an attenuation of their stressor-related anxiety/distress, feel confident that their home base is secure (i.e., experience felt security), and feel validated and cared for (but perhaps not understood), they are likely to have negative views of their own abilities to cope with and resolve problems. They may also feel smothered (if they perceive that their partners have provided too much unneeded support), guilty (if they perceive they are taking advantage of their partners, the partners are self-sacrificing, or they are not feeling grateful for the unneeded assistance), and indebted (if they perceive they should but cannot reciprocate what their partners have done for them). These concerns may lead recipients to have ambivalent perceptions of their partners and relationships. Recipients may experience feelings of intimacy and trust in their relationships, yet they may be ambivalent about their satisfaction with the relationships. These are mixed outcomes that are indicative of suboptimal states of both well-being and dependence.

Over time, recipients of compulsively overinvolved support provision may experience some of the benefits of responsive safe haven support, such as perceiving that the home base is secure or feeling that it is beneficial to seek support from others. However, overindulgent support provision is likely to produce some negative outcomes over time, including greater clinging to and dependence on partners, poor coping with stressors, poor regulation of the recipients' own emotions, and intense distress if the partners are even temporarily inaccessible. Because of their overreliance on

Safe Haven Processes: Response in Times of Adversity

Secure Base Processes: Response to Exploration Opportunities

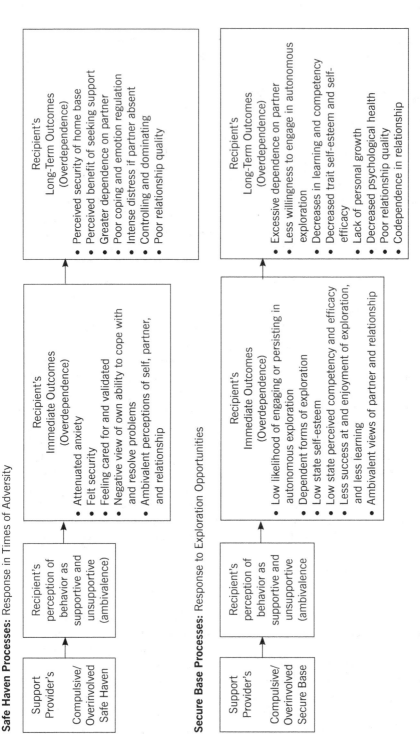

FIGURE 8.2. Proposed links between compulsively overinvolved support provider behavior and recipient perceptions and outcomes.

their partners, recipients may become increasingly controlling and dominating in their relationships, and they may insist that their partners stay
nearby and not pursue their own goals. This may result in poor relationship
quality in which partners have unequal status (e.g., one person does all the
giving), and it may take a toll on the health and well-being of the support
provider. See Figure 8.2 for a summary of proposed outcomes.

These long-term consequences are also theorized to influence recipients' responses to future life stressors and future exploration opportunities. For example, perceptions of the benefit of seeking support from others, combined with poor coping and emotion regulation and a controlling/
dominating interpersonal style, may lead recipients to seek support for life
stressors and exploration opportunities in an overly entitled manner. Individuals who have developed overdependence resulting from a history of
compulsively overinvolved caregiving may expect others to resolve their
stressors for them (even those they can handle themselves), and they may
expect others to do much of their exploration or goal pursuit either for
them or with them.

Compulsively Overinvolved Support in Secure Base Contexts

In secure base contexts, compulsively overinvolved support provider behavior may occur either in response to a partner's support-seeking/exploration
behavior or spontaneously in response to the presence of a partner's exploration opportunity. This type of support provider behavior can include (1)
being available for assistance during exploration (during which availability
may be imposed on the recipient); (2) frequent interference in the partner's
exploration (e.g., taking over the activity, inserting oneself in the partner's
exploration activities, providing assistance that is not needed or requested);
and (3) discouragement of autonomous exploration. The discouragement
of autonomous exploration displayed by a compulsive caregiver is likely to
be exhibited in a concerned manner. For example, discouragement may be
shown by being overprotective, by invoking fear in the partner regarding
potential dangers and hazards of exploration, by wanting to be involved in
all of the partner's activities, and/or by clinging to the partner and communicating one's own need to have the partner stay close to the home base.

A recipient of these behaviors should also have ambivalent perceptions
of the behaviors as being both supportive (in the sense that the partner conveys caring and concern, has supportive intent, and may have assisted him
or her) and unsupportive (in the sense that the support behavior is out of
synchrony with the recipient's needs, interferes with exploration attempts,
or is not helpful in promoting healthy autonomy). These compulsive behaviors and ensuing perceptions should result in immediate outcomes indicative of a lack of healthy dependence. First, recipients should be unlikely to
engage and persist in autonomous exploration. When they do explore, it is

likely to be a dependent form of exploration that involves stronger desires for assistance from and involvement of their partners. Second, because they engage in dependent forms of exploration (or no exploration at all), recipients are likely to experience lower levels of state self-esteem, perceived self-efficacy, perceived competency, and confidence in their own abilities. Third, recipients ought to experience less success at exploration, because their exploration is disrupted and they do not feel capable of successful autonomous exploration (and therefore put less effort into it). As a result, they are less likely to learn and discover during their explorations. Fourth, because of their partners' interference in and discouragement of autonomous exploration, recipients should report less enjoyment of it, greater guilt when they do engage in it, and less willingness to explore autonomously in the future. However, recipients may view dependent or joint exploration as less threatening, more enjoyable, or as an opportunity to obtain intimacy with their partners. Fifth, although recipients may perceive their home base as secure, their views of their partners may depend on the degree to which they feel assisted versus stifled by the partners.

To test some of these predictions, we examined immediate outcomes of intrusive or interfering behaviors during laboratory exploration activities (Feeney, 2004; Feeney & Thrush, 2010). As expected, interference was a major inhibitor of exploration. Spouse interference predicted less persistence, poorer performance (even when the interference involved providing answers to challenging tasks), and less enthusiasm during the tasks. Recipients of interfering behaviors also showed an ambivalent behavioral pattern: Although they expressed greater concern about their spouses' watching their explorations, they also sought greater task assistance from them. Interestingly, they were receptive to both solicited and unsolicited task assistance, and they were simultaneously rejecting of both solicited and unsolicited task assistance.

We suspect that the ambivalent behavioral pattern observed for explorers with interfering spouses reflects a fundamental tension they experience in most exploration contexts. On the one hand, people with interfering partners may have come to believe that they are incapable of successful independent exploration. These self-doubts may make them receptive to both solicited and unsolicited task assistance, and may lead them to seek assistance despite a concern about their partners' involvement. On the other hand, because spouse interference is also likely to feel demeaning and to impede their goals and efforts, it makes sense that recipients are simultaneously rejecting of both solicited and unsolicited task assistance.

Other studies have revealed that (1) support providers who were intrusive during a discussion of their partners' personal goals had partners who tended to modify and minimize the importance of their original goals; (2) recipients of experimentally manipulated intrusive support messages from their spouses viewed the messages as frustrating and insensitive, and they perceived the spouses as both intrusive/interfering and helpful (providing further evidence of ambivalent feelings toward their spouses); and (3) intrusive/interfering support provision during exploration was predictive of decreases in state self-esteem (Feeney, 2004; Feeney & Thrush, 2010). These results for adults are consistent with research showing that parental interference in children's exploratory activities is associated with negative outcomes for children, including disrupted concentration, less persistence and enthusiasm during exploration, more passivity, more negative emotion, less competence, and less curiosity (e.g., Ainsworth, Bell, & Stayton, 1974; Cassidy & Berlin, 1994; Egeland & Farber, 1984; Main, 1983; Matas, Arend, & Sroufe, 1978).

Over time, the recipients of compulsively overinvolved support provision are likely to become overly dependent on their partners and less willing to engage in autonomous exploration. They may become less willing to venture away from their secure base (their partners) to pursue autonomous goals because they have developed fears and concerns about autonomous exploration, or because they have grown accustomed to having their partners do everything for them. The overdependence on their partners and resulting lack of exploration may lead to decreases in learning/discovery (development of competencies), and therefore to decreases in perceived self-efficacy, perceived competency, confidence in the recipients' own abilities, and trait self-esteem. Overdependence and lack of exploration may also result in decreased psychological health over time (e.g., lower life satisfaction, greater depression) because the recipients are not living up to their full potential and growing as individuals. The relationship may be characterized by increases in conflict over time, especially if the recipients grow more demanding or feel stifled by their partners. This consistently overinvolved support pattern may also contribute to the development of codependence within the relationship, in which the compulsively overinvolved partner may depend on the recipient to fill his or her need to compulsively care for others, and the recipient may in turn depend on the partner to do things for him or her that the recipient can accomplish unaided (see Figure 8.2 for a summary).

Negative/Demeaning Behavior

Negative and demeaning support provider behavior in safe haven and/or secure base support contexts should undermine optimal dependence by creating a defensive or compulsive self-reliance in the recipients. We next describe processes involving negative/demeaning support provider behavior that have implications for an unhealthy lack of dependence on others, as depicted in Figure 8.3.

Negative/Demeaning Behavior in Safe Haven Contexts

When attachment needs are activated, negative/demeaning support provider behavior may occur either in response to a partner's support seeking (e.g., expressions of distress) or spontaneously in response to the presence of a partner's life stressor. This type of behavior can include (1) encouraging suppression of feelings (or disallowing them) and discouraging the expression of distress or vulnerability; (2) rejecting a recipient's bids for support; (3) being critical, harsh, cruel, or contemptuous of a recipient's distress or vulnerability; (4) blaming the recipient for his or her misfortune; (5) making the recipient feel weak, pathetic, or abnormal for being distressed; (6) providing support that is controlling in nature; (7) giving assistance in a way that communicates the recipient is burdensome or incompetent; (8) expressing anger or frustration in response to the recipient's distress or request for support; (9) blaming the recipient for the support provider's own negative response to the stressor; and (10) forcing the recipient to accept the support provider's views about the stressor by disallowing a different perspective.

Recipients of this behavior in safe haven support contexts are likely to perceive it not only as unsupportive, but also as unkind, hurtful, frightening, or threatening. These behaviors and perceptions should result in immediate outcomes reflecting an inability to depend on others in times of need. Recipients should experience intensified feelings of anxiety, distress, and fear, as well as intensified feelings of insecurity in relation to their partners. They should not feel understood, validated, cared for, or valued/accepted by their partners, and they are likely to experience negative self-perceptions (e.g., perceptions that they are not lovable and unworthy of care and support from others). Recipients may also perceive that their home base is not only insecure, but may be threatening and dangerous, which should lead them to experience immediate decreases in relationship satisfaction, intimacy, and trust. Recipients may view interactions with their partners as negative and stressful, and perceive that seeking support from the partners is risky and costly—which may cause them to view problems as worse than they are.

Over time, recipients of negative/demeaning behaviors during times of stress are likely to exhibit increasingly intense reactivity to stressors; they may also experience chronically elevated stress responses such as increased allostatic load (McEwen & Stellar, 1993) because they cannot rely on others in times of need, and because their partners may themselves have become life stressors. Merely anticipating that one's partner will be unavailable in times of stress and expecting negative support exchanges should heighten the stressfulness of an already negative event (Pierce et al., 1997). As a result, such recipients should develop a defensive independence (underdependence on others) when coping with stress and solving problems. They should become reluctant to express their needs to others (Collins & Feeney,

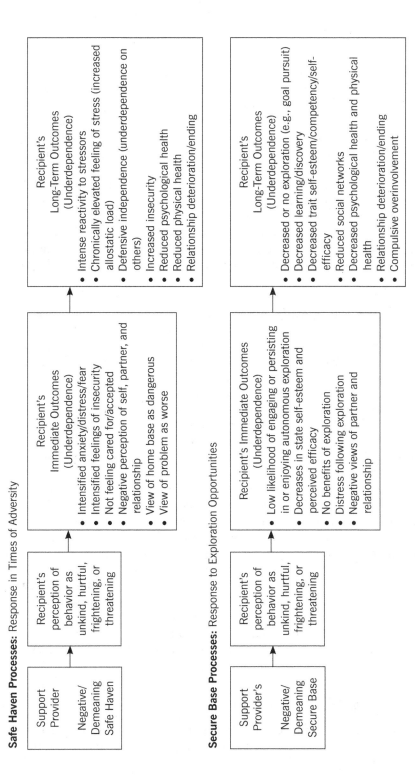

FIGURE 8.3. Proposed links between negative/demeaning support provider behavior and recipient perceptions and outcomes.

217

2000). Over time, they may experience decreases in perceptions of their own self-worth and decreases in feelings of security. Recipients may also experience deteriorating psychological and physical health, as well as worsening relationship quality over time because they may begin to psychologically detach themselves from their partners. The hostility exhibited in this support pattern is likely to contribute to relationship dissolution (e.g., Carrere & Gottman, 1999; Gottman, Coan, Carrere, & Swanson, 1998; Gottman & Levenson, 2000). See Figure 8.3 for a summary.

Consistent with these predictions, prior research has shown that recipients of unresponsive forms of support express their needs only indirectly, if at all (Collins & Feeney, 2000), and that negative/hostile support interactions predict slower cardiovascular recovery after experiencing a stressor (Fritz, Nagurney, & Helgeson, 2003) and poorer immune function (i.e., increased proinflammatory cytokine production and slower wound healing) (Kiecolt-Glaser et al., 2005). Overall, research indicates that negative social support interactions are strongly related to adverse outcomes over time (e.g., Bolger, DeLongis, Kessler, & Schilling, 1989; Coyne & DeLongis, 1986; Cutrona, 1996; Lakey, Tardiff, & Drew, 1994; Pagel, Erdly, & Becker, 1987; Robles & Kiecolt-Glaser, 2003; Rook, 1984; Vinokur & van Ryn, 1993), and that invalidating or negative exchanges exert a powerful negative impact on individuals and relationships that outweighs the beneficial impact of positive exchanges (e.g., Rook, 1984). These findings are consistent with evidence indicating that interpersonal conflicts are by far the most upsetting of all daily stressors (Bolger et al., 1989), and that negative social interactions increase psychological symptoms by inducing a less favorable evaluation of both the self and others (Lakey et al., 1994).

These immediate and long-term outcomes of negative support exchanges are indicative of a deteriorated state of both personal and relational well-being, and convey to recipients that they cannot depend or rely on others, even in times of extreme need. This in turn should influence responses to future life stressors and exploration opportunities in a way that promotes an unhealthy lack of dependence on others. For example, recipients of negative/demeaning partner behaviors may come to view dependence as a weakness, refuse to request or accept support from others in times of need (yet experience stressors more intensely because of their inability to do so), become unaccepting of others' dependence needs (or compulsively overinvolved in responding to others' needs), and fear venturing out to engage in autonomous exploration.

Negative/Demeaning Behavior in Secure Base Contexts

In secure base contexts, negative/demeaning support provider behavior may occur either in response to a partner's support seeking for exploration or exploration behavior, or spontaneously in response to the presence of a partner's exploration opportunity. This type of behavior can include (1) a lack of availability for facilitating exploration, (2) negative and controlling interference in the partner's exploration, or (3) active discouragement of the partner's exploration. This behavior may take the form of expressing criticism, anger, or disapproval in response to a partner's exploration opportunities; controlling his or her engagement in autonomous exploration; having the partner engage in exploration for the support provider's own benefit; taking over a partner's exploration activity in a negative or demeaning manner; minimizing the importance of the recipient's exploration opportunities; criticizing or belittling the recipient, and making him or her feel incapable of engaging in successful exploration; and instilling fear about autonomous exploration.

Recipients of this behavior should perceive it as unkind, hurtful, or threatening, and these behaviors and perceptions are expected to result in immediate outcomes reflecting an inability to depend on significant others in exploration contexts. First, recipients should be unlikely to engage in exploration or persist at or enjoy uninhibited exploration if they do engage in it, and they are unlikely to view exploration as worth the effort and risk involved. Second, recipients should experience decreases in *state* self-esteem, perceived self-competence, perceived self-efficacy, and self-confidence regarding exploration. Third, they are unlikely to benefit from exploration by learning/discovering and increasing their competencies, and they are less likely to perform well in exploration activities, given their inability to focus on the activities. They ought to experience more distress and more negative moods (e.g., frustration, sadness, disappointment) following exploration attempts. Finally, recipients should feel dissatisfied with their partners and relationships. These are immediate outcomes that are indicative of a deteriorated state of well-being, fueled by an inability to depend appropriately on others in exploration contexts.

Some initial evidence for these predictions was obtained in an observational study in which recipients explored in the presence of their spouses (Feeney & Thrush, 2010). A lack of spouse encouragement and availability (and spouse interference) predicted poorer performance and less enthusiasm during exploration; lower levels of persistence at exploration; decreases in positive mood and increases in negative mood from before to after the exploration; decreases in state self-esteem from before to after the exploration; and negative postexploration perceptions of the self, the spouse, and the exploration activity. In another study, spouses who were coded by observers as being unsupportive, discouraging of, and uncomfortable with their partners' goals were viewed by their partners as being insensitive, self-focused, and disappointing (Feeney, 2004). Further research that specifically assesses negative/demeaning behaviors in exploration contexts is still needed to establish its effects.

Over time, the recipients of negative/demeaning support behaviors in response to exploration opportunities should experience decreases in genuine exploration (or no exploration at all). In addition, they should show decreases (or no change) over time in learning, discovery, productivity, and the acquisition of new skills. As a result of their partners' negative/demeaning behaviors and their own lack of exploration, recipients should experience erosion of *trait* self-esteem, perceived self-competence, perceived self-efficacy, and confidence over time. In addition, the extended social networks of recipients may decrease or deteriorate over time, as a lack of exploration may prevent them from establishing and maintaining social contacts. These interpersonal processes surrounding a lack of secure base support ought to result in decreased psychological health over time (e.g., increased depression, anxiety, and anger/hostility, and decreased life satisfaction), as well as decreases in physical health (because recipients are less likely to engage in the types of behaviors that contribute to better health and well-being).

Finally, perceiving a partner as undermining the pursuit of personal goals should impair relationship satisfaction by posing a threat to the accomplishment of highly valued goal states (Brunstein et al., 1996; Kaplan & Maddux, 2002). There is likely to be little or no intimacy or confiding about dreams and goals; there should be little or no trust in the relationship; and there is likely to be increasing volatility in which negative interactions outweigh positive ones, leading to relationship dissolution (Gottman et al., 1998; Gottman & Levenson, 2000). A recipient may withdraw from the relationship literally or psychologically, or may over time become compulsively overinvolved with the partner (the source of rejection) in an attempt to maintain calm/peace in the relationship and gain a sense of approval or acceptance. These long-term consequences should result in a defensive self-reliance that influences responses to future exploration opportunities and life stressors. Defensively self-reliant individuals are less likely to seek support for attachment needs or for exploration, and less likely to risk depending on others who might be able to provide a responsive safe haven and secure base.

Neglectful/Disengaged Behavior

Neglectful/disengaged support provider behavior in safe haven and/or secure base support contexts is also likely to hinder one's ability to establish a healthy dependence on others, and it is also likely to result in defensive self-reliance, albeit for different reasons than in the case of negative/demeaning support provider behavior. We now describe processes involving neglectful/disengaged support provider behavior that have implications for a suboptimal lack of dependence on others, as depicted in Figure 8.4.

Safe Haven Processes: Response in Times of Adversity

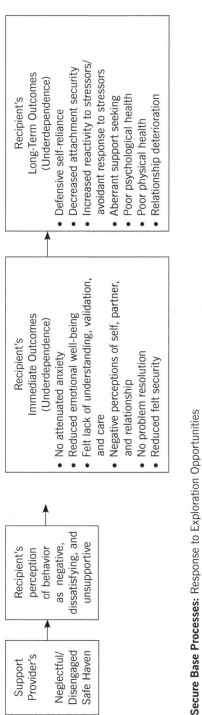

Secure Base Processes: Response to Exploration Opportunities

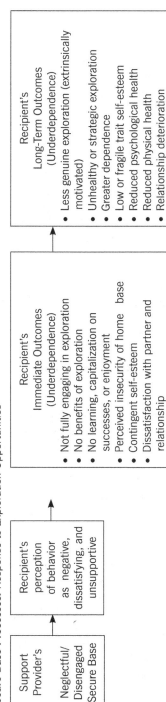

FIGURE 8.4. Proposed links between neglectful/disengaged support provider behavior and recipient perceptions and outcomes.

Neglectful/Disengaged Behavior in Safe Haven Contexts

In safe haven contexts, neglectful/disengaged support provider behavior may occur either in response to a partner's support seeking (e.g., expressions of distress) or spontaneously in response to the presence of a partner's life stressor. This type of behavior can include (1) not attending to the recipient's expression of emotion or bids for support, (2) focusing only on one's own needs and neglecting those of the recipient, (3) being uninterested in the problems or concerns of the recipient, (4) not engaging in conversations about the recipient's problems or concerns, (5) being inattentive to the recipient's cues and signals, or (6) not providing any active form of support.

Recipients of such behavior should perceive it as negative, dissatisfying, and unsupportive, and they are likely to perceive that they are on their own and must deal with life's stressors independently. These behaviors and perceptions should result in immediate outcomes reflecting an inability to depend on others in times of need. Recipients should be less likely to experience attenuation of their anxiety and distress, and instead they may experience decreases in emotional well-being (e.g., greater anxiety, depression). They may not feel understood, validated, or cared for, and they may develop negative self-perceptions because of the lack of care they perceive. They might also feel dissatisfied with their relationships and experience decreases in feelings of intimacy and trust. Additional immediate outcomes of neglectful/disengaged partner behavior may include either no improved problem resolution or worse problem solving, especially if a recipient copes by disengaging from a problem. Neglectful/disengaged partner behavior also should lead recipients to perceive that their home base is insecure. These are all immediate outcomes that should have implications for these individuals' ability to develop optimal levels of dependence on others.

These predictions are consistent with research showing that (1) individuals who were waiting to begin a stressful procedure were less calmed when their partners avoided or downplayed their concerns (Simpson et al., 1992); (2) individuals who had been exposed to an inattentive/neglectful partner in a virtual world reported greater anxiety, less positive self-evaluations, and decreased relationship satisfaction immediately afterward, and they kept greater distance between themselves and the partner during an immediately subsequent (but unrelated) task in the virtual world (Kane et al., 2012); (3) individuals who received no support from their partners (manipulated experimentally) were in a less positive mood after a stressful speech task, had lower self-esteem, and felt less satisfied with their relationships compared to those who received responsive support (Collins, Ford, Guichard, Kane, & Feeney, 2010); and (4) unsupportive interactions predicted slower cardiovascular recovery after experiencing a stressor (Fritz et al., 2003). These findings suggest that neglectful/disengaged support provision can immediately begin to erode both physical and emotional closeness between partners, as well as the well-being of a recipient.

Over time, recipients of neglectful/disengaged partner behavior in safe haven contexts may show a defensive self-reliance in coping and solving problems, and may perceive that turning to others for support and depending on others is not a helpful strategy. They are likely to report decreased attachment security over time, and they may either experience increased reactivity to stressors or show an increasingly avoidant response to stressors along with an avoidant style of coping. Because recipients of unresponsive support do not directly express their needs (Collins & Feeney, 2000), recipients of neglect may eventually engage in aberrant forms of support seeking (e.g., eating disorders, substance use, sexual infidelity) to draw the attention of their partners and elicit supportive behaviors (Bowlby, 1979).

Consistent neglect/disengagement over time should also predict decrements in psychological health, because important attachment needs are not being met (Bowlby, 1969/1982, 1988). Physical health also may be adversely affected over time because the neglected individuals' increased reactivity to stressors, avoidant coping style, decreased mental health, and aberrant coping behaviors (e.g., eating problems, drug or alcohol use) are likely to have deleterious health consequences. Finally, neglect or disengagement should take a toll on a relationship over time. Research has shown that a partner's consistent failure to provide responsive support (including dismissing behaviors during support interactions) can become a major source of disruption in relationships due to the emotional detachment this failure creates, which in turn predicts relationship dissolution (Barbee et al., 1993; Barbee & Cunningham, 1995). All of these negative long-term consequences arise because of the inability of a recipient to depend appropriately on a partner in times of need. See Figure 8.4 for a summary.

Neglectful/Disengaged Behavior in Secure Base Contexts

In secure base contexts, neglectful/disengaged support provider behavior may occur either in response to a partner's support-seeking/exploration behavior or spontaneously in response to the presence of a partner's exploration opportunity. This type of behavior can include (1) a lack of availability (e.g., being unavailable to assist with obstacles during exploration or to facilitate exploration, failing to respond to the partner's needs during exploration); (2) noninterference in the partner's exploration, albeit in a detached way that includes not noticing or attending to exploration successes; and (3) an uncaring and uninvolved acceptance of exploration in which the partner is not discouraged or held back from exploring, but there is no attention to or encouragement of exploration behavior.

Recipients of such behavior should also perceive it as negative, dissatisfying, and unsupportive, and they are likely to perceive that they are "on their own" in their explorations of the world. These behaviors and perceptions ought to result in immediate outcomes reflective of a lack of healthy dependence on others. Recipients may engage in exploration as a means of finding a connection that is missing for them. However, they are unlikely to explore in a passionate, fully engaged manner (or persist at especially challenging explorations) because they perceive that their home base is insecure. Because of the perceived insecurity of their home base, and the resulting attentional toll this is likely to take on exploration behavior, recipients are unlikely to reap the full benefits of exploration in terms of learning and discovery, capitalizing on exploration successes, and enjoying exploration. Their state self-esteem, perceived self-efficacy, perceived competence, and self-confidence are likely to be contingent on successes or failures during exploration (Crocker, Brook, Niiya, & Villacorta, 2006; Crocker & Knight, 2005; Park & Crocker, 2005; Park, Crocker, & Kiefer, 2007). Finally, recipients are unlikely to feel valued and accepted, and will consequently feel dissatisfied with their partners and relationships.

Consistent with these predictions, prior research has shown that a lack of spouse availability and encouragement during exploration is associated with poorer performance during exploration, less persistence at exploration, less enthusiasm during exploration activities, decreases in positive mood and increases in negative mood after engaging in exploration, decreases in state self-esteem, and negative perceptions of exploration (Feeney & Thrush, 2010). In a study that examined links between secure base behavior and exploration in discussions of personal goals (Feeney, 2004), support providers who were coded by observers as avoiding discussion of their partners' goals had partners who did not discuss their goals openly, did not confidently explore avenues for achieving their goals, were not receptive to support attempts (when they occurred), and avoided discussion of the goals.

Over time, recipients of neglecting/disengaged behavior in secure base contexts may engage in less genuine exploration that is more extrinsically motivated (e.g., done to gain others' approval or acceptance, to fill relational voids; Deci & Ryan, 2000; Ryan & Deci, 2000), and it may involve engaging in forms of exploration that are detrimental to the relationship, such as exploring alternative partners. Alternatively, recipients may become less willing to venture from their home base to take on challenges or risks because of the insecurity of their home base. They may strategically choose exploration activities that match those of their partners, to gain proximity to them in a context in which proximity is acceptable to the partners. Although this type of partner behavior is thought to produce a forced independence, recipients should become more dependent (and less independent) over time, consistent with research showing that a lack of partner availability predicts decreases in independent functioning over time (Feeney, 2007).

Because recipients may pursue exploration for reasons other than genuine interest, may engage in unhealthy forms of exploration, and are likely to feel contingently accepted by their partners, they ought to experience poorer psychological health and lower relationship satisfaction, intimacy, and trust over time. Recipients also are likely to have either low or fragile trait self-esteem, particularly if it is based on successes at independent exploration. If recipients engage in aberrant forms of exploration (e.g., seeking extramarital relationships, drug abuse), relationship dissolution and deterioration in physical health are likely outcomes.

Conclusions and Caveats

Our goal in this chapter has been to consider optimal dependence in close relationships from an attachment-theoretical perspective. We have elaborated on attachment-theoretical propositions and emphasized that (1) relational dependence is important for both personal and relationship functioning; (2) there is an optimal level of dependence that one should strive for in close relationships; and (3) the quality of relational support in both safe haven and secure base contexts influences the extent to which one can develop and maintain optimal levels of dependence.

Our discussion has focused primarily on the role of attachment figures in creating optimal or suboptimal levels of dependence in relationships. However, support recipients also play a significant role in creating healthy or unhealthy levels of dependence in relationships. For example, recipients may transfer unhealthy beliefs and interaction patterns (based on prior experiences with unresponsive attachment figures) into new attachment relationships where those beliefs and patterns are no longer adaptive and preclude the establishment of healthy dependence (even with responsive partners). In addition, a person's broader network of significant others (e.g., other family members) may play a substantial role in determining the influence of an attachment figure's behavior on the ultimate outcomes for the individual. Even within a central relationship, partners may be responsive in both safe haven and secure base contexts, responsive in only one context, or responsive in neither context. Although there is evidence for some of the predictions regarding optimal dependence from an attachment perspective, many others await future investigation. A program of research establishing important consequences of optimal and suboptimal dependence in relationships (in both safe haven and secure base contexts) is an area ripe for future theoretical and empirical attention.

References

Ainsworth, M. D. (1982). Attachment: Retrospect and prospect. In C. M. Parkes & J. Stevenson-Hinde (Eds.), *The place of attachment in human behavior* (pp. 3–30). New York: Basic Books.

Ainsworth, M. D., Bell, S. M., & Stayton, D. (1974). Infant–mother attachment and social development: Socialization as a product of reciprocal responsiveness to signals. In M. P. M. Richard (Ed.), *The integration of a child into a social world* (pp. 99–135). New York: Cambridge University Press.

Ainsworth, M. D., Blehar, M. C., Waters, E., & Wall, S. (1978). *Patterns of attachment: A psychological study of the Strange Situation.* Hillsdale, NJ: Erlbaum.

Allen, J. P., & Land, D. (1999). Attachment in adolescence. In J. Cassidy & P. R. Shaver (Eds.), *Handbook of attachment: Theory, research, and clinical applications* (pp. 319–335). New York: Guilford Press.

Allen, K. M., Blascovich, J., Tomaka, J., & Kelsey, R. M. (1991). Presence of human friends and pet dogs as moderators of autonomic responses to stress in women. *Journal of Personality and Social Psychology, 61,* 582–589.

Barbee, A. P., & Cunningham, M. R. (1995). An experimental approach to social support communications: Interactive coping in close relationships. *Communication Yearbook, 18,* 381–413.

Barbee, A. P., Cunningham, M. R., Winstead, B. A., Derlega, V. J., Gulley, M. R., Yankeelov, P. A., et al. (1993). Effects of gender role expectations on the social support process. *Journal of Social Issues, 49,* 175–190.

Belsky, J., Rovine, M., & Taylor, D. G. (1984). The Pennsylvania Infant and Family Development Project: III. The origins of individual differences in infant–mother attachment: Maternal and infant contributions. *Child Development, 55,* 718–728.

Blair, S. N., Cheng, Y., & Holder, J. S. (2001). Is physical activity or physical fitness more important in defining health benefits? *Medicine and Science in Sports and Exercise, 33,* 379–399.

Bolger, N., DeLongis, A., Kessler, R. C., & Schilling, E. A. (1989). Effects of daily stress on negative mood. *Journal of Personality and Social Psychology, 57,* 808–818.

Bornstein, R. F. (2005). Dependency across the life span. In R. F. Bornstein (Ed.), *The dependent patient: A practitioner's guide* (pp. 39–55). Washington, DC: American Psychological Association.

Bornstein, R. F., & Languirand, M. A. (2003). *Healthy dependency: Leaning on others without losing yourself.* New York: Newmarket Press.

Bowlby, J. (1969/1982). *Attachment and loss: Vol. 1. Attachment.* New York: Basic Books.

Bowlby, J. (1973). *Attachment and loss: Vol. 2. Separation: Anxiety and anger.* New York: Basic Books.

Bowlby, J. (1979). On knowing what you are not supposed to know and feeling what you are not supposed to feel. *Canadian Journal of Psychiatry, 24,* 403–408.

Bowlby, J. (1980). *Attachment and loss: Vol. 3. Loss: Sadness and depression.* New York: Basic Books.

Bowlby, J. (1988). *A secure base.* New York: Basic Books.

Brunstein, J. C. (1993). Personal goals and subjective well-being: A longitudinal study. *Journal of Personality and Social Psychology, 65,* 1061–1070.

Brunstein, J. C., Dangelmayer, G., & Schultheiss, O. C. (1996). Personal goals and social support in close relationships: Effects on relationship mood and marital satisfaction. *Journal of Personality and Social Psychology, 71,* 1006–1019.

Brunstein, J. C., Schultheiss, O. C., & Grassman, R. (1998). Personal goals and emotional well-being: The moderating role of motive dispositions. *Journal of Personality and Social Psychology, 75,* 494–508.

Buhrmester, D., Furman, W., Wittenberg, M. T., & Reis, H. T. (1988). Five domains of interpersonal competence in peer relationships. *Journal of Personality and Social Psychology, 55,* 991–1008.

Carnelley, K. B., Pietromonaco, P. R., & Jaffe, K. (1996). Attachment, caregiving, and relationship functioning in couples: Effects of self and partner. *Personal Relationships, 3,* 257–278.

Carrere, S., & Gottman, J. M. (1999). Predicting divorce among newlyweds from the first three minutes of a marital conflict discussion. *Family Process, 38,* 293–301.

Cassidy, J., & Berlin, L. J. (1994). The insecure/ambivalent pattern of attachment: Theory and research. *Child Development, 65,* 971–991.

Coan, J., Schaefer, H. S., & Davidson, R. J. (2006). Lending a hand: Social regulation of the neural response to threat. *Psychological Science, 17,* 1032–1039.

Cohen, S., Doyle, W. J., Turner, R., Alper, C. M., & Skoner, D. P. (2003). Sociability and susceptibility to the common cold. *Psychological Sciences, 14,* 389–395.

Cohen, S., & Pressman, S. D. (2006). Positive affect and health. *Current Directions in Psychological Science, 15,* 122–125.

Cohen, S., & Wills, T. A. (1985). Stress, social support, and the buffering hypothesis. *Psychological Bulletin, 98,* 310–357.

Collins, N. L., & Feeney, B. C. (2000). A safe haven: An attachment theory perspective on support-seeking and caregiving in adult romantic relationships. *Journal of Personality and Social Psychology, 78,* 1053–1073.

Collins, N. L., & Feeney, B. C. (2004). An attachment theory perspective on closeness and intimacy. In D. J. Mashek & A. P. Aron (Eds.), *Handbook of closeness and intimacy* (pp. 163–187). Mahwah, NJ: Erlbaum.

Collins, N. L., & Feeney, B. C. (2005, May). *Attachment processes in intimate relationships: Support-seeking and caregiving behavior in daily interaction.* Paper presented at the meeting of the American Psychological Society, Los Angeles.

Collins, N. L., Kane, H. S., Guichard, A. C., & Ford, M. B. (2008). *Will you be there when I need you?: Perceived partner responsiveness shapes support-seeking behavior and motivations.* Unpublished manuscript, University of California, Santa Barbara.

Collins, N. L., Ford, M. B., Guichard, A. C., Kane, H. S., & Feeney, B. C. (2010). Responding to need in intimate relationships: Social support and caregiving processes in couples. In M. Mikulincer & P. R. Shaver (Eds.), *Prosocial motives, emotions, and behavior: The better angels of our nature* (pp. 367–389). Washington, DC: American Psychological Association.

Coyne, J. C., & DeLongis, A. (1986). Going beyond social support: The role of social relationships in adaptation. *Journal of Consulting and Clinical Psychology, 54,* 454–460.

Crocker, J., Brook, A. T., Niiya, Y., & Villacorta, M. (2006). The pursuit of self-esteem: Contingencies of self-worth and self-regulation. *Journal of Personality, 74,* 1749–1771.

Crocker, J., & Knight, K. M. (2005). Contingencies of self-worth. *Current Directions in Psychological Science, 14*, 200–203.

Cutrona, C. E. (1986). Behavioral manifestations of social support: A microanalytic investigation. *Journal of Personality and Social Psychology, 51*, 201–208.

Cutrona, C. E. (1990). Stress and social support: In search of optimal matching. *Journal of Social and Clinical Psychology, 9*, 3–14.

Cutrona, C. E. (1996). *Social support in couples.* Thousand Oaks, CA: Sage.

Cutrona, C. E., Cohen, B. B., & Igram, S. (1990). Contextual determinants of the perceived supportiveness of helping behaviors. *Journal of Social and Personal Relationships, 7*, 553–562.

Cutrona, C. E., & Russell, D. (1990). Type of social support and specific stress: Toward a theory of optimal matching. In I. G. Sarason, B. R. Sarason, & G. R. Pierce (Eds.), *Social support: An interactional view* (pp. 319–366). New York: Wiley.

Deci, E. L., & Ryan, R. M. (2000). The "what" and "why" of goal pursuits: Human needs and the self-determination of behavior. *Psychological Inquiry, 11*, 227–268.

Ditzen, B., Neumann, I. D., Bodenmann, G., von Dawans., B., Turner, R. A., Ehlert, U., et al. (2007). Effects of different kinds of couple interaction on cortisol and heart rate responses to stress in women. *Psychoneuroendocrinology, 32*, 565–574.

Dunkel-Schetter, C., Folkman, S., & Lazarus, R. (1987). Correlates of social support receipt. *Journal of Personality and Social Psychology, 53*, 71–80.

Edens, J. L., Larkin, K. T., & Abel, J. L. (1992). The effect of social support and physical touch on cardiovascular reactions to mental stress. *Journal of Psychosomatic Research, 36*, 371–382.

Egeland, B., & Farber, E. (1984). Infant–mother attachment: Factors related to its development and changes over time. *Child Development, 55*, 753–771.

Elliot, A. J., & Reis, H. T. (2003). Attachment and exploration in adulthood. *Journal of Personality and Social Psychology, 85*, 317–331.

Emmons, R. A. (1986). Personal strivings: An approach to personality and subjective well-being. *Journal of Personality and Social Psychology, 51*, 1058–1068.

Emmons, R. A., & King, L. A. (1988). Conflict among personal strivings: Immediate and long-term implications for psychological and physical well-being. *Journal of Personality and Social Psychology, 54*, 1040–1048.

Feeney, B. C. (2004). A secure base: Responsive support of goal strivings and exploration in adult intimate relationships. *Journal of Personality and Social Psychology, 87*, 631–648.

Feeney, B. C. (2007). The dependency paradox in close relationships: Accepting dependence promotes independence. *Journal of Personality and Social Psychology, 92*, 268–285.

Feeney, B. C., & Collins, N. L. (2001). Predictors of caregiving in adult intimate relationships: An attachment theoretical perspective. *Journal of Personality and Social Psychology, 80*, 972–994.

Feeney, B. C., & Collins, N. L. (2004). Interpersonal safe haven and secure base caregiving processes in adulthood. In W. S. Rholes & J. A. Simpson (Eds.), *Adult attachment: Theory, research, and clinical implications* (pp. 300–338). New York: Guilford Press.

Feeney, B. C., & Collins, N. L. (2014). A new look at social support: A theoretical perspective on thriving through relationships. *Personality and Social Psychology Review.* Advance online publication.

Feeney, B. C., & Lemay, E. P. (2012). Surviving relationship threats: The role of emotional capital. *Personality and Social Psychology Bulletin, 38,* 1004–1017.

Feeney, B. C., & Thrush, R. L. (2010). Relationship influences on exploration in adulthood: The characteristics and function of a secure base. *Journal of Personality and Social Psychology, 98,* 57–76.

Feeney, B. C., & Van Vleet, M. (2010). Growing through attachment: The interplay of attachment and exploration in adulthood. *Journal of Social and Personal Relationships, 27,* 226–234.

Feeney, J. A. (1996). Attachment, caregiving, and marital satisfaction. *Personal Relationships, 3,* 401–416.

Fine, M., & Glendinning, C. (2005). Dependence, independence or inter-dependence?: Revisiting the concepts of "care" and "dependency." *Aging and Society, 25,* 601–621.

Fincham, F. D., & Bradbury, T. N. (1990). Social support in marriage: The role of social cognition. *Journal of Social and Clinical Psychology, 9,* 31–42.

Fishman, E., Turkheimer, E., & DeGood, D. (1995). Touch relieves stress and pain. *Journal of Behavioral Medicine, 18,* 69–79.

Fitzsimons, G. M., & Fishbach, A. (2010). Shifting closeness: Interpersonal effects of personal goal progress. *Journal of Personality and Social Psychology, 98,* 535–549.

Fitzsimons, G. M., & Shah, J. Y. (2008). How goal instrumentality shapes relationship evaluations. *Journal of Personality and Social Psychology, 95,* 319–337.

Fontana, A. M., Diegnan, T., Villeneuve, A., & Lepore, S. J. (1999). Nonevaluative social support reduces cardiovascular reactivity in young women during acutely stressful performance situations. *Journal of Behavioral Medicine, 22,* 75–91.

Fritz, H. L., Nagurney, A. J., & Helgeson, V. S. (2003). Social interactions and cardiovascular reactivity during problem disclosure among friends. *Personality and Social Personality Bulletin, 29,* 713–725.

Gable, S. L., Gonzaga, G. C., & Strachman, A. (2006). Will you be there for me when things go right?: Supportive responses to positive event disclosures. *Journal of Personality and Social Psychology, 91,* 904–917.

Gable, S. L., Reis, H. T., Impett, E. A., & Asher, E. R. (2004). What do you do when things go right?: The intrapersonal and interpersonal benefits of sharing positive events. *Journal of Personality and Social Psychology, 87,* 228–245.

Gore, J. S., & Cross, S. E. (2006). Pursuing goals for us: Relationally autonomous reasons in long-term goal pursuit. *Journal of Personality and Social Psychology, 90,* 848–861.

Gottman, J. M., Coan, J., Carrere, S., & Swanson, C. (1998). Predicting marital happiness and stability from newlywed interactions. *Journal of Marriage and the Family, 60,* 5–22.

Gottman, J. M., & Levenson, R. W. (2000). The timing of divorce: Predicting when a couple will divorce over a 14-year period. *Journal of Marriage and the Family, 62,* 737–745.

Grewen, K., Anderson, B., Girdler, S., & Light, K. C. (2003). Warm partner contact is related to lower cardiovascular reactivity. *Behavioral Medicine, 29,* 123–130.

Hawley, P. H. (1999). The ontogenesis of social dominance: A strategy-based evolutionary perspective. *Developmental Review, 19,* 97–132.

Jaremka, L., Kane, H. S., Guichard, A. C., Ford, M. B., & Collins, N. L. (2010). *Perceived partner responsiveness and the development and maintenance of felt-security in intimate relationships.* Unpublished manuscript, University of California, Santa Barbara.

Kamarck, T. W., Manuck, S. B., & Jennings, J. R. (1990). Social support reduces cardiovascular reactivity to psychological challenge: A laboratory model. *Psychosomatic Medicine, 52,* 42–58.

Kane, H. S., Jaremka, L. M., Guichard, A. C., Ford, M. B., Collins, N. L., & Feeney, B. C. (2007). Feeling supported and feeling secure: How one partner's attachment style predicts the other partner's perceived support and relationship satisfaction. *Journal of Social and Personal Relationships, 24,* 535–555.

Kane, H. S., McCall, C., Collins, N. L., & Blascovich, J. (2012). Mere presence is not enough: Responsive support in a virtual world. *Journal of Experimental Social Psychology, 48,* 37–44.

Kaplan, M., & Maddux, J. E. (2002). Goals and marital satisfaction: Perceived support for personal goals and collective efficacy for collective goals. *Journal of Social and Clinical Psychology, 21,* 157–164.

Katz, J., Beach, S. R. H., & Anderson, P. (1996). Self-enhancement versus self-verification: Does spousal support always help? *Cognitive Therapy and Research, 20,* 345–360.

Kiecolt-Glaser, J. K., Loving, T. J., Stowell, J. R., Malarkey, W. B., Lemeshow, S., Dickinson, S. L., et al. (2005). Hostile marital interactions, proinflammatory cytokine production, and wound healing. *Archives of General Psychiatry, 62,* 1377–1384.

Kotler, T. (1985). Security and autonomy within marriage. *Human Relations, 38,* 299–321.

Kunce, L. J., & Shaver, P. R. (1994). An attachment-theoretical approach to caregiving in romantic relationships. In K. Bartholomew & D. Perlman (Eds.), *Advances in personal relationships* (Vol. 5, pp. 205–237). London: Jessica Kingsley.

La Guardia, J. G., Ryan, R. M., Couchman, C. E., & Deci, E. L. (2000). Within-person variation in security of attachment: A self-determination theory perspective on attachment, need fulfillment, and well-being. *Journal of Personality and Social Psychology, 79,* 367–384.

Lakey, B., Tardiff, T. A., & Drew, J. B. (1994). Negative social interactions: Assessment and relations to social support, cognition, and psychological distress. *Journal of Social and Clinical Psychology, 13,* 42–62.

Little, T. D. (1998). Sociocultural influences on the development of children's action-control beliefs. In J. Heckhausen & C. S. Dweck (Eds.), *Motivation and self-regulation across the lifespan* (pp. 281–315). New York: University Press.

Little, T. D., Hawley, P. H., Heinrich, C. C., & Marsland, K. (2002). Three views of the agentic self: A developmental synthesis. In E. L. Deci & R. M. Ryan (Eds.), *Handbook of self-determination research* (pp. 389–404). Rochester, NY: University of Rochester Press.

Lynch, J. J., Thomas, S. A., Paskewitz, D. A., Katcher, A. H., & Weir, L. O. (1977). Human contact and cardiac arrhythmia in a coronary care unit. *Psychosomatic Medicine, 39,* 188–192.

Main, M. (1983). Exploration, play, and cognitive functioning related to infant–mother attachment. *Infant Behavior and Development, 6,* 167–174.

Marvin, R., Cooper, G., Hoffman, K., & Powell, B. (2002). The Circle of Security Project: Attachment-based intervention with caregiver–preschool child dyads. *Attachment and Human Development, 4,* 107–124.

Matas, L., Arend, R., & Sroufe, L. A. (1978). Continuity of adaptation in the second year: The relationship between quality of attachment and later competence. *Child Development, 49,* 547–556.

McEwen, B. S., & Stellar, E. (1993). Stress and the individual: Mechanisms leading to disease. *Archives of Internal Medicine, 153,* 2093–2101.

Moore, D. (1987). Parent–adolescent separation: The construction of adulthood by late adolescents. *Developmental Psychology, 23,* 298–307.

Noom, M. M., Dekovic, M., & Meeus, W. H. J. (1999). Autonomy, attachment and psychosocial adjustment during adolescence: A double-edged sword? *Journal of Adolescence, 22,* 771–783.

Omodei, M. M., & Wearing, A. J. (1990). Need satisfaction and involvement in personal projects: Toward an integrative model of subjective well-being. *Journal of Personality and Social Psychology, 59,* 762–769.

Pagel, M. D., Erdly, W. W., & Becker, J. (1987). Social networks: We get by with (and in spite of) a little help from our friends. *Journal of Personality and Social Psychology, 53,* 793–804.

Palys, T. S., & Little, B. R. (1983). Perceived life satisfaction and the organization of personal project systems. *Journal of Personality and Social Psychology, 44,* 1221–1230.

Park, L. E., & Crocker, J. (2005). Interpersonal consequences of seeking self-esteem. *Personality and Social Psychology Bulletin, 31,* 1587–1598.

Park, L. E., Crocker, J., & Kiefer, A. K. (2007). Contingencies of self-worth, academic failure, and goal pursuit. *Personality and Social Psychology Bulletin, 33,* 1503–1517.

Pierce, G. R., Baldwin, M. W., & Lydon, J. E. (1997). A relational schema approach to social support. In G. R. Pierce, B. Lakey, I. G. Sarason, & B. R. Sarason (Eds.), *Sourcebook of social support and personality* (pp. 19–47). New York: Plenum Press.

Pressman, S. D., & Cohen, S. (2005). Does positive affect influence health? *Psychological Bulletin, 131,* 925–971.

Rasmussen, P. R. (2005). The dependent prototype. In P. R. Rasmussen (Ed.), *Personality-guided cognitive-behavioral therapy* (pp. 215–234). Washington, DC: American Psychological Association.

Reis, H. T., & Shaver, P. (1988). Intimacy as an interpersonal process. In S. Duck (Ed.), *Handbook of personal relationships: Theory, research, and interventions* (pp. 367–389). Chichester, UK: Wiley.

Robles, T. F., & Kiecolt-Glaser, J. K. (2003). The physiology of marriage: Pathways to health. *Physiology and Behavior, 79,* 409–416.

Rook, K. S. (1984). The negative side of social interaction: Impact on psychological well-being. *Journal of Personality and Social Psychology, 45,* 1097–1108.

Ruehlman, L. S., & Wolchik, S. A. (1988). Personal goals and interpersonal support and hindrance as factors in psychological distress and well-being. *Journal of Personality and Social Psychology, 55,* 293–301.

Ryan, R. M., & Deci, E. L. (2000a). Self-determination theory and the facilitation of intrinsic motivation, social development, and well-being. *American Psychologist, 55,* 68–78.

Ryan, R. M., & Deci, E. L. (2000b). The darker and brighter sides of human existence: Basic psychological needs as a unifying concept. *Psychological Inquiry, 11,* 319–338.

Ryan, R. M., & Deci, E. L. (2004). Autonomy is no illusion: Self-determination theory and the empirical study of authenticity, awareness, and will. In J. Greenberg, S. L. Koole, & T. Pyszczynski (Eds.), *Handbook of experimental existential psychology* (pp. 449–479). New York: Guilford Press.

Simpson, J. A., & Rholes, W. S. (2010). Attachment and relationships: Milestones and future directions. *Journal of Social and Personal Relationships, 27,* 173–180.

Simpson, J. A., Rholes, W. S., & Nelligan, J. S. (1992). Support seeking and support giving within couples in an anxiety-provoking situation: The role of attachment styles. *Journal of Personality and Social Psychology, 62,* 434–446.

Simpson, J. A., Winterheld, H. A., Rholes, W. S., & Oriña, M. M. (2007). Working models of attachment and reactions to different forms of caregiving from romantic partners. *Journal of Personality and Social Psychology, 93,* 466–477.

Snydersmith, M. A., & Cacioppo, J. T. (1992). Parsing complex social factors to determine component effects: I. Autonomic activity and reactivity as a function of human association. *Journal of Social and Clinical Psychology, 11,* 263–278.

Solomon, M. (1994). *Lean on me: The power of positive dependency in intimate relationships.* New York: Simon & Schuster.

Sutton, A. (2001). Dependence and dependability: Winnicott in a culture of symptom intolerance. *Psychoanalytic Psychotherapy, 15,* 1–19.

Van Vleet, M., & Feeney, B. C. (2012). *Long-term consequences afforded by secure base support among newlyweds.* Paper presented at the conference for the International Association for Relationship Research, Chicago.

Vinokur, A. D., & van Ryn, M. (1993). Social support and undermining in close relationships: Their independent effects on the mental health of unemployed persons. *Journal of Personality and Social Psychology, 65,* 350–359.

Warburton, D. E. R., Nicol, C. W., & Bredin, S. S. D. (2006). Health benefits of physical activity: The evidence. *Canadian Medical Association Journal, 174,* 801–809.

Whitcher, S. J., & Fisher, J. D. (1979). Multidimensional reaction to therapeutic touch in a hospital setting. *Journal of Personality and Social Psychology, 37,* 87–96.

Winstead, B. A., & Derlega, V. J. (1985). Benefits of same-sex friendships in a stressful situation. *Journal of Social and Clinical Psychology, 3,* 378–384.

Yetim, U. (1993). Life satisfaction: A study based on the organization of personal projects. *Social Indicators Research, 29,* 277–289.

Zaleski, Z. (1987). Behavioral effects of self-set goals for different time ranges. *International Journal of Psychology, 22,* 17–38.

9

Adult Attachment Style and Parenting

Jason D. Jones
Jude Cassidy
Phillip R. Shaver

For almost three decades, attachment scholars have been studying how parents' adult attachment relates to their own parenting and the quality of their relationships with their children. This line of research has traditionally been viewed as mainly residing within the purview of developmental and clinical attachment researchers, who typically employ the Adult Attachment Interview (AAI; George, Kaplan, & Main, 1984, 1996) to assess parents' *current state of mind with respect to attachment*. However, since the mid-1990s, attachment researchers within the social/personality tradition have been investigating how self-reported adult *attachment styles* relate to various facets of parenting. Recently we reviewed over 60 published studies that examined the relation between parents' self-reported attachment styles and parenting; we found that attachment styles are related to various aspects of parenting across a range of contexts and child ages (from infancy to early adulthood; Jones, Cassidy, & Shaver, 2014).

The main goals of the present chapter are to (1) summarize our review of the theoretical and empirical links between parents' self-reported attachment styles and parenting, (2) highlight our own work in this area of research, and (3) discuss the prospects for future research. We begin by discussing Bowlby's (e.g., 1969/1982, 1988) theoretical ideas about relations between the attachment and caregiving behavioral systems. We then briefly discuss the birth of adult attachment research in the 1980s, and describe the two main approaches to measuring individual differences in adult attachment (i.e., the AAI and self-reports). The link between attachment styles and parenting was not the main focus of the first attachment style researchers (Hazan & Shaver, 1987); thus we explain how both theory and subsequent attachment style research provide a basis for expecting this link. We then review the empirically established associations between attachment styles and three aspects of parenting—parental behaviors, emotions, and cognitions—and discuss important factors to consider when interpreting the findings in this literature. Next, we describe our current work focusing on the links between attachment styles and caregiving in parents of adolescents. Finally, we propose directions for future research.

Theory Concerning Adult Attachment and Parental Caregiving

During his career, Bowlby focused mainly on attachment in infancy, but he conceptualized attachment as a lifespan process that affects thoughts, feelings, and behaviors in relationships "from the cradle to the grave" (1979, p. 129). Although he did not write extensively about caregiving, his conception of interacting behavioral systems—including the attachment and caregiving systems—and his proposal that cognitive representations of early relationships provide templates for future relationships provide theoretical foundations for studying the links between adult attachment and parenting.

Two Behavioral Systems: Attachment and Caregiving

Bowlby adopted the ethological concept of the *behavioral system* to characterize innate motivational systems and their development over the lifespan. A behavioral system is a species-universal set of actions (e.g., seeking proximity to a caregiver or providing care to a needy other) activated by specific internal and external stimuli that lead to, or predispose, a specific biologically relevant outcome. Such behavioral systems are assumed to have evolved because they organize behavior in ways that increase the likelihood of survival and reproductive success (Bowlby, 1969/1982; Stevenson-Hinde, 1994). Although these behavioral systems are assumed to be innate, Bowlby argued that their development is influenced by experiences and contexts.

One such system, the *attachment behavioral system*, organizes infant behavior around the goal of seeking and maintaining proximity to an attachment figure (usually a child's principal caregiver). The main function of the attachment system in infancy is to protect young, vulnerable infants from danger (e.g., predation), which increases the probability that they will survive to reproductive age and succeed in passing on their genes. Although the attachment system is perhaps most evident early in life when one is most vulnerable, Bowlby believed that it continues to influence behavior across

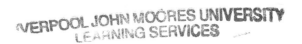

the lifespan. As such, a parent's attachment system is likely to influence parenting, even though a parent's bond to a young child is not itself conceptualized as an attachment (Ainsworth, 1989). Thus *both* child and parent possess attachment behavioral systems that influence thoughts, feelings, and behaviors in the parent–child relationship, but in notably different ways.

The primary behavioral system thought to organize parenting behaviors, emotions, and cognitions is the *caregiving system*. The behaviors organized by the caregiving system protect offspring from danger, reduce offspring distress, and promote offspring growth. Although Bowlby did not write about the caregiving system in great detail, he did note that parenting behavior could "usefully be approached from the same ethologically inspired [i.e., behavioral systems] viewpoint" (1988, pp. 4–5). Subsequent attachment scholars have written extensively about the nature of the caregiving system and its interactions with other behavioral systems (George & Solomon, 2008; Solomon & George, 1996).

Bowlby (1969/1982, 1988) viewed a parent's caregiving behavior as complementing his or her child's attachment behavior; that is, in the context of a well-functioning parent–child relationship, the child's attachment system and the parent's caregiving system work in synchrony. The two systems share a goal—proximity between infant and attachment figure (particularly under conditions of threat or danger)—and serve common functions: protection and survival of offspring. For example, when there is physical distance between a child and an attachment figure and a threat arises, the child's attachment system motivates him or her to seek proximity to the attachment figure, and the parent's caregiving system motivates the parent to seek proximity to and provide solace and protection to the child (Cassidy, 1999).

However, synchrony between the child's attachment system and the parent's caregiving system is not guaranteed. Building on ethologists' observation that the increased activation of one behavioral system often reduces the activation of another, Bowlby (1969/1982) described how increased activation of the infant's attachment system typically results in reduced activation of the infant's exploration system. Similarly, increased activation of a parent's attachment system may result in reduced activation of his or her caregiving system. In such cases, the parent's own attachment-related needs and strategies may interfere with the ability to respond appropriately to the child's needs. Similarly, dispositional attachment patterns, established over the period of childhood and adolescence, may affect the general quality of parents' care for their children.

Internal Working Models of Relationships

A central proposition of attachment theory is that infants develop experience-based mental representations, or *internal working models* (IWMs), of the self, attachment figures, and relationships (see Bretherton & Munholland, 2008, for a review). According to theory, these IWMs serve as templates for current and future relationships, and as such are one of the mechanisms by which early attachment experiences influence later relationships, including the parent–child relationship. Importantly, individual differences in the nature and quality of IWMs emerge as a function of the type of care received from attachment figures. Thus an infant who receives sensitive and responsive care from an attachment figure will likely form representations of the self as worthy of care, and of attachment figures as people who can be relied upon in times of need. On the other hand, an infant whose attachment-related needs are responded to only inconsistently or in a rejecting manner will likely form representations of the self as unworthy of care, and of attachment figures as unavailable or inconsistently available. These representations then affect thoughts, feelings, and behaviors in subsequent relationships, including ones with offspring.

Attachment in Adulthood

During the 1980s, two independent lines of research were initiated to explore the nature of attachment in adulthood. Main and her colleagues (George et al., 1984; Main, Kaplan, & Cassidy, 1985) developed an interview procedure, the AAI, to assess current state of mind with respect to attachment, inferred from the linguistic properties (e.g., coherence) of responses to questions about early attachment experiences, recent losses, and current relationships with one's parents and children. AAI transcripts are coded in detail and then assigned to one of three primary categories (secure, dismissing, preoccupied) that parallel the infant categories in Ainsworth's Strange Situation procedure (Ainsworth, Blehar, Waters, & Wall, 1978; see Hesse, 2008, for a discussion of the AAI categories). Many studies have found that an adult's state of mind with respect to attachment in the AAI is related to his or her child's attachment classification in the Strange Situation and to parenting behavior that partially mediates this connection (see van IJzendoorn, 1995, and Madigan et al., 2006, for meta-analyses).

Also in the 1980s, two social psychologists (Hazan & Shaver, 1987) suggested that there are adolescent and adult parallels of Ainsworth's infant attachment categories—which they labeled *attachment styles*— that influence a person's experiences and behavior in romantic relationships. They found that these styles could be assessed with self-report measures, and subsequent psychometric research showed that the three (or four, according to some researchers) adult attachment styles are better captured by dimensional than by categorical measures (Brennan, Clark, & Shaver, 1998). Following Ainsworth et al.'s (1978) diagram of two dimensions underlying Strange Situation categories, the two adult dimensions are generally labeled attachment-related *anxiety* and *avoidance*; more recently (e.g., Fraley, Heffernan, Vicary, & Brumbaugh, 2011; Mikulincer & Shaver, 2007), these dimensions have been considered to reflect thoughts, feelings, and behaviors in relationships with close others more broadly (i.e., not with romantic partners only). Avoidance reflects a tendency to deactivate the attachment system and is characterized by discomfort with intimacy, dependency, and emotional disclosure in close relationships. Anxiety, on the other hand, reflects the tendency to hyperactivate the attachment system and is characterized by a strong desire for closeness in relationships and intense fears of rejection and abandonment (Shaver & Mikulincer, 2002). A high score on either of these two dimensions reflects greater attachment insecurity, whereas low scores on both dimensions reflect greater attachment security.

A large body of research indicates that adult attachment styles predict variation in caregiving behavior within couple relationships (e.g., Feeney & Collins, 2001; Kunce & Shaver, 1994; Rholes, Simpson, & Oriña, 1999; Simpson, Rholes, & Nelligan, 1992; Simpson, Rholes, & Phillips, 1996). For example, anxious attachment in such relationships is associated with caregiving that is intrusive, controlling, and out of synchrony with a relationship partner's needs. Avoidant attachment, on the other hand, is associated with tepid, unsupportive, or insensitive caregiving. Low scores on both insecurity dimensions (indicating attachment security) are positively related to indicators of availability, sensitivity, and responsiveness.

In addition to the findings regarding couple relationships, findings from other areas of research suggest that attachment styles may influence caregiving in parent–child relationships. For example, greater insecurity has been found to predict maladaptive responses to distress and difficulties with emotion regulation (e.g., Mikulincer & Florian, 1998; Mikulincer & Shaver, 2007), as well as reduced empathy, compassion, and forgiveness (Mikulincer et al., 2001; Mikulincer, Shaver, Gillath, & Nitzberg, 2005; Shaver, Mikulincer, Lavy, & Cassidy, 2009). Parents who have difficulty regulating their own emotions, and who respond to others with insufficient empathy, compassion, and forgiveness, may struggle with the challenges and stresses of child rearing.

Although the AAI and self-report measures of attachment style derive from the same theoretical tradition and are described as measures of "adult attachment," they differ in many respects and are not strongly related to each other (see Roisman, Holland, et al., 2007, for a meta-analysis). As mentioned above, the AAI is coded with special reference to the coherence of a person's discourse when discussing early attachment relationships, whereas self-report measures of attachment style (e.g., Experiences in Close Relationships; Brennan et al., 1998) ask more directly about a person's experiences in recent close relationships. However, despite these differences and the weak relation between the two kinds of measures, the AAI and attachment style measures are similarly associated with a variety of attachment-related constructs such as emotion regulation (Mikulincer & Shaver, 2007), romantic relationship functioning (e.g., Simpson, Rholes, Oriña, & Grich, 2002), and social information processing (Dykas & Cassidy, 2011). To date, there has been little effort to integrate what is known about the use of self-report measures of adult attachment style to predict cognitive, emotional, and behavioral aspects of parenting. This chapter, as well as our review paper (Jones et al., 2014), performs that service.

Review and Analysis of the Empirical Evidence

Several factors make reviewing this literature complicated. First, there is variability across studies in the way parental attachment style was operationalized: Some researchers used dimensional measures of avoidance, anxiety, or security, whereas others used categorical measures of three or four attachment categories. Some authors did not differentiate between insecure subtypes or dimensions, whereas others did, making it difficult to interpret the consistency or inconsistency of findings across studies. Second, many studies included only women; several included both men and women; and a few included only men. Not every study that included both men and women reported comparisons between them.

Parents' Self-Reported Attachment Styles and Their Parenting Behaviors

These studies can be placed into one of four parenting behavior categories: (1) parental sensitivity, responsiveness, and supportiveness; (2) hostility and conflict behavior; (3) child abuse/maltreatment; and (4) overall parental functioning and miscellaneous parenting behaviors.

Parental Sensitivity, Responsiveness, and Supportiveness

Attachment-related avoidance has been consistently associated with less sensitive, responsive, and supportive parental behavior (Berlin et al., 2011; Edelstein et al., 2004; Goodman, Quas, Batterman-Faunce, Riddlesberger, & Kuhn, 1997; Mills-Koonce et al., 2011; Rholes, Simpson, & Blakely, 1995, Study 1; Selcuk et al., 2010). Studies have revealed both main effects of avoidance on parenting behavior and interactions between avoidance and characteristics of the parent or child. For example, Rholes et al. found a main effect of avoidance on maternal supportiveness, as well as a significant avoidance × child behavior interaction in predicting less supportive behavior. In contrast, Edelstein et al. found no significant main effect of avoidance on parenting behavior, but found that the link was moderated by the level of child distress: Avoidance was negatively related to parental responsiveness only when children were highly distressed.

The empirical links between attachment-related anxiety and parental sensitivity and responsiveness have been less consistent than the links between avoidance and these parental qualities. Only two studies have reported significant links between anxiety and less sensitive and responsive maternal behavior (Goodman et al., 1997; Selcuk et al., 2010). For example, Goodman et al. found that maternal anxiety was negatively associated with providing physical comfort to a distressed child following a painful medical procedure.

Hostility and Conflict Behavior

Rholes et al. (1995, Study 1) found no significant association between mothers' attachment styles and observed hostility toward their children. However, parental attachment styles have been found to relate to the degree of conflict in parent–child interactions and to the ways in which parents behave when engaged in conflict with their children. Selcuk et al. (2010) found that maternal anxiety, but not avoidance, was associated with greater observed conflict in mother–child interactions. In addition, two studies found that insecure parental attachment styles were related to less supportive and constructive parental behavior during parent–child conflicts (e.g., more anger and yelling, less problem solving, less collaborating; Feeney, 2006; La Valley & Guerrero, 2010). Feeney found that the links between attachment style and conflict behavior were somewhat different for mothers and fathers. For mothers, avoidance and anxiety were related to less constructive conflict behavior, whereas only anxiety mattered for fathers.

Child Maltreatment and Corporal Punishment

Six studies suggest that insecure parental attachment styles are related to increased risk for child maltreatment. For example, parents with insecure attachment styles were overrepresented in a sample of maltreating parents whose children were removed from the home (59% insecure, compared to 44% insecure in a community sample reported by Hazan & Shaver, 1987; Cramer & Kelly, 2010). In this sample of abusive parents, the fearful attachment category was the most frequently endorsed insecure style. In addition, insecure parents scored higher than secure parents did on indices of child abuse risk (Howard, 2010; Moncher, 1996; Rodriguez, 2006). The subtype of insecurity related to abuse risk was, however, inconsistent across these studies. Moncher and Rodriguez found that both maternal anxiety and avoidance were associated with higher abuse risk. On the other hand, in a sample of fathers, Howard found that anxious, but not avoidant, fathers were at higher risk for abuse than secure fathers. Finally, two studies found that insecure maternal attachment styles were weakly related to greater use of corporal punishment (i.e., spanking; Berlin et al., 2011; Coyl, Newland, & Freeman, 2010).

Overall Parental Functioning and Miscellaneous Parenting Behaviors

Researchers have also examined how attachment styles relate to various other aspects of parental behavior that do not fall neatly into a single subcategory of parenting behavior. In general, these studies suggest that insecure parental attachment styles are associated with more negative parental behaviors, including less consistent parental behavior (Coyl et al., 2010; Kilmann, Vendemia, Parnell, & Urbaniak, 2009), less parental involvement (Coyl et al., 2010), less caring behavior (Feeney, 2002), lower parental acceptance (Kilmann et al., 2009; but see Meredith & Noller, 2003, for null findings), more intrusiveness (Mills-Koonce et al., 2011; but see Berlin et al., 2011, for null findings), greater psychological control (Kilmann et al., 2009), lower-quality maternal teaching behavior (Rholes et al., 1995, Study 1), less engagement in activities with children thought to promote positive development (Green, Furrer, & McAllister, 2007), greater socialization of avoidant coping strategies (Abaied & Rudolph, 2010), more authoritarian and more permissive parenting (Millings, Walsh, Hepper, & O'Brien, 2013), and more negative ratings of overall functioning as a parent (Cohen, Zerach, & Solomon, 2011). As with the other subdomains of parental behavior, there was variability in which subtype or dimension of insecurity better predicted a particular aspect of parental behavior.

Summary of Research on Parenting Behavior

Taken together, the studies reviewed in this section suggest that parental attachment styles have implications for a variety of both observed and self-reported parenting behaviors. The broad range of parenting behaviors associated with parental attachment styles is impressive, but what may be most intriguing to attachment researchers is the link between attachment styles and parental sensitivity and responsiveness. Parental sensitivity and responsiveness are at the core of attachment theory and are thought to be among the most important predictors of child attachment security (Ainsworth et al., 1978; De Wolff & van IJzendoorn, 1997). The findings showing that parental insecurity is related to less sensitive, supportive, and responsive parental behavior mesh nicely with the results of studies finding links between insecure attachment styles and less sensitive and supportive caregiving in romantic relationships (e.g., Feeney & Collins, 2001; Rholes et al., 1999; Simpson et al., 1992, 1996). Furthermore, the link between self-reported attachment styles and parental sensitivity meshes with the well-documented association between parents' state of mind with respect to attachment in the AAI and parental sensitivity/responsiveness (van IJzendoorn, 1995). Nonetheless, additional studies are needed to replicate and further clarify the link between attachment styles and parental sensitivity.

Parents' Attachment Styles and Their Emotions Related to Parenting

Studies examining the links between attachment styles and parental emotions have focused on seven areas: (1) desire to have children; (2) feelings of closeness to children; (3) parental satisfaction; (4) coping with pregnancy and parenthood; (5) parental stress; (6) maternal separation anxiety; and (7) miscellaneous parenting emotions.

Desire to Have Children

Five studies found that attachment-related avoidance was related, among both male and female nonparents, to a weaker desire to have children (Rholes et al., 1995, Study 2; Rholes, Simpson, Blakely, Lanigan, & Allen, 1997, Studies 1 and 2; Rholes, Simpson, & Friedman, 2006; Wilson, Rholes, Simpson, & Tran, 2007). Only one study, using an all-male sample, found that anxiety was inversely related to the desire to have children (Scharf & Mayseless, 2011). Finally, Nathanson and Manohar (2012) found that insecurity was negatively associated with the desire to have children, but these authors did not distinguish between the subtypes of insecurity.

Feelings of Closeness to Children

Compared to secure mothers, insecure mothers report feeling less close to their children, both prenatally (Priel & Besser, 2000; Mikulincer & Florian, 1999c, Studies 1 and 2) and after childbirth (Rholes et al., 1995, Study 1; Wilson et al., 2007). In general, the findings are more consistent for avoidance than for anxiety. Only one of these studies included fathers: Wilson et al. found no significant links between fathers' attachment styles and feelings of closeness to children.

Parental Satisfaction

Six studies on this topic have yielded inconsistent results. Four found that avoidance was related to lower parental satisfaction (Cohen & Finzi-Dottan, 2005; Cohen et al., 2011; Rholes et al., 2006; Vieira, Ávila, & Matos, 2012), but in one study this effect emerged only for mothers (Cohen &

Finzi-Dottan, 2005), and in another the effect of avoidance on satisfaction was indirect through work–family conflict (Vieira et al., 2012). The findings related to anxiety are harder to interpret, with Cohen et al. (2011) finding a negative relation between anxiety and satisfaction, Rholes et al. (2006) finding no association, and Vieira et al. (2012) finding a positive direct effect of anxiety on satisfaction. However, Vieira et al. found that anxiety was indirectly related to lower parental satisfaction via higher work–family conflict. Lau and Peterson (2011) found no significant association between attachment style and parental satisfaction. Finally, La Valley and Guerrero (2010) found that security was related to greater parental satisfaction.

Coping with Pregnancy and Parenthood

The results of several studies suggest that secure mothers are better able than insecure mothers to cope with pregnancy, the transition to parenthood, and parenting stresses (Alexander, Feeney, Hohaus, & Noller, 2001; Berant, Mikulincer, & Florian, 2001a, 2001b; Mikulincer & Florian, 1998, Studies 1–4; Mikulincer & Florian, 1999c, Study 2; Trillingsgaard, Elklit, Shevlin, & Maimburg, 2011). Specifically, secure mothers reported less psychological distress during pregnancy and early parenthood, felt more equipped to handle pregnancy and the transition to parenthood, reported less fear and anxiety about their own health and the health of the fetus during pregnancy, and reported more adaptive coping strategies than insecure mothers did. Following a pattern that is strikingly consistent with the larger literature on attachment styles and coping with stress (Mikulincer & Florian, 1998; Mikulincer & Shaver, 2007), security was associated with greater support seeking and problem-focused coping; avoidance was related to more distancing coping; and anxiety was related to greater emotion-focused coping when dealing with stressors related to pregnancy and parenthood.

Parental Stress

Eleven studies yielded significant associations between attachment style and parental stress (Alexander et al., 2001; Fernandes, Muller, & Rodin, 2012; Howard, 2010; Kor, Mikulincer, & Pirutinsky, 2012; Kwako, Noll, Putnam, & Trickett, 2010; Mills-Koonce et al., 2011; Nygren, Carstensen, Ludvigsson, & Frostell, 2012; Rholes et al., 2006; Trillingsgaard et al., 2011; Vasquez, Durik, & Hyde, 2002; Vieira et al., 2012). The majority found that both avoidance and anxiety were related to greater parenting stress. Studies that examined the effect of parent gender generally found no differences (Kor et al., 2012; Nygren et al., 2012; Rholes et al., 2006; Vasquez et al., 2002).

Maternal Separation Anxiety

Three studies found that adult attachment insecurity was related to greater maternal separation anxiety (Mayseless & Scher, 2000; Scher & Mayseless, 1994; Vasquez et al., 2002). Two of these studies (Mayseless & Scher, 2000; Scher & Mayseless, 1994) found that only avoidance directly predicted greater separation anxiety, whereas Vasquez et al. found that mothers high in both avoidance and anxiety (i.e., fearful) reported the greatest separation anxiety.

Miscellaneous Parental Emotions

Four studies examined facets of parental emotions that do not fall neatly into one of our subcategories. In one study, Leerkes and Siepak (2006) presented female undergraduates with separate videos of infants expressing fear and anger, and then asked them to identify the infants' emotions and rate their own emotional responses to the videos. Higher scores on avoidance were related to less accurate identification of infant fear, and higher scores on both avoidance and anxiety were associated with mistaking fear for another emotion (e.g., sadness). In addition, avoidance was related to being amused by infant fear.

Consistent with the general tendency of anxious individuals to be jealous and to want more of their relationship partners' attention (Collins & Read, 1990; Hazan & Shaver, 1987), Wilson et al. (2007) found that anxiety (but not avoidance) was related to both men's and women's feelings of jealousy toward unborn infants (6 weeks before childbirth) as competitors for their partners' love and attention. Also, in a study of stepmothers, Ceglian and Gardner (2000) found that anxious stepmothers felt less appreciated and respected by stepchildren than avoidant stepmothers did, whereas avoidant stepmothers reported more resentment toward stepchildren than anxious stepmothers did. Finally, Scher and Dror (2003) found that more anxious mothers reported greater feelings of hostility toward their infants, but that attachment style was unrelated to feelings of pleasure from being a parent.

Summary of Research on Parental Emotions

The studies reviewed in this section support the link between parents' self-reported attachment styles and various facets of parental emotion. This body of work contributes importantly to the literature on links between adult attachment and parenting in ways that have not been adequately addressed by AAI studies. AAI researchers have tended to focus on associations between adult attachment and observed parental behavior (e.g.,

Adam, Gunnar, & Tanaka, 2004; Cohn, Cowan, Cowan, & Pearson, 1992), but have not devoted much attention to emotions related to specific aspects of parenting (e.g., stress, desire to have children). It would be interesting to examine how parental states of mind assessed by the AAI relate to these specific parental feelings and to compare the findings with those in the attachment style literature.

Given the well-documented link between parental emotions and parenting outcomes (Dix, 1991), future research should examine how various parental emotions mediate and moderate associations between attachment styles and parenting behavior. In addition, researchers should go beyond self-reports of parental emotion and include physiological and behavioral indices of emotion. For example, how do parental attachment styles relate to physiological responses during interactions with children or in response to child distress?

Parents' Self-Reported Attachment Styles and Their Cognitions Related to Parenting

Studies examining the links between attachment styles and parental cognitions have focused on four areas: (1) perceptions of parenthood and of oneself as a parent; (2) perceptions of current and future children; (3) perceptions of the parent–child relationship and family functioning; and (4) cognitive responses to infant distress.

Perceptions of Parenthood and of Oneself as a Parent

Self-reported attachment security is consistently associated with a generally more positive outlook on parenthood—part of what Rholes et al. (1997) have referred to as "working models of parenthood" (Berant et al., 2001a, 2001b; Mikulincer & Florian, 1998, Study 2; Nathanson & Manohar, 2012; Rholes et al., 1997, Study 1; Vasquez et al., 2002). That is, secure parents perceive parenthood as less threatening and concerning, and secure fathers view parenthood as more rewarding. In addition, in samples of nonparents, insecurity is related to more negative attitudes toward child rearing and to expecting child care to be more stressful and aggravating (Nathanson & Manohar, 2012; Rholes et al., 1997, Study 1; yet see Scharf & Mayseless, 2011, who did not find a link between attachment style and expected parental satisfaction). Although not all of these studies examined the subtypes or dimensions of insecure attachment, the ones that did mostly found that both avoidance and anxiety were related to more negative views of parenthood.

Studies examining individuals' perceptions of themselves as current or future parents have found that insecurity is associated with less self-reported competence in the parental role, less confidence in the ability to relate to children and to parent effectively, less emphasis on children's attaining developmental goals, less knowledge of child development, and more unrealistic expectations of being a "perfect" parent (Caldwell, Shaver, Li, & Minzenberg, 2011; Howard, 2010; Kilmann et al., 2009; Kohlhoff & Barnett, 2013; Rholes et al., 1995, Study 2; Scharf & Mayseless, 2011; Scher & Mayseless, 1994; Snell, Overbey, & Brewer, 2005). However, the subtype of insecurity predicting each of these parenting cognitions was inconsistent across studies. Nonparents who reported greater insecurity also reported that they expected to be less warm and more strict with future children (Nathanson & Manohar, 2012; Rholes et al., 1997, Study 1). These links emerged in relation to both avoidance and anxiety for both men and women (Rholes et al., 1997, Study 1).

Perceptions of Current and Future Children

Studies examining perceptions of current and prospective children have yielded inconsistent results. Four studies found no relation between parents' attachment styles and perceptions of their current (Lench, Quas, & Edelstein, 2006; Mayseless & Scher, 2000; Meredith & Noller, 2003) or future (Scharf & Mayseless, 2011) children. On the other hand, three studies found that insecure attachment styles were related to more negative perceptions of current child temperament (e.g., less adaptable, more fearful; Pesonen, Räikkönen, Keltikangas-Järvinen, Strandberg, & Järvenpää, 2003; Pesonen, Räikkönen, Strandberg, Keltikangas-Järvinen, & Järvenpää, 2004; Priel & Besser, 2000). In general, these studies found that both avoidance and anxiety were associated with more negative perceptions of infant temperament. In addition, Scher and Mayseless (1997) found that maternal avoidance, but not anxiety, predicted an increase in negative perceptions of infant temperament from 3 to 9 months. Finally, Rholes et al. (1997, Study 2) found that nonparents' avoidance, but not anxiety, was related to more negative expectations of future child attachment behavior.

In addition to these findings on perceptions of child temperament and behavior, Rholes et al. (2011) found that parental anxiety, but not avoidance, was associated with perceiving an infant as interfering with the parents' romantic relationship. This fits with the general tendency of anxious individuals to desire more attention from close others (Collins & Read, 1990; Hazan & Shaver, 1987); it also meshes with the finding that anxiety is related to feelings of jealousy toward infants (Wilson et al., 2007). Finally, greater parental avoidance has been linked to less optimistic expectations for child outcomes (Lench et al., 2006). That is, more avoidant parents view their children as more likely to experience negative life events (e.g., become seriously ill) and less likely to experience positive life events (e.g., stay healthy).

Perceptions of the Parent–Child Relationship and Family Functioning

Both avoidance and anxiety have been linked with more negative perceptions of the parent–child relationship (e.g., feeling disliked by one's child;
Berlin et al., 2011). Related to overall family functioning, two studies found
that parental security was associated with higher ratings of family cohesion and adaptability (Mikulincer & Florian, 1999a; Finzi-Dottan, Cohen,
Iwaniec, Sapir, & Wiezman, 2006; but see Mikulincer & Florian, 1999b,
for null results). In addition, Kor et al. (2012) found that parents' avoidance and anxiety were related to greater emotional distance among family
members and greater family chaos (i.e., lower organization and control).
Finally, Kohn et al. (2012) found that higher parental anxiety was related
to perceiving family responsibilities as overwhelming and to perceptions of
greater work–family conflict in both mothers and fathers. Avoidance was
also related to perceiving family responsibilities as overwhelming and to
more work–family conflict, but only among fathers.

Cognitive Responses to Infant Distress

Leerkes and Siepak (2006) asked female college students to view videos of
infants expressing anger and fear, and then assessed participants' attributions for why the infant in each video was crying. Avoidance was positively
associated with negative/internal attributions for infant fear (e.g., "the
infant is spoiled or difficult") and negatively associated with situation/emo-
tion attributions for infant anger (e.g., "the baby is upset by the situation").
On the other hand, anxiety was positively associated with temporary/
physical attributions for infant fear and anger (e.g., "the baby is hungry
or tired"). These findings, in conjunction with the results from this study
related to emotional responses to infant distress (reported above), suggest
that avoidance is associated with rather maladaptive responses to infant
distress. That is, more avoidant women attribute infant distress to negative
stable characteristics of the infant, rather than to situational factors, and
respond to infant fear with amusement. The findings related to anxiety are
more difficult to interpret. The authors suggest that the combination of
mistaking fear for another negative emotion and attributing infant distress
to temporary, physical factors may reflect a pattern of responding that is
out of synchrony with the needs of the infant (e.g., feeding a frightened
infant rather than providing comfort).

Summary of Research on Parental Cognitions

Taken together, these studies suggest that insecure parental attachment
styles are related to more negative parenting cognitions. The findings make
a novel and important contribution to understanding the links between

adult attachment and parenting. As mentioned in the summary of parental emotions, AAI researchers have tended to focus mainly on the relation between adult attachment and parenting behavior, and for the most part have not examined how AAI states of mind relate to parental cognitions. An interesting question for future research is whether states of mind in the AAI are related to specific parental cognitions (e.g., working models of parenthood) in the same way that self-reported attachment styles are (see Scharf & Mayseless, 2011, for some initial evidence).

Several important cognitive aspects of parenting have yet to be examined in relation to parental attachment styles—for example, parental mind-mindedness (Meins, 1997), reflective function (Slade, 2005), and parental insightfulness (Oppenheim & Koren-Karie, 2009), which are important predictors of parenting behavior and child outcomes. Future research should examine how parents' attachment styles relate to these cognitions. In addition, future research should examine parental cognitions as mediators and moderators of the link between parental attachment styles and parenting behavior. For example, do negative attributions for child distress mediate the link between insecure attachment styles and insensitive parenting behavior?

Additional Considerations

Across all three broad parenting domains reviewed here, the empirical evidence suggests that self-reported attachment security is associated with more positive parenting characteristics and outcomes, whereas self-reported attachment insecurity is associated with more negative parenting characteristics and outcomes. Thus the conclusion that parents' self-reported adult attachment styles can be used profitably to study thoughts, feelings, and behaviors in parent–child relationships seems to be justified by the available empirical evidence. However, there are several important factors to consider if one intends to understand the more nuanced aspects of this literature.

First, although it is true that insecurity is related to more negative parenting behaviors, emotions, and cognitions, the literature is less consistent in terms of how the specific subtypes or dimensions of insecurity relate to particular parenting outcomes. Attachment-related avoidance and anxiety reflect very different approaches to close relationships; therefore, some aspects of parenting may be particularly influenced by avoidance rather than anxiety or vice versa, and this may account for some of the variability in findings. For example, most attachment researchers would probably expect the desire to have children (i.e., the desire for a close relationship characterized by intense emotion and dependency) to be particularly low for avoidant individuals, who value their independence and are uncomfortable with intimacy, and this is what the literature shows. In contrast, other aspects of parenting—such as jealousy toward an infant for "stealing" a romantic partner's time and affection, or perceiving an infant as interfering with the parents' romantic relationship—may be more strongly associated with anxiety than avoidance (see Collins & Read, 1990, and Hazan & Shaver, 1987, for relevant research within adult relationships), and this expectation too is borne out in the literature. Still other aspects, such as parental stress, may be associated with both avoidance and anxiety, because both dimensions of insecurity are associated with emotion regulation and coping difficulties (Mikulincer & Florian, 1998; Mikulincer & Shaver, 2007). The literature supports this prediction and also shows that anxious and avoidant parents differ in the ways they cope with parenting stress (Berant et al., 2001a; Mikulincer & Florian, 1998, Studies 2–4; Mikulincer & Florian, 1999c, Study 2). In future studies, researchers should give careful a priori thought to how the subtypes of insecurity will relate to a particular aspect of parenting.

Second, in some cases, findings related to the same parenting construct were inconsistent across studies. Two potential explanations for this variability include differences in how attachment style was measured and diversity of samples across studies. There is considerable variability in how attachment style was measured across studies. Researchers have used a variety of dimensional attachment style measures that, although similar, are not identical. Of perhaps greater importance is the issue of comparing findings from studies that used categorical measures with findings from studies based on dimensional measures. In accord with the psychometric evidence indicating that adult attachment is better conceptualized in terms of dimensions than of categories (Brennan et al., 1998; Roisman, Fraley, & Belsky, 2007), we encourage researchers studying links between attachment style and parenting to use dimensional measures.

The studies reviewed in this chapter were conducted in 10 countries, with diverse samples characterized by differing life circumstances (e.g., parents vs. nonparents; parents of infants vs. parents of older children; parents of sick vs. healthy children; single vs. married parents; parents of low vs. middle socioeconomic status). This diversity could account for some of the variability across studies. Future research should involve giving greater consideration to sample-specific characteristics that could influence results, and should include discussion of how results are consistent or inconsistent with prior research conducted with different samples.

Another important factor to consider is parent gender. The links between attachment style and aspects of parenting sometimes, but not always, differed for mothers and fathers (or for female and male nonparents). Similar to the larger literature on parenting, research in this area has tended to exclude fathers. In particular, studies examining attachment styles and *observed* parenting behavior have been completely limited to mothers (Edelstein et al., 2004, included four fathers). Given the evidence for sex differences in attachment styles (Del Giudice, 2011), which vary across cultures, and the initial evidence reported in this review for potential differences in how attachment styles relate to some aspects of parenting as a function of parent gender, future research should include both mothers and fathers, and any gender differences should be reported.

A Focus on Adolescence

Our extensive review of the literature on attachment styles and parenting has revealed that virtually all of the studies to date have focused on parents of young children or college-age children. Noticeably lacking in this area of research are studies examining links between attachment styles and parenting in samples of parents of adolescents. Thus we have begun a line of research to address this gap in the literature.

In an initial study of adolescents (mean age = 16 years) and their parents (Jones & Cassidy, 2014), we examined how mothers' and fathers' attachment styles related to observed parental secure base provision and adolescent secure base use in the context of a parent–adolescent conflict discussion task. We also examined how parents' attachment styles related to parent-reported hostile behavior toward their adolescents and to adolescents' perceptions of their parents, and tested whether these variables mediated the link between parental attachment styles and secure base use. Parental attachment styles were related to observed adolescent secure base use, but not to parental secure base provision; yet the pattern of findings differed for mothers and fathers. At the bivariate level, maternal avoidance, but not anxiety, was negatively related to adolescent secure base use. Furthermore, maternal avoidance was indirectly related to less adolescent secure base use through greater mother-reported hostile behavior toward the adolescents and through adolescents' negative perceptions of their mothers (i.e., a composite indicating less secure base availability, less warmth, less understanding, and more hostility). For fathers, attachment anxiety, but not avoidance, was indirectly related to less adolescent secure base use through greater father-reported hostility toward the adolescents.

In a second study with parents and adolescents (mean age = 14 years), we (Jones, Ehrlich, Lejuez, & Cassidy, 2014) examined how parental attachment styles related to mothers', fathers', and adolescents' perceptions of the degree to which parents were knowledgeable about their adolescents' whereabouts and activities—a variable well known to predict adolescent risk behavior and delinquency (e.g., Stattin & Kerr, 2000). For both mothers and fathers, attachment anxiety and avoidance were negatively correlated with their own reports of parental knowledge. With regard to adolescents' reports of parental knowledge, the pattern of results differed for mothers and fathers: Maternal avoidance (but not anxiety) and paternal anxiety (but not avoidance) were negatively associated with adolescents' perceptions of parental knowledge.

In a third study (Jones, Brett, Ehrlich, Lejuez, & Cassidy, 2014), we examined the prospective association between mothers' attachment styles and their self-reported responses to their adolescents' (mean age = 15 years) negative emotions 2 years later. Furthermore, we examined whether mothers' emotion regulation difficulties mediated this link. We found that maternal avoidance and anxiety were both indirectly related to more harsh, more distressed, and less supportive responses to adolescents' negative emotions through maternal difficulties with emotion regulation. In addition, we found a significant direct effect of mothers' avoidance on more harsh responses to their adolescents' negative emotions 2 years later.

In sum, consistent with the findings of studies conducted with parents of much younger and much older children, these three studies suggest that parental attachment styles are related to caregiving among parents of adolescents. However, these three studies also reveal the complexity of these links. More work is needed to clarify whether these links are better construed as direct or indirect, and whether the answer to this question depends on the type of parenting construct measured. In addition, given the similarities and differences in results we found as a function of parent gender, future work should include both mothers and fathers. Finally, given our failure to replicate previous studies that reported links between parental attachment styles and *observed* parental behavior toward young children (e.g., Edelstein et al., 2004; Mills-Koonce et al., 2011; Rholes et al., 1995, Study 1; Selcuk et al., 2010), future studies should include observations of parent–adolescent interactions to determine whether these links will emerge in different samples or in a different observational task.

Future Directions

Throughout this chapter, we have mentioned many future directions for this area of research. Below, we suggest several additional avenues for future research.

One issue that remains to be investigated is whether individual differences in attachment style relate to differences in physiological and neurobiological responses to stimuli relevant to caregiving. Several studies have found that variation in state of mind in the AAI is related to differences in neural responses to infant cues, as well as to differences in peripheral oxytocin response to infant contact (Riem, Bakermans-Kranenburg, van IJzendoorn, Out, & Rombouts, 2012; Strathearn, 2011; Strathearn, Fonagy, Amico, & Montague, 2009). Given that attachment styles are related to differences in physiological and neuroendocrine responding during romantic partner interactions (Gouin et al., 2009; Powers, Pietromonaco,

Gunlicks, & Sayer, 2006), it is possible that they also relate to neurobiological responses to one's children.

Future research should include greater consideration of the role of parents' romantic relationship quality in regard to the links between attachment styles and parenting. It has long been recognized that marital relationships both influence and are influenced by parent–child relationships (e.g., Belsky, 1981). Given substantial evidence for strong associations between adult attachment styles and romantic relationship quality (Mikulincer & Shaver, 2007), as well as evidence for links between marital quality and the quality of parent–child relationships (see Erel & Burman, 1995, for a meta-analysis), future research should examine the additive and interactive influences of attachment styles and marital quality on parenting (see Rholes et al., 1995, Study 1, for some initial evidence).

Future research should examine not only how parental attachment styles relate to parenting, but also how the experience of parenthood may change parents' attachment styles. The transition to parenthood is a major life event that likely leads individuals to reflect upon, reevaluate, and possibly change their orientation toward close relationships (Bowlby, 1988; Simpson, Rholes, Campbell, & Wilson, 2003). Furthermore, researchers should consider how characteristics of the parents, of the parents' romantic relationship, and of the child relate to changes in parents' attachment styles across the transition to parenthood.

Another issue is experimentation. Much of the attachment style literature is based on studies in which contexts, stressors, subliminal security or insecurity primes, and experimental tasks for couples are manipulated, and the interaction of the manipulations and attachment styles is assessed. Similar research techniques could be used in studies of parent–child relationships.

Finally, research on adult attachment and parenting would benefit greatly from increased collaboration among researchers from the social and developmental attachment research traditions. The modest empirical association between the AAI and self-report attachment style measures indicates that one measure is not simply a substitute for the other. Yet both seem to be reliably associated with various facets of parenting. Therefore, researchers should strive to include *both* the AAI and self-report measures of attachment style in their studies. It should be particularly easy for researchers already administering the AAI to add a brief self-report attachment style measure to their studies.

Acknowledgments

Preparation of this chapter was supported by awards to Jason D. Jones from the National Institute on Drug Abuse (No. F31 DA033848), and to Phillip R. Shaver from the Fetzer Institute.

References

Abaied, J. L., & Rudolph, K. D. (2010). Contributions of maternal adult attachment to socialization of coping. *Journal of Social and Personal Relationships, 27,* 637–657.

Adam, E. K., Gunnar, M. R., & Tanaka, A. (2004). Adult attachment, parent emotion, and observed parenting behavior: Mediator and moderator models. *Child Development, 75,* 110–122.

Ainsworth, M. D. S. (1989). Attachments beyond infancy. *American Psychologist, 44,* 709–716.

Ainsworth, M. D. S., Blehar, M. C., Waters, E., & Wall, S. (1978). *Patterns of attachment: A psychological study of the Strange Situation.* Hillsdale, NJ: Erlbaum.

Alexander, R., Feeney, J., Hohaus, L., & Noller, P. (2001). Attachment style and coping resources as predictors of coping strategies in the transition to parenthood. *Personal Relationships, 8,* 137–152.

Belsky, J. (1981). Early human experience: A family perspective. *Developmental Psychology, 17,* 3–23.

Berant, E., Mikulincer, M., & Florian, V. (2001a). The association of mothers' attachment style and their psychological reactions to the diagnosis of infant's congenital heart disease. *Journal of Social and Clinical Psychology, 20,* 208–232.

Berant, E., Mikulincer, M., & Florian, V. (2001b). Attachment style and mental health: A 1-year follow-up study of mothers of infants with congenital heart disease. *Personality and Social Psychology Bulletin, 27,* 956–968.

Berlin, L. J., Whiteside-Mansell, L., Roggman, L. A., Green, B. L., Robinson, J., & Spieker, S. (2011). Testing maternal depression and attachment style as moderators of Early Head Start's effects on parenting. *Attachment and Human Development, 13,* 49–67.

Bowlby, J. (1969/1982). *Attachment and loss: Vol. 1. Attachment.* New York: Basic Books.

Bowlby, J. (1979). *The making and breaking of affectional bonds.* London: Tavistock.

Bowlby, J. (1988). *A secure base: Parent–child attachment and healthy human development.* New York: Basic Books.

Brennan, K. A., Clark, C. L., & Shaver, P. R. (1998). Self-report measurement of adult romantic attachment: An integrative overview. In J. A. Simpson & W. S. Rholes (Eds.), *Attachment theory and close relationships* (pp. 46–76). New York: Guilford Press.

Bretherton, I., & Munholland, K. A. (2008). Internal working models in attachment relationships: Elaborating a central construct in attachment theory. In J. Cassidy & P. R. Shaver (Eds.), *Handbook of attachment: Theory, research, and clinical applications* (2nd ed., pp. 102–130). New York: Guilford Press.

Caldwell, J. G., Shaver, P. R., Li, C., & Minzenberg, M. J. (2011). Childhood maltreatment, adult attachment, and depression as predictors of parental self-efficacy in at-risk mothers. *Journal of Aggression, Maltreatment and Trauma, 20,* 595–616.

Cassidy, J. (1999). The nature of the child's ties. In J. Cassidy & P. R. Shaver

(Eds.), *Handbook of attachment: Theory, research, and clinical applications* (pp. 3–20). New York: Guilford Press.

Ceglian, C., & Gardner, S. (2000). Attachment style and the "wicked stepmother" spiral. *Journal of Divorce and Remarriage, 34,* 111–129.

Cohen, E., Zerach, G., & Solomon, Z. (2011). The implication of combat-induced stress reaction, PTSD, and attachment in parenting among war veterans. *Journal of Family Psychology, 25,* 688–698.

Cohen, O., & Finzi-Dottan, R. (2005). Parent–child relationships during the divorce process: From attachment theory and intergenerational perspective. *Contemporary Family Therapy: An International Journal, 27,* 81–99.

Cohn, D. A., Cowan, P. A., Cowan, C. P., & Pearson, J. (1992). Mothers' and fathers' working models of childhood attachment relationships, parenting styles, and child behavior. *Development and Psychopathology, 4,* 417–431.

Collins, N. L., & Read, S. J. (1990). Adult attachment, working models, and relationship quality in dating couples. *Journal of Personality and Social Psychology, 58,* 644–663.

Coyl, D. D., Newland, L. A., & Freeman, H. (2010). Predicting preschoolers' attachment security from parenting behaviours, parents' attachment relationships and their use of social support. *Early Child Development and Care, 180,* 499–512.

Cramer, P., & Kelly, F. D. (2010). Attachment style and defense mechanisms in parents who abuse their children. *Journal of Nervous and Mental Disease, 198,* 619–627.

Del Giudice, M. (2011). Sex differences in romantic attachment: A meta-analysis. *Personality and Social Psychology Bulletin, 37,* 193–214.

De Wolff, M., & van IJzendoorn, M. H. (1997). Sensitivity and attachment: A meta-analysis on parental antecedents of infant attachment. *Child Development, 68,* 571–591.

Dix, T. (1991). The affective organization of parenting: Adaptive and maladaptive processes. *Psychological Bulletin, 110,* 3–25.

Dykas, M. J., & Cassidy, J. (2011). Attachment and the processing of social information across the life span: Theory and evidence. *Psychological Bulletin, 137,* 19–46.

Edelstein, R. S., Alexander, K., Shaver, P. R., Schaaf, J. M., Quas, J. A., Lovas, G. S., et al. (2004). Adult attachment style and parental responsiveness during a stressful event. *Attachment and Human Development, 6,* 31–52.

Erel, O., & Burman, B. (1995). Interrelatedness of marital relations and parent–child relations: A meta-analytic review. *Psychological Bulletin, 118,* 108–132.

Feeney, B. C., & Collins, N. L. (2001). Predictors of caregiving in adult intimate relationships: An attachment theoretical perspective. *Journal of Personality and Social Psychology, 80,* 972–994.

Feeney, J. A. (2002). Early parenting and parental attachment: Links with offspring's attachment and perceptions of social support. *Journal of Family Studies, 8,* 5–23.

Feeney, J. A. (2006). Parental attachment and conflict behavior: Implications for offspring's attachment, loneliness, and relationship satisfaction. *Personal Relationships, 13,* 19–36.

Fernandes, C., Muller, R., & Rodin, G. (2012). Predictors of parenting stress in patients with haematological cancer. *Journal of Psychosocial Oncology, 30,* 81–96.

Finzi-Dottan, R., Cohen, O., Iwaniec, D., Sapir, Y., & Weizman, A. (2006). The child in the family of a drug-using father: Attachment styles and family characteristics. *Journal of Social Work Practice in the Addictions, 6,* 89–111.

Fraley, R. C., Heffernan, M. E., Vicary, A. M., & Brumbaugh, C. C. (2011). The Experiences in Close Relationships—Relationship Structures Questionnaire: A method for assessing attachment orientations across relationships. *Psychological Assessment, 23,* 615–625.

George, C., Kaplan, N., & Main, M. (1984). *Adult Attachment Interview protocol.* Unpublished manuscript, University of California at Berkeley.

George, C., Kaplan, N., & Main, M. (1996). *Adult Attachment Interview protocol* (3rd ed.). Unpublished manuscript, University of California at Berkeley.

George, C., & Solomon, J. (2008). The caregiving system: A behavioral systems approach to parenting. In J. Cassidy & P. R. Shaver (Eds.), *Handbook of attachment: Theory, research, and clinical applications* (2nd ed., pp. 833–856). New York: Guilford Press.

Goodman, G. S., Quas, J. A., Batterman-Faunce, J. M., Riddlesberger, M. M., & Kuhn, J. (1997). Children's reactions to and memory for a stressful event: Influence of age, anatomical dolls, knowledge, and parental attachment. *Applied Developmental Science, 1,* 54–75.

Gouin, J., Glaser, R., Loving, T. J., Malarkey, W. B., Stowell, J., Houts, C., et al. (2009). Attachment avoidance predicts inflammatory responses to marital conflict. *Brain, Behavior, and Immunity, 23,* 898–904.

Green, B. L., Furrer, C., & McAllister, C. (2007). How do relationships support parenting?: Effects of attachment style and social support on parenting behavior in an at-risk population. *American Journal of Community Psychology, 40,* 96–108.

Hazan, C., & Shaver, P. R. (1987). Romantic love conceptualized as an attachment process. *Journal of Personality and Social Psychology, 52,* 511–524.

Hesse, E. (2008). The Adult Attachment Interview: Protocol, method of analysis, and empirical studies. In J. Cassidy & P. R. Shaver (Eds.), *Handbook of attachment: Theory, research, and clinical applications* (2nd ed., pp. 552–598). New York: Guilford Press.

Howard, K. S. (2010). Paternal attachment, parenting beliefs and children's attachment. *Early Child Development and Care, 180,* 157–171.

Jones, J. D., Brett, B. E., Ehrlich, K. B., Lejuez, C. W., & Cassidy, J. (2014). Maternal attachment style and responses to adolescents' negative emotions: The mediating role of maternal emotion regulation. *Parenting: Science and Practice.* Advance online publication.

Jones, J. D., & Cassidy, J. (2014). Parental attachment style: Examination of links with parent secure base provision and adolescent secure base use. *Attachment and Human Development, 16,* 437–461.

Jones, J. D., Cassidy, J., & Shaver, P. R. (2014). Parents' self-reported attachment styles: A review of links with parenting behaviors, emotions, and cognitions. *Personality and Social Psychology Review.* Advance online publication.

Jones, J. D., Ehrlich, K. B., Lejuez, C. W., & Cassidy, J. (2014). *Parental knowledge of adolescent activities: Links with parental attachment style and adolescent substance use.* Manuscript submitted for publication.

Kilmann, P. R., Vendemia, J. C., Parnell, M. M., & Urbaniak, G. C. (2009). Parent characteristics linked with daughters' attachment styles. *Family Therapy, 36,* 83–94.

Kohlhoff, J., & Barnett, B. (2013). Parenting self-efficacy: Links with maternal depression, infant behaviour and adult attachment. *Early Human Development, 89,* 249–256.

Kohn, J. L., Rholes, W. S., Simpson, J. A., Martin, A., Tran, S., & Wilson, C. L. (2012). Changes in marital satisfaction across the transition to parenthood: The role of adult attachment orientations. *Personality and Social Psychology Bulletin, 38,* 1506–1522.

Kor, A., Mikulincer, M., & Pirutinsky, S. (2012). Family functioning among returnees to Orthodox Judaism in Israel. *Journal of Family Psychology, 26,* 149–158.

Kunce, L. J., & Shaver, P. R. (1994). An attachment-theoretical approach to caregiving in romantic relationships. In K. Bartholomew & D. Perlman (Eds.), *Advances in personal relationships: Vol. 5. Attachment processes in adulthood* (pp. 205–237). London: Jessica Kingsley.

Kwako, L. E., Noll, J. G., Putnam, F. W., & Trickett, P. K. (2010). Childhood sexual abuse and attachment: An intergenerational perspective. *Clinical Child Psychology and Psychiatry, 15,* 407–422.

Lau, W., & Peterson, C. C. (2011). Adults and children with Asperger syndrome: Exploring adult attachment style, marital satisfaction and satisfaction with parenthood. *Research in Autism Spectrum Disorders, 5,* 392–399.

La Valley, A. G., & Guerrero, L. K. (2010). Perceptions of conflict behavior and relational satisfaction in adult parent–child relationships: A dyadic analysis from an attachment perspective. *Communication Research, 39,* 48–78.

Leerkes, E., & Siepak, K. (2006). Attachment linked predictors of women's emotional and cognitive responses to infant distress. *Attachment and Human Development, 8,* 11–32.

Lench, H. C., Quas, J. A., & Edelstein, R. S. (2006). My child is better than average: The extension and restriction of unrealistic optimism. *Journal of Applied Social Psychology, 36,* 2963–2979.

Madigan, S., Bakermans-Kranenburg, M. J., van IJzendoorn, M. H., Moran, G., Pederson, D. R., & Benoit, D. (2006). Unresolved states of mind, anomalous parental behavior, and disorganized attachment: A review and meta-analysis of a transmission gap. *Attachment and Human Development, 8,* 89–111.

Main, M., Kaplan, N., & Cassidy, J. (1985). Security in infancy, childhood, and adulthood: A move to the level of representation. In I. Bretherton & E. Waters (Eds.), Growing points of attachment theory and research. *Monographs of the Society for Research in Child Development, 50*(1–2, Serial No. 209), 66–104.

Mayseless, O., & Scher, A. (2000). Mother's attachment concerns regarding spouse and infant's temperament as modulators of maternal separation anxiety. *Journal of Child Psychology and Psychiatry, 41,* 917–925.

Meins, E. (1997). *Security of attachment and the social development of cognition.* Hove, UK: Psychology Press.

Meredith, P., & Noller, P. (2003). Attachment and infant difficultness in postnatal depression. *Journal of Family Issues, 24,* 668–686.

Mikulincer, M., & Florian, V. (1998). The relationship between adult attachment styles and emotional and cognitive reactions to stressful events. In J. A. Simpson & W. S. Rholes (Eds.), *Attachment theory and close relationships* (pp. 143–165). New York: Guilford Press.

Mikulincer, M., & Florian, V. (1999a). The association between spouses' self-reports of attachment styles and representations of family dynamics. *Family Process, 38,* 69–83.

Mikulincer, M., & Florian, V. (1999b). The association between parental reports of attachment style and family dynamics, and offspring's reports of adult attachment style. *Family Process, 38,* 243–257.

Mikulincer, M., & Florian, V. (1999c). Maternal–fetal bonding, coping strategies, and mental health during pregnancy: The contribution of attachment style. *Journal of Social and Clinical Psychology, 18,* 255–276.

Mikulincer, M., Gillath, O., Halevy, V., Avihou, N., Avidan, S., & Eshkoli, N. (2001). Attachment theory and reactions to others' needs: Evidence that activation of the sense of attachment security promotes empathic responses. *Journal of Personality and Social Psychology, 81,* 1205–1224.

Mikulincer, M., & Shaver, P. R. (2007). *Attachment in adulthood: Structure, dynamics, and change.* New York: Guilford Press.

Mikulincer, M., Shaver, P. R., Gillath, O., & Nitzberg, R. A. (2005). Attachment, caregiving, and altruism: Boosting attachment security increases compassion and helping. *Journal of Personality and Social Psychology, 89,* 817–839.

Millings, A., Walsh, J., Hepper, E., & O'Brien, M. (2013). Good partner, good parent: Responsiveness mediates the link between romantic attachment and parenting style. *Personality and Social Psychology Bulletin, 39,* 170–180.

Mills-Koonce, W., Appleyard, K., Barnett, M., Deng, M., Putallaz, M., & Cox, M. (2011). Adult attachment style and stress as risk factors for early maternal sensitivity and negativity. *Infant Mental Health Journal, 32,* 277–285.

Moncher, F. J. (1996). The relationship of maternal adult attachment style and risk of physical child abuse. *Journal of Interpersonal Violence, 11,* 335–350.

Nathanson, A. I., & Manohar, U. (2012). Attachment, working models of parenting, and expectations for using television in childrearing. *Family Relations: An Interdisciplinary Journal of Applied Family Studies, 61,* 441–454.

Nygren, M., Carstensen, J., Ludvigsson, J., & Frostell, A. (2012). Adult attachment and parenting stress among parents of toddlers. *Journal of Reproductive and Infant Psychology, 30,* 289–302.

Oppenheim, D., & Koren-Karie, N. (2009). Infant–parent relationship assessment: Parents' insightfulness regarding their young children's internal worlds. In C. R. Zeanah (Ed.), *Handbook of infant mental health* (3rd ed., pp. 266–280). New York: Guilford Press.

Pesonen, A., Räikkönen, K., Keltikangas-Järvinen, L., Strandberg, T., & Järvenpää, A. (2003). Parental perception of infant temperament: Does parents' joint attachment matter? *Infant Behavior and Development, 26,* 167–182.

Pesonen, A., Räikkönen, K., Strandberg, T., Kelitikangas-Järvinen, L., & Järvenpää, A. (2004). Insecure adult attachment style and depressive symptoms:

Implications for parental perceptions of infant temperament. *Infant Mental Health Journal, 25,* 99–116.

Priel, B., & Besser, A. (2000). Adult attachment styles, early relationships, antenatal attachment, and perceptions of infant temperament: A study of first-time mothers. *Personal Relationships, 7,* 291–310.

Powers, S. I., Pietromonaco, P. R., Gunlicks, M., & Sayer, A. (2006). Dating couples' attachment styles and patterns of cortisol reactivity and recovery in response to a relationship conflict. *Journal of Personality and Social Psychology, 90,* 613–628.

Rholes, W. S., Simpson, J. A., & Blakely, B. S. (1995). Adult attachment styles and mothers' relationships with their young children. *Personal Relationships, 2,* 35–54.

Rholes, W. S., Simpson, J. A., Blakely, B. S., Lanigan, L., & Allen, E. A. (1997). Adult attachment styles, the desire to have children, and working models of parenthood. *Journal of Personality, 65,* 357–385.

Rholes, W. S., Simpson, J. A., & Friedman, M. (2006). Avoidant attachment and the experience of parenting. *Personality and Social Psychology Bulletin, 32,* 275–285.

Rholes, W. S., Simpson, J. A., Kohn, J. L., Wilson, C. L., Martin, A., Tran, S., et al. (2011). Attachment orientations and depression: A longitudinal study of new parents. *Journal of Personality and Social Psychology, 100,* 567–586.

Rholes, W. S., Simpson, J. A., & Oriña, M. (1999). Attachment and anger in an anxiety-provoking situation. *Journal of Personality and Social Psychology, 76,* 940–957.

Riem, M. E., Bakermans-Kranenburg, M. J., van IJzendoorn, M. H., Out, D., & Rombouts, S. B. (2012). Attachment in the brain: Adult attachment representations predict amygdala and behavioral responses to infant crying. *Attachment and Human Development, 14,* 533–551.

Rodriguez, C. M. (2006). Emotional functioning, attachment style, and attributions as predictors of child abuse potential in domestic violence victims. *Violence and Victims, 21,* 199–212.

Roisman, G. I., Fraley, R., & Belsky, J. (2007). A taxometric study of the Adult Attachment Interview. *Developmental Psychology, 43,* 675–686.

Roisman, G. I., Holland, A., Fortuna, K., Fraley, R., Clausell, E., & Clarke, A. (2007). The Adult Attachment Interview and self-reports of attachment style: An empirical rapprochement. *Journal of Personality and Social Psychology, 92,* 678–697.

Scharf, M., & Mayseless, O. (2011). Buds of parenting in emerging adult males: What we learned from our parents. *Journal of Adolescent Research, 26,* 479–505.

Scher, A., & Dror, E. (2003). Attachment, caregiving, and sleep: The tie that keeps infants and mothers awake. *Sleep and Hypnosis, 5,* 27–37.

Scher, A., & Mayseless, O. (1994). Mothers' attachment with spouse and parenting in the first year. *Journal of Social and Personal Relationships, 11,* 601–609.

Scher, A., & Mayseless, O. (1997). Changes in negative emotionality in infancy: The role of mother's attachment concerns. *British Journal of Developmental Psychology, 15,* 311–321.

Selcuk, E., Günaydin, G., Sumer, N., Harma, M., Salman, S., Hazan, C., et al. (2010). Self-reported romantic attachment style predicts everyday maternal caregiving behavior at home. *Journal of Research in Personality, 44,* 544–549.

Shaver, P. R., & Mikulincer, M. (2002). Attachment-related psychodynamics. *Attachment and Human Development, 4,* 133–161.

Shaver, P. R., Mikulincer, M., Lavy, S., & Cassidy, J. (2009). Understanding and altering hurt feelings: An attachment-theoretical perspective on the generation and regulation of emotions. In A. L. Vangelisti (Ed.), *Feeling hurt in close relationships* (pp. 92–122). New York: Cambridge University Press.

Simpson, J. A., Rholes, W. S., Campbell, L., & Wilson, C. L. (2003). Changes in attachment orientations across the transitions to parenthood. *Journal of Experimental Social Psychology, 39,* 317–331.

Simpson, J. A., Rholes, W. S., & Nelligan, J. S. (1992). Support seeking and support giving within couples in an anxiety-provoking situation: The role of attachment styles. *Journal of Personality and Social Psychology, 62,* 434–446.

Simpson, J. A., Rholes, W. S., Oriña, M., & Grich, J. (2002). Working models of attachment, support giving, and support seeking in a stressful situation. *Personality and Social Psychology Bulletin, 28,* 598–608.

Simpson, J. A., Rholes, W. S., & Phillips, D. (1996). Conflict in close relationships: An attachment perspective. *Journal of Personality and Social Psychology, 71,* 899–914.

Slade, A. (2005). Parental reflective functioning: An introduction. *Attachment and Human Development, 7,* 269–281.

Snell, W. R., Overbey, G. A., & Brewer, A. (2005). Parenting perfectionism and the parenting role. *Personality and Individual Differences, 39,* 613–624.

Solomon, J., & George, C. (1996). Defining the caregiving system: Toward a theory of caregiving. *Infant Mental Health Journal, 17,* 183–197.

Stattin, H., & Kerr, M. (2000). Parental monitoring: A reinterpretation. *Child Development, 71,* 1072–1085.

Stevenson-Hinde, J. (1994). An ethological perspective. *Psychological Inquiry, 5,* 62–65.

Strathearn, L. (2011). Maternal neglect: Oxytocin, dopamine and the neurobiology of attachment. *Journal of Neuroendocrinology, 23,* 1054–1065.

Strathearn, L., Fonagy, P., Amico, J., & Montague, P. (2009). Adult attachment predicts maternal brain and oxytocin response to infant cues. *Neuropsychopharmacology, 34,* 2655–2666.

Trillingsgaard, T., Elklit, A., Shevlin, M., & Maimburg, R. D. (2011). Adult attachment at the transition to motherhood: Predicting worry, health care utility and relationship functioning. *Journal of Reproductive and Infant Psychology, 29,* 354–363.

van IJzendoorn, M. (1995). Adult attachment representations, parental responsiveness, and infant attachment: A meta-analysis on the predictive validity of the Adult Attachment Interview. *Psychological Bulletin, 117,* 387–403.

Vasquez, K., Durik, A. M., & Hyde, J. (2002). Family and work: Implications of adult attachment styles. *Personality and Social Psychology Bulletin, 28,* 874–886.

Vieira, J., Ávila, M., & Matos, P. (2012). Attachment and parenting: The mediating role of work–family balance in Portuguese parents of preschool children. *Family Relations: An Interdisciplinary Journal of Applied Family Studies, 61*, 31–50.

Wilson, C. L., Rholes, W. S., Simpson, J. A., & Tran, S. (2007). Labor, delivery, and early parenthood: An attachment theory perspective. *Personality and Social Psychology Bulletin, 33*, 505–518.

Attachment Theory in Organizational Settings

Ramona L. Paetzold

According to Mikulincer and Shaver (2007), social-psychological approaches to attachment theory show that it addresses important psychodynamic issues beyond close personal relationships, including those present in important organizational processes and outcomes. Bowlby himself described attachment theory as being relevant "from the cradle to the grave" (1973, p. 203), noting that the lack of appropriately supportive and protective caregivers when growing up can have far-reaching effects. He described individuals who, early in life, lack good-quality care as "hav[ing] no confidence that a caretaking figure will ever be truly available and dependable," further mentioning that their world is "seen as comfortless and unpredictable; and they respond either by shrinking from it or by doing battle with it" (1973, p. 208).

Organizations are complex and inherently interpersonal entities, requiring workers to negotiate lateral and hierarchical relationships, learn role identities, communicate and coordinate activities in interdependent settings, balance work and family issues, engage in self-regulation, and meet organizational norms to become valued and contributing organizational members. And as Hazan and Shaver (1990) have shown, adult romantic attachment style is predictably linked to work orientations, attitudes, and motivations. It is not surprising, therefore, that a growing literature on the role of attachment theory in organizations has accumulated within the last 15–20 years. Attachment theory has been shown to account for variance in organizational variables over and above that of the Big Five traits (Neustadt,

Charorro-Premuzic, & Furnham, 2011; Noftle & Shaver, 2006; Richards & Schat, 2011), measures of which are the most widely used assessments of personality in organizational behavior research (e.g., Barrick & Mount, 1991; Christiansen & Tett, 2013; Judge, Heller, & Mount, 2002).

This chapter begins with an overview of the justifications that have been provided for considering attachment theory as relevant to organizational relationships and processes. Next, the chapter addresses the myriad problems with measurement of attachment style, noting that the methods used are often parallel but distinct from those that have evolved in developmental and social psychology. Third, the bulk of the chapter reviews the substantial body of research that has included attachment style as an important consideration for understanding organizational phenomena. The chapter concludes with suggestions to extend the role that attachment theory may play in organizational research.

Conceptual Rationales for Including Attachment Theory in Organizational Research

There are several theoretical justifications for linking attachment style to the workplace. Hazan and Shaver (1990) saw work as paralleling play in infants and children. Other researchers have noted that many organizational relationships are dyadic in nature, such as leader–follower or supervisor–subordinate, which are similar to parent–child (e.g., Game, 2008; Davidovitz, Mikulincer, Shaver, Izsak, & Popper, 2007). These relationships are argued to allow for proximity seeking in times of need, a safe haven where social support can be obtained, and a secure base from which the follower/subordinate can explore and learn. This is particularly true for workplace relationships in which there is regular interaction, such as in supervisory relationships (Game, 2008).

Some researchers see even fairly distal relationships as providing *attachment dynamics*, allowing organizations to supplement individual needs for belonging and social involvement that may not be met in other close dyadic relationships (e.g., Mayseless & Popper, 2007). For example, leaders such as CEOs—whom employees don't know personally and who are unfamiliar with their employees—may be part of attachment dynamics by symbolically providing a sense of security (say, by appearing close and familiar through media self-disclosures). Or employees may have less need for attachment figures because, when distressed, they can use institutional processes such as grievance systems, help lines, and other human resource services for instrumental support (Mayseless & Popper, 2007).

One avenue for bringing attachment theory to work that has not been explicitly explored is the use of *group-level attachment*, a concept first proposed and measured by Smith, Murphy, and Coats (1999). Work settings or entire organizations can serve as groups, which can vary in size, cohesion, and entitativity. Smith et al. (1999) demonstrated, using their Social Group Attachment Scale, that group-level attachment style is distinct from romantic relationship attachment style and from group identification. Thus a combination of the two types of attachment style could be useful for understanding attachment theory's role in organizations.

Measurement Issues and Organizational Research

How to measure attachment style for organizational research is an unresolved issue that can make comparability of studies difficult. There is still considerable reliance on categorical measures, including Hazan and Shaver's (1990) three prototypes (referred to as H&S in this chapter) and Bartholomew and Horowitz's (1991) Relationship Questionnaire (RQ). The H&S classification allows participants to classify themselves as secure, anxious/ambivalent, or avoidant. The RQ leads to four prototypic forms for attachment style: secure, preoccupied (similar to anxious/ambivalent), dismissing/avoidant, and fearful/avoidant. Social psychologists have largely abandoned these in favor of dimensional measures of anxiety and avoidance—for example, the Adult Attachment Questionnaire (AAQ; Simpson, 1990; Simpson, Rholes, & Phillips, 1996) and more recently the Experiences in Close Relationships (ECR) scale (Brennan, Clark, & Shaver, 1998), which have been accepted as assessing (relatively) orthogonal factors underlying the adult attachment style construct. Low scores on anxiety and avoidance imply attachment security for these dimensional measures. In organizational research, there are multiple dimensional measures, typically looking at the relationship between the respondent and "work" or others at work. The most similar to the ECR is the Experience of Relationships Scale (ERS; Richards & Schat, 2011), which is directly adapted from the ECR by changing the word "partner" to "others" or "other people."

Another alternative, the Adult Attachment in the Workplace (AAW) scale (Neustadt, Chamorro-Premuzic, & Furnham, 2006, 2011), is based on Collins and Read's (1990) 18-item Adult Attachment Scale (AAS) but changes the language about romantic partners to "my boss" and about "people" to "others at work" and "work colleagues." Whereas the AAS separates avoidance into two highly correlated subfacets understood to be related to avoidance and a separate subfacet representing anxiety (Mikulincer & Shaver, 2007), the AAW represents two oblique factors (Secure/ Autonomous, or SAAW, and Insecure, or IAW) that the authors interpret as representing security and insecurity. Sample items on the SAAW subscale include "I find it relatively easy to get close to others at work" and "I do not often worry about being left in the lurch at work"; sample items on the IAW subscale are "I often worry that people will not want to stay on my work team" and "I get nervous when anyone at work confides too much." Thus it appears that each dimension of the AAW combines elements of anxiety (i.e., worrying about rejection/abandonment) and avoidance (i.e., handling issues of physical/psychological closeness), posing problems for interpretation.

One often-used self-report scale is substantially different from others in the organizational literature. The Self-Reliance Inventory (SRI; Quick, Joplin, Nelson, & Quick, 1992) appears to have been developed at about the same time as early dimensional scales in the social-psychological literature. It generates three factors: Counterdependence (dismissing), Overdependence (preoccupied), and Interdependence (secure) (Joplin, Nelson, & Quick, 1999; Little, Nelson, Wallace, & Johnson, 2011). The SRI contains items such as "Needing someone is a sign of weakness" (Counterdependence), "My desire to be close to my coworkers sometimes scares them away" (Overdependence), and "I can usually take care of my own work but I don't mind getting help if I need it" (Interdependence) (Little et al., 2011). Although an early version of the SRI has been validated and recommended for use by organizational researchers (Hinkin, 1995), a question remains as to how this scale can be compared to two-dimensional scales focusing on anxiety and avoidance, where security represents being low in either or both.

Throughout this chapter, the ECR (either the short or the long form) has been used to measure attachment style unless another measure is designated.

Attachment Theory and Organizational Research

Today's workplaces often demand cooperative teamwork, increased interdependence, prosocial behaviors, and high-quality relationships among employees. At the same time, job satisfaction, job performance, and factors that affect them continue to be of utmost importance to organizational researchers. This section of the chapter reviews the role that attachment theory plays throughout a series of often interrelated workplace or organizational constructs. To some extent, areas of specialization have grown up separately around these key concepts, and the chapter tends to reflect those. First, workplace group and dyadic processes are examined. The remaining portion of this section of the chapter explores constructs from more of an individual perspective, which, according to Murphy (1996), can be reflected in either the employee's experiences in the workplace (e.g., attitudes, attributions) or task- and non-task-related behaviors in the workplace. These latter constructs are therefore divided along those lines.

Work Group and Team Processes

In general, attachment styles have been predictably linked to affect and cognitions toward groups, perceptions of social support from groups, satisfaction with groups, group functioning, and plans for group exit. In their study of social groups, Smith et al. (1999) found that members high in anxiety experienced more negative affect toward, and lower levels of social support from, their groups. Members high in avoidance, on the other hand, experienced lower positive affect, perceived less social support, and provided exit intentions for the group. These findings parallel Rom and Mikulincer's (2003) results concerning work groups in both laboratory and field (military) settings. Using a 10-item attachment style scale developed by Mikulincer, Florian, and Tolmacz (1990), they found that people with higher levels of anxiety had stronger negative emotions, more negative memories about group interactions, and more negative self-appraisals resulting from group interactions; saw group activities as threatening; had lower perceptions of self-efficacy in the group; and performed poorly on group tasks (based on self-report and observers' ratings). Higher levels of avoidance were related to more negative appraisals of and lack of closeness to group members, increased dismissal of any potential benefits from group interactions, endorsement of self-reliance goals, and lower levels of task and socioemotional functioning. Unexpectedly, more avoidant group members also experienced greater recall of negative memories of group interactions; according to Rom and Mikulincer (2003), this indicates that suppression of feelings of distress is difficult in settings where a high level of interdependence (e.g., a team-based setting) is required.

Although group cohesion was related to improved group functioning, it did not improve task functioning for more avoidant individuals, who appeared not to benefit from the support or security cohesion represented. Group cohesion may in fact signal a high level of interdependence that should be threatening to more avoidant people's needs for self-reliance (Mikulincer & Shaver, 2007). Cohesion did attenuate the negative relationship between anxiety and self-perception of task functioning, so that group cohesion seemed to provide a buffer by allowing support for more anxious individuals to engage in task performance.

Rom (2008), also using Mikulincer et al.'s (1990) attachment style scale, examined the attachment-related mental representations of group members, where the groups could be more properly referred to as *teams*. In other words, they were role-delineated, highly structured, and task-oriented, with high levels of interdependence required for task performance (e.g., Crawford & LePine, 2013). Rom's study of undergraduates who had "command-and-control" team experience in the military revealed that avoidance was significantly related to lower instrumental content and to lower positive and higher negative content regarding teams. Persons higher in anxiety demonstrated lower cognitive complexity in their team mental representations, while those with higher avoidance had lower levels of mental differentiation. In combination, these results suggest that insecurity is related to lower perceptions of team performance and/or dismissal of the importance of team-based interactions.

Finally, Daus and Joplin (1999), using the SRI with undergraduates who, in small groups, performed consensus-based ranking tasks, found that groups composed of members who were more counterdependent had lower levels of group satisfaction (and satisfaction with the emergent leader, who was determined by both group leaders and a research assistant). Average group-level attachment style also interacted with group-level coping strategies to have an impact on group performance. Lower performance was associated with high average group counterdependence paired with high levels of group members' coping avoidance. High average group levels of counterdependence coupled with a group's greater likelihood to use positive reappraisal also was associated with lower group satisfaction, satisfaction with the leader, and with the task.[1] Daus and Joplin (1991) also investigated the effects of *leader* attachment and coping styles on group performance, finding that higher levels of leader counterdependence interacted with the leader's avoidant coping style to predict lower group performance, as did higher levels of leader overdependence paired with a leader's lack of using positive reappraisal as a coping style.

Leaders and Followers

Using Freud's work as a basis, organizational researchers have drawn parallels between parent–child and leader–follower relationships (Keller, 2003; Keller & Cacioppe, 2001; Popper & Amit, 2009; Popper, Mayseless, & Castelnovo, 2000; Towler, 2005). The early focus was on transformational (i.e., more relational) leaders, because they tend to provide strong investments of emotional and instrumental resources in their followers; they are responsive and sensitive to followers' needs; and they give followers individualized attention in the spirit of empowering them to build self-esteem and individual autonomy. Transformational leaders also model prosocial behaviors, being empathetic and nurturing (Popper & Mayseless, 2003). Thus transformational leaders are sensitive, responsive caregivers who provide their followers with a sense of security that enables followers to self-actualize. By contrast, more personalized (i.e., less relational) leaders follow their own personal vision and self-interests; provide one-way

---

[1] It should be noted that because Daus and Joplin (1999) were apparently unaware of Smith et al.'s (1999) work, they did not consider a group-based measure of attachment orientation, but averaged individual group members' scores to represent a group-level attachment style.

communication; are more detached, more self-oriented, and less empathetic; and can be prone to narcissism (Shalit, Popper, & Zakay, 2010). Popper et al. (2000), using the SRI, found that transformational leadership characteristics were correlated with having a secure attachment style. Moss (2009), using the AAQ, found that leaders (supervisors) of more anxiously attached individuals were less transformational, suggesting an effect for followers on leadership style.

Motives for becoming leaders have also been demonstrated to vary across attachment styles, as shown by Davidovitz, Mikulincer, Shaver, Izsak, and Popper (2007). Greater anxiety was linked to seeing leadership as an opportunity to have needs for acceptance met, while more avoidant persons sought to be leaders to distance themselves from followers and viewed leadership as an opportunity to demonstrate their autonomy and toughness. Attachment insecurity in general reduced the probability than at individual would have prosocial motives for leadership and was associated with more personalized forms of leadership. Greater anxiety was related to control-related motives, whereas greater avoidance was associated with lower task-oriented motives (possibly a way of avoiding the interdependence necessary for task performance). Thus higher security was linked to having motives related to being prosocial, being supportive, and in general being more of a transformational leader.

This does not mean that followers necessarily prefer leaders who are more secure, more transformational (relational), or less personalized. For example, Mikulincer and Florian (1995), using the H&S attachment measure, found that individuals with either a secure or an avoidant attachment style were viewed as more suitable for officer roles by their military peers. Thus even avoidant leaders may be viewed as capable of providing instrumental forms of leadership, at least in military settings. Furthermore, followers' attachment styles help to predict their leadership preferences. Shalit et al. (2010) compared preferences for personalized leaders over socialized leaders, and found (based on use of the H&S measure) that among college students who viewed videos comparing candidates for a CEO position, secure students preferred more socialized leaders over personalized leaders, while avoidant students had just the opposite preference. Berson, Dan, and Yammarino (2006) found, again using the H&S prototypes, that secure followers emphasize more relationship-oriented qualities in their ideal leaders than do either ambivalent or avoidant followers. Using the RQ in a study of adult workers in a retail organization, Boatwright, Lopez, Sauer, VanDerWege, and Huber (2010) demonstrated that workers who were preoccupied reported stronger preferences for relational forms of leadership as ideal than did workers who were dismissing/avoidant. Secure workers also more strongly preferred relationship leadership than did dismissing/avoidant workers. Thus it appears that secure followers, who can work well with others and will rely on leadership from appropriate others when it is needed, and preoccupied followers, who exhibit more dependence on others and require support and comforting to manage anxiety, prefer a relational style of interacting with a leader/supervisor, whereas dismissing/avoidant followers, who strongly value autonomy and independence and cope with distress through distancing, apparently do not. While results on leadership preferences across these studies are somewhat mixed, it appears that relational or transformational leaders are preferred by followers who are not more avoidant. This finding can perhaps be explained by Davidovitz et al. (2007), who found that followers who were high in avoidance viewed leaders as having less ability to lead in both task- and emotion-focused situations. More avoidant followers also tended to view themselves as having lower instrumental and socioemotional functioning within teams.

Most studies indicate advantages for having more secure leaders. Davidovitz et al. (2007) found that when followers assessed leader performance, they saw leaders higher in avoidance as having lower efficacy in handling emotion-focused situations, and perceived leaders higher in anxiety as having lower efficacy in handling task-focused situations. Officers having higher avoidance were also viewed as having military units with less cohesion. Leader attachment style was related to follower self-ratings of functioning as well: High leader avoidance was negatively associated with follower self-ratings of socioemotional functioning, while high leader anxiety was positively associated with such self-ratings. These effects for leader and follower were additive, so that the pairing of a leader high on avoidance with followers high on avoidance led to fewer contributions from followers to a positive emotional climate and the lowest amount of unit cohesion of any leader–follower pairing. This suggests that leader–follower congruence in attachment styles—a model proposed by Keller (2003) for beneficial attachment-related leadership—does not appear to hold for avoidance.

Research has also shown that leader avoidance tends to have particularly deleterious effects on the health and well-being of followers. In a longitudinal study, Davidovitz et al. (2007) assessed mental health outcomes of followers when the leader had the opportunity to serve as a security-providing attachment figure during a stressful period of combat training. When a leader was high on avoidance, his followers saw him as less sensitive and responsive than if a leader was lower in avoidance; in addition, a soldier's own anxiety or avoidance was associated with perceptions that the leader was not a good security provider. At the level of the unit, higher leader avoidance was related to the deterioration of the mental health of the soldiers in the unit. Within the unit, soldiers who were more highly avoidant also saw greater declines in their mental health. Officer avoidance interacted with soldier insecurity, so that more insecure soldiers (either anxious or avoidant) experienced greater reductions in mental health than others. Furthermore, the soldiers' assessments of the officer's ability to be a secure attachment figure mediated the relationship between the officer's attachment style and changes in the soldiers' mental health levels. After only 2 months, leader avoidance was directly related to follower mental health, which was lower for insecure followers than for those who were more secure. Followers who were more secure managed to maintain a higher level of mental health after the 2-month period, regardless of the insecurity of their leader. This buffering of the followers' own attachment style appeared to disappear after 4 months, however, so that negative effects of the leader's avoidance were present for all soldiers, regardless of their own attachment style.

The relationship between leaders and followers has also been studied through the lens of *leader–member exchange* (LMX), which focuses on the process of dyadic relationship development via role and social exchange theories (Wayne, Shore, & Linden, 1997). For example, Towler and Stuhl-macher (2013), in a study of career-oriented working women, found that although anxiety was not related to the quality of employee relationships with supervisors (via LMX), avoidance was negatively related to LMX quality; these results support the notion that more avoidant persons do not make investments in their relationships with supervisors, perhaps as a means of maintaining distance and autonomy. In addition, having good-quality relationships with supervisors (for employees low in avoidance) was associated with less work conflict. However, Towler and Stuhlmacher (2013) did not consider the role of supervisor attachment style in determining LMX quality.

Richards and Hackett (2012)—using the ERS to measure both supervisor and subordinate attachment styles in a sample obtained through the StudyResponse project (Stanton & Weiss, 2002), and using the *actor–partner independence model* (APIM) for data analysis—found that LMX quality perceptions were negatively related to both anxiety and avoidance in an actor (i.e., there was a lack of trust, there was too much clinginess in the relationship, and individuation was hindered), but there were no partner effects. However, low levels of anxiety in actors and partners interacted to predict higher perceived levels of LMX quality, with quality deteriorating as a function of the difference between levels of anxiety in actors and partners (leaders and their subordinates). Thus there was support for a congruence effect for anxiety in LMX quality (Keller, 2003), but because there was no significant interaction for avoidance, congruence was not supported for that attachment style.

Richards and Hackett (2012) also found that cognitive and behavioral strategies such as reappraisal and suppression moderated the connection between attachment styles and LMX quality, due to either reducing the emotional impact of a situation (appraisal) or changing behavioral response to a felt emotion (suppression). A higher quality of LMX was found in dyads with highly anxious partners, when both supervisors and subordinates used reappraisal to reframe threats that triggered the attachment system (e.g., negative treatment at work, presence of work stressors). Reappraisal was not an effective strategy for avoidant dyadic partners, however, perhaps because avoidant denial prevented them from using it. Suppression of negative emotions was also an effective strategy for highly anxious dyadic partners. For highly avoidant partners, there was a significant partner effect (not an actor effect), such that LMX quality was significantly higher when these supervisor and subordinate pairs used suppression to regulate their emotions. These results regarding regulatory strategies also support Keller's (2003) notion that there is congruency in anxiety pairings, but not for partners who are avoidant.

Although not using the LMX framework, Game (2008) examined supervisor–subordinate dyadic models by looking at the differential effects of global and specific models of attachment styles. She found that supervisor-specific avoidance, but not anxiety, was related to negative relationship attributions, above and beyond the role that global attachment styles played. In this research, global attachment styles were measured with a version of the ECR adapted to the workplace (e.g., "others" instead of "my partner"); specific attachment styles were measured with a combination of items from the ECR and the Client Attachment to Therapist Scale (Mallinckrodt, Gant, & Coble, 1995), reworded to refer to supervisors. Supervisor-specific avoidance was also positively related to anger and distress within supervisory relationships, beyond the contribution of global attachment styles, and this association was partially mediated by negative attributions about the supervisory relationship. Furthermore, there was no buffering effect for global attachment styles in these relationships; in fact, when global anxiety was lower (higher global security), the relationship between supervisor-specific anxiety and anger was stronger. Anger toward the supervisor appeared to be high, regardless of the level of supervisor-specific anxiety, but particularly when global anxiety levels were high. Game's (2008) work provides the first indication that when researchers are assessing outcomes for dyadic relationships in organizations, it may be important to consider the different roles that global and specific attachment styles play.

Attitudes in and Experience of the Workplace

Stress, Health, and Job Burnout

Attachment styles also play an important role in the experience of stress and health outcomes related to work, as well as job burnout. Early research (Joplin et al., 1999) found that having a secure attachment style (as assessed with the SRI) was positively related to both physical and psychological well-being, whereas insecure attachment styles had the opposite effect (both counterdependence and overdependence were positively associated with psychological symptoms, anxiety and insomnia, and social dysfunction).

Although results vary across studies, research in general has demonstrated some negative effects of insecure attachment styles on workplace well-being. Schirmer and Lopez (2001) found that employee anxiety predicted higher levels of work stress intensity and physical/psychological symptoms such as depression, but there was a significant interaction with levels of supervisory support. With low supervisory support, highly anxious employees reported marginally higher stress levels than did those lower in anxiety, but with high levels of support, there was no significant link between anxiety and stress. Avoidance was unrelated to stress and symptomology. The authors also used the RQ, finding no difference in work stress among anxious, secure, and dismissing/avoidant employees.

Clearer effects have also been established between employee attachment insecurity and job burnout. For example, Simmons, Gooty, Nelson, and Little (2009) found that having a secure attachment style (as measured by the Interdependence subscale of the SRI) was negatively related to burnout (measured as emotional exhaustion, physical fatigue, and cognitive weariness), although security was positively associated with feelings of hope. Negative appraisals of contextual workplace factors may be the critical link between attachment insecurity and burnout. Ronen and Mikulincer (2009) studied nonmanagerial Israeli employees from a large variety of business organizations to determine whether perceptions of team cohesion and organizational fairness mediated the insecurity–burnout connection. Anxiety and avoidance were both positively linked to job burnout, with perceptions of organizational fairness completely mediating the association between avoidance and burnout.[2] Avoidance was associated with lowered perceptions of organizational fairness, which in turn was positively related to job burnout. Also, lower levels of perceived team cohesion partially mediated the association between anxiety and burnout. This study demonstrates that attachment styles negatively bias appraisal of contextual workplace factors, thus both directly and indirectly contributing to job burnout. Similarly, Ronen and Baldwin (2010), using the same burnout measure, demonstrated in a longitudinal study that perceptions of social rejection mediated the relation between anxiety and perceived stress, as well as the connection between anxiety and prospective job burnout. Being hypersensitive to perceived social rejection from others at work (i.e., work colleagues) predicted higher levels of perceived stress and job burnout 1 month later.

Furthermore, the attachment styles of supervisors or managers, as well

---

[2]Here, burnout was assessed with the Maslach Burnout Inventory—General Scale (Schaufeli, Leiter, Maslach, & Jackson, 1996), which measures emotional exhaustion, cynicism, and professional effectiveness.

as their caregiving styles, have an impact on employee levels of job burnout. Ronen and Mikulincer (2012) found that not only were subordinates' reports of job burnout related to their own attachment avoidance and anxiety (with higher burnout being associated with higher levels of insecurity), but their job burnout levels were also directly related to their direct managers' levels of anxiety (but not avoidance). There also was an interaction between managers' avoidance and subordinate anxiety, however, such that managers' level of avoidance had a negative impact on the self-appraised efficacy of subordinates who scored relatively low on attachment anxiety (i.e., relatively secure subordinates perceived themselves as less capable when their managers were more avoidant). Subordinates who were higher in anxiety did not report that their efficacy levels were affected by direct manager avoidance. Managerial caregiving style fully mediated the connection between managers' anxiety level and subordinate job burnout, such that managers higher in anxiety tended to use more hyperactivated caregiving styles, which accounted for subordinate job burnout. Managers with deactivated caregiving styles did not affect subordinates' reports of job burnout. Thus one form of nonoptimal managerial caregiving—being coercive and/or intrusive—completely explained the relationship between a manager's anxiety and a subordinate's associated job burnout.

In addition to differences in experience of job burnout, employees use different coping strategies to handle it. In a set of studies focused on different cultural groups of individuals living within Israel, Pines (2004) found that different attachment styles were related to different ways of coping with the emotional exhaustion dimension of burnout. Using Mikulincer et al.'s (1990) measure of attachment styles, Pines found a negative link between attachment security and burnout, and a positive correlation between both avoidance and anxiety and burnout, among Israeli nurses, Hungarian nurses, an Arab sample living in Israel, and an Israeli national sample (with anxiety being the best predictor of burnout for this last group). Furthermore, in terms of coping with burnout, security was related to viewing burnout in a more positive light and was negatively correlated with ignoring it. Anxiety was negatively related to solving issues related to burnout and seeing positive aspects of burnout, but was positively related to negative coping strategies such as ignoring it, obsessing over it, using drugs, and avoiding the situation. Avoidance was negatively correlated with talking about burnout problems and positively related to avoiding and leaving the situation.

Work Engagement

Work engagement is often represented by two constructs: *vigor* at work and *dedication* (Schaufeli, Salanova, González-Romá, & Bakker, 2002). Little et al. (2011) have defined vigor as a "positive affective state in a work context that combines elements of an emotion and a mood state" (p. 467), and that provides physical and emotional energy as well as mental alertness for performing the job. Dedication, on the other hand, represents a sense of purpose and pride at work (Moss, 2009).

Using the AAQ, Moss (2009) found that vigor and dedication were both inversely correlated with anxiety and avoidance. In a more specialized study of vigor based on the SRI, Little et al. (2011) found that security was positively related to vigor, and, like Moss (2009), found that both counterdependence and overdependence were negatively related to vigor at work. They interpreted these results as being consistent with the characteristics of anxiety and avoidance. For example, counterdependent workers may engage in defense mechanisms of denial or repression to avoid activation of their attachment systems, which in turn may deplete their resource availability for work. Overdependent individuals may be in a state of hyperactivation, with heightened levels of distress and rumination that leave few resources available for vigor at work. In total, these results indicate that employees higher in attachment security may be less engaged (or more disengaged) from work, which is consistent with the findings on job burnout (which may be loosely interpreted as a form of work disengagement).

Job Satisfaction

Studies have tended to show that more insecure workers tend to be dissatisfied with at least some aspects of their jobs (e.g., lack of recognition, coworkers, overall job) (Hardy & Barkham, 1994; Hazan & Shaver, 1990; Ronen & Mikulincer, 2012; Sumer & Knight, 2001). Both moderators and mediators have been investigated to explain the link between attachment insecurity and job dissatisfaction. In a survey study of employees, Schirmer and Lopez (2001), who incorporated both the RQ and the ECR into their research, found that avoidance interacted with supervisory support to predict levels of job satisfaction. In particular, under low levels of support, workers who were more highly avoidant (ECR) reported higher job satisfaction than did those who were lower in avoidance, but under high levels of support, the group means were the same.[3] Towler and Stuhlmacher (2013), in their study of working women, found that the association between avoidance and job dissatisfaction was fully mediated by LMX.[4] Avoidance was negatively related to LMX, which was positively related to job satisfaction, such that more secure women reported higher levels of job satisfaction as a result of having higher-quality relationships with their

---

[3] The RQ, however, did not detect differences in job satisfaction among preoccupied, secure, and dismissing/avoidant workers.

[4] Anxiety was not related to any of the mediators, and thus not to job satisfaction in the mediation model.

supervisors. These two studies indicate the role that supervisory support and the quality of supervisory relationships can play in determining job satisfaction. More avoidant individuals are more satisfied without much support from supervisors (an interaction effect), but because they tend to have poor-quality relationships with their supervisors (as viewed through an LMX lens), they tend to be less satisfied with their jobs (a mediation effect). In other words, highly avoidant employees tend to prefer that their supervisors allow them to work unaided, but relational leadership, as provided through LMX, does not permit that outcome.

Managerial/supervisory attachment styles are also related to subordinate–employee job satisfaction levels. Ronen and Mikulincer (2012) found that a manager's anxiety was negatively related to his or her subordinates' job satisfaction level, and that the hyperactivated caregiving associated with the level of managerial anxiety accounted for the lowered job satisfaction of the subordinates. Managers' avoidance bore no connection to the job satisfaction of their subordinates, however, and no dyadic interactions of attachment styles predicted the job satisfaction levels of subordinates.

Work–Family Issues

Work–family balance (or work–family conflict) continues to be a major area of organizational research, with models of the work–family interface becoming increasingly complex over time (Ferguson, Carlson, Zivnuska, & Whitten, 2012). Research in this area largely supports a *spillover* model, indicating that work experiences flow into family life (and vice versa) (Kinnunen, Feldt, Geurts, & Pulkkinen, 2006). Crossover effects based on workplace support for not only the employee, but also the spouse/partner and children, can also be important in work–family issues (Ransford, Crouter, & McHale, 2008).

Attachment research related to work–family issues is in the early stages, with most of the focus on just an employee's attachment style, and without sufficient consideration of a partner's roles or the presence of children. For example, Sumer and Knight (2001), using the RQ, reported support for the spillover model based on a measure they developed to assess work–family linkage (the Work–Family Linkage Questionnaire). On this measure, preoccupied employees reported higher levels of negative spillover from home to work than did secure or dismissing/avoidant employees (with fearful/avoidant employees not differing from secure or dismissing/avoidant ones). Secure employees were more likely to experience positive spillover from family to work than were any of the other three groups. They were also more likely to have positive spillover from work to family (compared to dismissing and fearful employees), but they did not differ from preoccupied employees on this dimension. In addition, preoccupied employees were less likely than all other groups to experience segmentation (independence of work and family lives), which indicates that such workers may use both life aspects as a means of getting their safety and other needs met.

Towler and Stuhlmacher (2013) found that having higher-quality home relationships (e.g., higher satisfaction with the partner/spouse, greater relationship cohesion)—which was related to higher levels of attachment security—was positively related to a woman's job satisfaction and lower levels of conflict in the workplace, such that being more secure was associated with more positive family–work spillover.

The most complex study to date was completed by Vasquez, Durik, and Hyde (2002), who conducted a longitudinal study to examine the experience of parenthood on work functioning. Using the RQ, they investigated mothers and fathers separately to determine how attachment styles related to variables such as marital rewards, parental stress, working hours, depression, and job satisfaction. At 1 year postpartum, secure and dismissing/avoidant mothers reported the least stress and greatest rewards from their family relationships, whereas fearful/avoidant mothers reported the most stress and fewest rewards. Depression was highest among fearful/avoidant mothers. There were no differences across the attachment style groups with regard to work functioning, however, so no spillover effects related to attachment styles were found. Among men, secure fathers tended to view family salience and parental role quality more positively and as less stressful than did fearful/avoidant fathers. Both preoccupied and fearful/avoidant fathers were more depressed than secure or dismissing/avoidant fathers. Work functioning varied across the attachment style groups, with secure fathers reporting fewer work-related concerns than either preoccupied or fearful/avoidant fathers (i.e., less negative family-work spillover). Secure fathers also reported less role overload than fearful/avoidant fathers (i.e., they reported better work–family balance).

Results were somewhat different at 4.5 years postpartum. At this follow-up, secure and dismissing/avoidant mothers were less stressed about their families and felt more rewarded in family relationships than fearful/avoidant mothers, just as at 1 year postpartum. Also, fearful/avoidant mothers at this stage reported fewer work rewards than did the other three attachment types, indicating greater negative family–work spillover for them. Differences between fearful/avoidant mothers and the other groups persisted with regard to depression, but the other three groups did not differ among themselves. For men, differences in family functioning were still present at 4.5 years postpartum, with fearful/avoidant fathers reporting the most stress and less family salience, and with secure fathers reporting the least stress and more family salience. There was no difference in depression levels among the four attachment style groups. With regard to work, however, preoccupied and fearful/avoidant fathers showed higher work-related concerns (more negative family–work spillover) and more role overload (less balance) than secure and dismissing/avoidant fathers did.

Even though Vasquez et al. (2002) provide indications of attachment-style-related support for the spillover model, several work-related outcome variables did not show significant differences across attachment styles. For example, work salience, the length of leave taken by mothers or fathers, and the number of hours worked did not vary across groups. Unexpectedly, neither dismissing/avoidant men nor women reported working a greater number of hours as a way to avoid family obligations, nor did dismissing/avoidant women take shorter maternity leaves. In general, on those variables for which there were significant differences, family and work outcomes were most positive for secure and more negative for fearful/avoidant parents, suggesting support for the spillover model of work–family balance/conflict.

Job Performance and Other Workplace Behaviors

Job Performance

There has been surprisingly little research on attachment styles and job performance, despite the construct's importance in the organizational behavior literature. Beginning with Hazan and Shaver (1990), however, there was evidence that job performance and workplace behaviors are linked to attachment styles. In the Hazan and Shaver work, secure employees reported higher levels of work success, but individuals who were anxious reported that they were unable to finish work tasks and meet work deadlines, suggesting poorer levels of work performance. Avoidant employees indicated that they persisted at work-related tasks, but tended to work alone, avoided receiving help, and gave themselves lower self-ratings on job performance, suggesting that their coworkers might similarly evaluate them.

Overall, higher levels of security are related to higher levels of job performance. Neustadt et al. (2011), using the AAW, found that individuals who scored higher on the SAAW dimension (i.e., were more secure) had higher levels of job performance, as indicated by managerial ratings provided by the organization. They further observed that this association was partially mediated by emotional self-efficacy. Simmons et al. (2009), using the Interdependence (secure) dimension of the SRI, found that more secure attachment was related to having more trust in the supervisor, which in turn was related to better employee task performance (although secure attachment did not have a direct effect on job performance).

Support Seeking

Again, little research has explicitly examined support-seeking behavior in the workplace, although work difficulties might be expected to activate the attachment system, even for individuals with lower levels of chronic activation. Using a convenience sample of different types of workers, Richards and Schat (2011), in a study using a StudyResponse project sample (Stanton & Weiss, 2002) and measuring attachment styles with the ERS, demonstrated that individuals higher in anxiety sought more emotional support from others. Although persons higher in anxiety are generally believed to fear rejection (and may therefore be less likely to seek support from collegial or supervisory relationships), this finding may result from work relationships' being designed to promote assistance, meaning that the possibility of rejection is attenuated and perceptions are not negatively biased. Employees higher in avoidance sought less instrumental and emotional support, consistent with other findings indicating that highly avoidant individuals prefer to work alone and are less satisfied with supervisory help. Furthermore, these associations held after the researchers controlled for the Big Five personality traits, trait affectivity, and level of organizational commitment.

Prosocial Behaviors

The construct most commonly used to measure prosocial behavior (support providing behavior) in the workplace is that of *organizational citizenship behaviors* (OCBs). OCBs are behaviors intended to help in the "maintenance and enhancement of the social and psychological context that supports task performance" (Organ, 1997, p. 91). These behaviors, therefore, are not task behaviors, but are generally viewed as discretionary and supportive of the organizational context (Motowidlo, 2000). OCBs are sometimes operationalized as two dimensions: OCB-I, which measures prosocial or supportive behaviors directed toward individuals within the organization, and OCB-O, which measures prosocial behaviors geared toward helping the organization (Coleman & Borman, 2000). Other researchers, however, sometimes use a five-dimensional measure for OCBs representing altruism, courtesy, sportsmanship, civic virtue, and conscientiousness (Niehoff & Moorman, 1993). Because these behaviors are generally viewed as voluntary, persons higher in attachment security should engage in more of them (Erez, Mikulincer, van IJzendoorn, & Kroonenberg, 2008).

A study by Desivilya, Sabag, and Ashton (2006) involving undergraduate employees and their reports of their OCBs found that both higher levels of anxiety and higher levels of avoidance were both associated with lower self-reports of OCBs. To explain this connection, the authors examined perceptions of *interactional justice* (a measure of organizational justice that assesses an employee's perceptions of fairness during interactions with his or her supervisor) as a potential moderator, but these perceptions did not moderate any of these relations. Richards and Schat (2011), using the ERS, found that OCB-O was negatively related to anxiety. This result was also supported by Little et al. (2011), using the SRI, who found that having an overdependent attachment style was negatively related to engaging in OCB-O. This relationship was also partially mediated by vigor, in that overdependence was negatively related to vigor and vigor was positively related to OCB-O. Thus it appears that anxiety may be positively related to OCB, but the relation between anxiety and OCB-I is not clearly established.

Using a somewhat different notion of social support, Geller and Bamberger (2009) found that for Israeli workers in call centers, higher levels of anxiety were related to lower levels of instrumental helping behavior. Avoidance was not associated with instrumental helping behavior, but this effect must be interpreted in the context of an interaction between attachment styles. Under higher levels of anxiety, the association between instrumental helping and avoidance was slightly, but not significantly, positive. At low levels of anxiety, however, the relationship between instrumental helping and avoidance was significantly negative. Workers who had more secure attachment styles provided the highest amount of instrumental help.

Antisocial Behavior

In the workplace, behaviors are sometimes viewed as counter to the best interests of the organization. Various labels have been attached to these behaviors: They are commonly termed *counterproductive work behaviors* (CWBs), *antisocial work behavior, workplace incivility,* or *workplace deviance* (Berry, Ones, & Sackett, 2007; Hershcovis, 2011). These constructs differ slightly in operationalization, but they all convey that the behaviors are undesirable and antithetical to the norms and goals of the organization. The attachment-style-related results are so far mixed. Richards and Schat (2011), using the ERS, found that anxiety was positively related, and avoidance was negatively related, to CWBs. Little et al. (2011), using the SRI, found instead that counterdependence positively predicted workplace deviance, with the relation being fully mediated by vigor at work (which was negatively related to deviance). They found no effects for either overdependence or interdependence (security).

Voluntary Turnover (Intentions)

Although extensive models of likelihood of turnover (i.e., employees' behavioral intentions to change jobs) exist in the organizational behavior literature (Lee, Mitchell, Sablynski, Burton, & Holtom, 2004), virtually no research has investigated the connection between attachment styles and turnover in organizations. Richards and Schat (2011), using the ERS, found that organizational commitment negatively predicted turnover intentions and that negative affect positively predicted such intentions, with attachment anxiety being related to turnover intentions above and beyond those significant predictors. Being more anxious predicted having a higher turnover intention. There was no relationship between turnover intentions and avoidance after the researchers controlled for other personality, attitudinal, and affective measures. Mikulincer and Shaver (2007), on the other hand, in a correlational study of high-tech workers, found that attachment insecurity was related to lower levels of organizational commitment, with avoidance being correlated with intentions to quit.

Summary and Future Research Directions

Overall, the results linking adult attachment styles to workplace or organizational processes and outcomes point to several disadvantages for insecurity. This is true across results for individuals, dyads, and teams/work groups, and the results also hold across categorical and various dimensional methods of assessing self-reported attachment styles. Thus the findings that secure employees are likely to be more satisfied, healthier, and more engaged with their work; higher performers on task-related and non-task-related jobs; less involved in deviant workplace behaviors; better team performers and team leaders; and more able to balance work and family issues appear to be quite robust. They parallel findings in the intimate relationship literature that individuals who are more secure are better caregivers and care receivers, suffer less depression and experience fewer negative emotions, and are more satisfied with their romantic relationships (see Mikulincer & Shaver, 2007, for a review). They also reflect Bowlby's (1973) view that secure individuals view the world as a more predictable place in which one can engage comfortably.

The robustness and consistency of the findings have practical issues for organizational attitudes toward this research. Although scholars have not called for employee selection based on attachment styles, they have suggested that employees might be able to "change" their attachment styles as a function of corrective experiences within the workplace, or perhaps even by having a secure style modeled (say, by a transformational leader). In general, attachment styles are relatively stable over time (e.g., Fraley, Vicary, Brumbaugh, & Roisman, 2011), although there is evidence that adult attachment styles are a function of not only early childhood caregiving experiences, but also subsequent close relationships and other life experiences (Fraley, Roisman, Booth-LaForce, Owen, & Holland, 2013). Whether attachment styles—either those representing orientations in relationships with specific individuals, or more global attachment styles—can be modified through workplace experiences is an unstudied and interesting question, one that would be of great interest to organizations.

In addition, the apparent robustness of these findings should not be construed as evidence that measurement of attachment styles is irrelevant. There are variations in the findings across different typologies or dimensions of insecurity, and these may be the result of differences in measurement. Although other design features such as types of participants, lab versus field settings, types of jobs or occupations, and organizational contexts may be responsible for some of the differential results, it is likely that the manner of assessment plays a role in outcome variation. First, it is clear that dimensional measures of attachment now constitute the accepted standard in social psychology, which underlies the study of organizational behavior. This suggests that dimensional measures are more appropriate for modern organizational research examining adult attachment styles, and that in particular, dimensional measures of avoidance and anxiety should be employed. Second, researchers need to investigate whether different dimensional measures lead to certain subtleties in outcomes. A nomological network for the role of attachment styles in organizational processes and outcomes requires that different methods of assessment be considered and compared. For example, what are the limits of romantic attachment styles for understanding organizational processes and outcomes? As noted by Mikulincer and Shaver (2007), the expansion of attachment styles to other social settings is in itself a controversial area of study and a source of tension between developmental and social psychologists. Are there organizational phenomena that cannot or should not be linked to romantic attachment styles? In addition, are there differential predictions or explanations when more organization-based attachment measures are used? Can group-related attachment styles provide further insights into the associations between attachment and workplace attitudes, experiences, and behaviors? And for dyadic workplace relationships, do more global attachment styles provide different insights than dyad-specific attachment considerations do?

One shortcoming of much of the research to date is that even in dyadic situations, the attachment style of only one dyad member is assessed. Because attachment styles are important for examining *interpersonal* processes, both members of a dyad should have their attachment styles measured and evaluated to assess dyadic processes and outcomes. Feedback loops based on each member's perceptions of the other are important in determining attitudes, emotions, and behaviors. The statistical methodology for examining dyadic data is more complex, but the gains in understanding easily offset the required use of hierarchical linear models (such as the APIM). For example, a fuller investigation of Keller's (2003) congruence model requires just such an analysis. In addition, the *formation* of attachment relationships in the workplace may best be understood through a dyadic approach. To date, no one has empirically examined how friendship bonds among work colleagues are formed, strengthened, and maintained via attachment processes.

Because of the focus on individual-difference measures (attachment styles), most of the research reviewed in this chapter has ignored the important role of organizational context. The research areas summarized above are more complex than the reviewed articles suggest; future research must examine the role that context plays in producing, exacerbating, or offsetting attachment theory effects. For example, results found among Israeli soldiers under situations of high stress may not apply to most American workplaces. Or some organizational contexts may provide such "strong situations" (e.g., highly unjust workplaces or workplaces dominated by high levels of discrimination) that they override even the otherwise beneficial effects of being more secure. Job description is another contextual variable that may also affect outcomes. For example, workers in call centers may be less likely than team workers to help each other complete tasks; attachment theory effects may therefore be stronger in one situation than the other. This suggests that context can be an important moderator of the antecedent role that attachment styles play in determining important organizational outcomes.

Greater attention also needs to be paid to mediators of the linkages between attachment styles and outcomes. Organizational attitudes, perceptions, and behaviors are complex interconnected phenomena, typically requiring mediation models to explain important pathways. Given that attachment styles have been demonstrated to be important antecedents of many workplace-related outcomes, the next step will be to insert attachment styles into these more complex mediation models to understand how views of self and other, as well as the behavioral dynamics associated with different attachment styles, affect organizational attitudes, perceptions, interpretations, experiences, and behaviors.

Many applied areas have yet to be examined from an attachment theory perspective. Fields such as constructive deviant behavior (whistleblowing, prosocial rule breaking), political workplace behavior (influence tactics), destructive leadership and abusive supervision, alternative dispute resolution (negotiation, mediation), person–organization fit, newcomer socialization (but see Nelson & Quick, 1991), and mentoring relationships are obvious areas where attachment styles would be expected to be relevant predictors. Moreover, types of employment (permanent, seasonal, temporary, full-time, part-time), compensation and benefits, training, top management teams, globalization, the boundaryless workplace, entrepreneurship, and other contemporary issues are all promising areas of study for social psychologists and organizational researchers/psychologists alike. For example, our work (Paetzold, Miner, & Carpenter, 2010) has shown that even bystanders' responses to sexual harassment of a coworker can be reliably explained by attachment theory, with more avoidant bystanders reporting less empathy for and less distress regarding the target of the harassment, including less willingness to help the target. More anxious bystanders, on the other hand, had greater empathy, felt more distress, and indicated a greater willingness to help the target. These results held even when bystander individual-difference measures such as trait empathy and negative affectivity were taken into account.

Finally, despite the important findings detailed in this chapter, there has been remarkably little research on the role of attachment theory in organizational studies in general. Every area of specialization covered in this chapter could benefit from a more extensive consideration of the role of attachment styles: Just as personality changed the way that researchers came to understand how employees interact in organizational settings (Christiansen & Tett, 2013), further work on attachment theory could add to the existing body of research and begin to revolutionize our current understanding of the roles played by employees in organizational processes and outcomes. It is hoped that this chapter will encourage researchers in both social psychology and organizational research/psychology to look beyond other individual-difference measures that are commonly used within the organizational context, and to explore more fully the role that attachment styles can—and most likely do—play.

References

Barrick, M. R., & Mount, M. K. (1991). The Big Five personality dimensions and job performance: A meta-analysis. *Personnel Psychology, 44,* 1–26.

Bartholomew, K., & Horowitz, L. M. (1991). Attachment styles among young adults: A test of a four-category model. *Journal of Personality and Social Psychology, 61,* 226–244.

Berry, C. M., Ones, D. S., & Sackett, P. R. (2007). Interpersonal deviance, organizational deviance, and their common correlates: A review and meta-analysis. *Journal of Applied Psychology, 92,* 410–424.

Berson, Y., Dan, O., & Yammarino, F. J. (2006). Attachment style and individual differences in leadership perceptions and emergence. *Journal of Social Psychology, 146,* 165–182.

Boatwright, K. J., Lopez, F. G., Sauer, E. M., VanDerWege, A., & Huber, D. M. (2010). The influence of adult attachment styles on workers' preferences for relational leadership behaviors. *Psychologist–Manager Journal, 13,* 1–14.

Bowlby, J. (1973). *Attachment and loss: Vol. 2. Separation: Anxiety and anger.* New York: Basic Books.

Brennan, K. A., Clark, C. L., & Shaver, P. R. (1998). Self-report measurement of adult romantic attachment: An integrative overview. In J. A. Simpson & W. S. Rholes (Eds.), *Attachment theory and close relationships* (pp. 46–76). New York: Guilford Press.

Christiansen, N., & Tett, R. (Eds.). (2013). *Handbook of personality at work.* New York: Routledge.

Coleman, V. I., & Borman, W. C. (2000). Investigating the underlying structure of the citizenship performance domain. *Human Resource Management Review, 10,* 25–44.

Collins, N. L., & Read, S. J. (1990). Adult attachment, working models, and relationship quality in dating couples. *Journal of Personality and Social Psychology, 58*, 644–663.

Crawford, E. R., & LePine, J. A. (2013). A configural theory of team processes: Accounting for the structure of taskwork and teamwork. *Academy of Management Review, 38*, 32–48.

Daus, C. S., & Joplin, J. R. W. (1999). Survival of the fittest: Implications for self-reliance and coping for leaders and team performance. *Journal of Occupational Health Psychology, 4*, 15–28.

Davidovitz, R., Mikulincer, M., Shaver, P. R., Izsak, R., & Popper, M. (2007). Leaders as attachment figures: Leaders' attachment orientations predict leadership-related mental representations and followers' performance and mental health. *Journal of Personality and Social Psychology, 93*, 632–650.

Desivilya, H. S., Sabag, Y., & Ashton, E. (2006). Prosocial tendencies in organizations: The role of attachment styles and organizational justice in shaping organizational citizenship behavior. *International Journal of Organizational Analysis, 14*, 22–42.

Erez, A., Mikulincer, M., van IJzendoorn, M. H., & Kroonenberg, P. M. (2008). Attachment, personality, and volunteering: Placing volunteerism in an attachment-theoretical framework. *Personality and Individual Differences, 44*, 64–74.

Ferguson, M., Carlson, D., Zivnuska, S., & Whitten, D. (2012). Support at work and home: The path to satisfaction through balance. *Journal of Vocational Behavior, 80*, 299–307.

Fraley, R. C., Roisman, G. I., Booth-LaForce, C., Owen, M. T., & Holland, A. S. (2013). Interpersonal and genetic origins of adult attachment styles: A longitudinal study from infancy to early adulthood. *Journal of Personality and Social Psychology, 104*, 817–838.

Fraley, R. C., Vicary, A. M., Brumbaugh, C. C., & Roisman, G. I. (2011). Patterns of stability in adult attachment: An empirical test of two models of continuity and change. *Journal of Personality and Social Psychology, 101*, 974–992.

Game, A. M. (2008). Negative emotions in supervisory relationships: The role of relational models. *Human Relations, 61*, 355–393.

Geller, D., & Bamberger, P. (2009). Bringing avoidance and anxiety to the job: Attachment style and instrumental helping behavior among co-workers. *Human Relations, 62*, 1803–1827.

Hardy, G. E., & Barkham, M. (1994). The relationship between interpersonal attachment styles and work difficulties. *Human Relations, 47*, 263–281.

Hazan, C., & Shaver, P. R. (1990). Love and work: An attachment-theoretical perspective. *Journal of Personality and Social Psychology, 59*, 270–280.

Hershcovis, M. S. (2011). Incivility, social undermining, bullying . . . oh my!: A call to reconcile constructs within workplace aggression research. *Journal of Organizational Behavior, 32*, 499–519.

Hinkin, T. R. (1995). A review of scale development practices in the study of organizations. *Journal of Management, 21*, 967–988.

Joplin, J. R. W., Nelson, D. L., & Quick, J. C. (1999). Attachment behavior and health: Relationships at work and home. *Journal of Organizational Behavior, 20*, 783–796.

Judge, T. A., Heller, D., & Mount, M. K. (2002). Five-factor model of personality and job satisfaction: A meta-analysis. *Journal of Applied Psychology, 87,* 530–541.

Keller, T. (2003). Parental images as a guide to leadership sensemaking: An attachment perspective on implicit leadership theories. *Leadership Quarterly, 14,* 141–160.

Keller, T., & Cacioppe, R. (2001). Leader–follower attachments: Understanding parental images at work. *Leadership and Organization Development Journal, 22,* 70–75.

Kinnunen, U., Feldt, T., Geurts, S., & Pulkkinen, L. (2006). Types of work–family interface: Well-being correlates of negative and positive spillover between work and family. *Scandinavian Journal of Psychology, 47,* 149–162.

Lee, T. W., Mitchell, T. R., Sablynski, C. J., Burton, J. P., & Holtom, B. C. (2004). The effects of job embeddedness on organizational citizenship, job performance, volitional absences, and voluntary turnover. *Academy of Management Journal, 47,* 711–722.

Little, L. M., Nelson, D. L., Wallace, J. C., & Johnson, P. D. (2011). Integrating attachment style, vigor at work, and extra-role performance. *Journal of Organizational Behavior, 32,* 464–484.

Mallinckrodt, B., Gant, D. L., & Coble, H. M. (1995). Attachment patterns in the psychotherapy relationship: Development of the Client Attachment to Therapist Scale. *Journal of Counseling Psychology, 42,* 307–317.

Mayseless, O., & Popper, M. (2007). Reliance on leaders and social institutions: An attachment perspective. *Attachment and Human Development, 9,* 73–93.

Mikulincer, M., & Florian, V. (1995). Appraisal of and coping with a real-life stressful situation: The contribution of attachment styles. *Personality and Social Psychology Bulletin, 21,* 406–414.

Mikulincer, M., Florian, V., & Tolmacz, R. (1990). Attachment styles and fear of personal death: A case study of affect regulation. *Journal of Personality and Social Psychology, 58,* 273–280.

Mikulincer, M., & Shaver, P. R. (2007). *Attachment in adulthood: Structure, dynamics, and change.* New York: Guilford Press.

Moss, S. (2009). Cultivating the regulatory focus of followers to amplify their sensitivity to transformational leadership. *Journal of Leadership and Organizational Studies, 15,* 241–259.

Motowidlo, S. J. (2000). Some basic issues related to contextual performance and organizational citizenship behavior in human resource management. *Human Resource Management Review, 10,* 115–126.

Murphy, K. R. (1996). Individual differences and behavior in organizations: Much more than *g*. In K. R. Murphy (Ed.), *Individual differences and behavior in organizations* (pp. 3–30). San Francisco: Jossey-Bass.

Nelson, D. L., & Quick, J. C. (1991). Social support and newcomer adjustment in organizations: Attachment theory at work? *Journal of Organizational Behavior, 12,* 543–554.

Neustadt, E., Chamorro-Premuzic, T., & Furnham, A. (2006). The relationship between personality traits, self-esteem, and attachments at work. *Journal of Individual Differences, 27,* 208–217.

Neustadt, E. A., Chamorro-Premuzic, T., & Furnham, A. (2011). Attachment at work and performance. *Attachment and Human Development, 13,* 471–488.

Niehoff, B. F., & Moorman, R. H. (1993). Justice as mediator of the relationship between methods of monitoring and organizational citizenship behavior. *Academy of Management Journal, 36,* 527–556.

Noftle, E., & Shaver, P. (2006). Attachment dimensions and the Big Five personality traits: Associations and comparative ability to predict relationship quality. *Journal of Research in Personality, 40,* 179–208.

Organ, D. W. (1997). Organizational citizenship behavior: It's construct clean-up time. *Human Performance, 10,* 85–97.

Paetzold, R. L., Miner, K. N., & Carpenter, N. C. C. (2010). *An attachment theory approach to bystander sexual harassment.* Paper presented at the annual meeting of the Academy of Management, Montreal, Quebec, Canada.

Pines, A. M. (2004). Adult attachment styles and their relationship to burnout: A preliminary, cross-cultural investigation. *Work and Stress, 18,* 66–80.

Popper, M., & Amit, K. (2009). Attachment and leader's development via experiences. *Leadership Quarterly, 20,* 749–763.

Popper, M., & Mayseless, O. (2003). Back to basics: Applying a parenting perspective to transformational leadership. *Leadership Quarterly, 14,* 41–65.

Popper, M., Mayseless, O., & Castelnovo, O. (2000). Transformational leadership and attachment. *Leadership Quarterly, 11,* 267–289.

Quick, J. C., Joplin, J. R., Nelson, D. L., & Quick, J. D. (1992). Behavioral responses to anxiety: Self-reliance, counterdependence, and overdependence. *Anxiety, Stress, and Coping, 5,* 41–54.

Ransford, C. R., Crouter, A. C., & McHale, S. M. (2008). Implications of work pressure and supervisor support for fathers', mothers' and adolescents' relationships and well-being in dual-earner families. *Community, Work and Family, 11,* 37–60.

Richards, D. A., & Hackett, R. D. (2012). Attachment and emotion regulation: Compensatory interactions and leader-member exchange. *Leadership Quarterly, 23,* 686–701.

Richards, D. A., & Schat, A. C. H. (2011). Attachment at (not to) work: Applying attachment theory to explain individual behavior in organizations. *Journal of Applied Psychology, 96,* 169–182.

Rom, E. (2008). Team-related mental representations: The role of individual differences. *Individual Differences Research, 6,* 289–302.

Rom, E., & Mikulincer, M. (2003). Attachment theory and group processes: The association between attachment style and group-related representations, goals, memories, and functioning. *Journal of Personality and Social Psychology, 84,* 1220–1235.

Ronen, S., & Baldwin, M. W. (2010). Hypersensitivity to social rejection and perceived stress as mediators between attachment anxiety and future burnout: A prospective analysis. *Applied Psychology: An International Review, 59,* 380–403.

Ronen, S., & Mikulincer, M. (2009). Attachment orientations and job burnout: The mediating roles of team cohesion and organizational fairness. *Journal of Social and Personal Relationships, 26,* 549–567.

Ronen, S., & Mikulincer, M. (2012). Predicting employees' satisfaction and burnout from managers' attachment and caregiving orientations. *European Journal of Work and Organizational Psychology, 21,* 828–849.

Schaufeli, W., Leiter, M. P., Maslach, C., & Jackson, S. E. (1996). MBI-General Survey. In C. Maslach, S. E. Jackson, & M. P. Leiter (Eds.), *Maslach Burnout Inventory manual* (3rd ed., pp. 6–42). Palo Alto, CA: Consulting Psychologists Press.

Schaufeli, W. B., Salanova, M., González-Romá, V., & Bakker, A. B. (2002). The measurement of engagement and burnout: A two sample confirmatory factor analytic approach. *Journal of Happiness Studies, 3*, 71–92.

Schirmer, L. L., & Lopez, F. G. (2001). Probing the social support and work strain relationship among adult workers: Contributions of adult attachment orientations. *Journal of Vocational Behavior, 59*, 17–33.

Shalit, A., Popper, M., & Zakay, D. (2010). Followers' attachment styles and their preference for social or for personal charismatic leaders. *Leadership and Organization Development Journal, 31*, 458–472.

Simmons, B. L., Gooty, J., Nelson, D., & Little, L. M. (2009). Secure attachment: Implications for hope, trust, burnout, and performance. *Journal of Organizational Behavior, 30*, 233–247.

Simpson, J. A. (1990). Influence of attachment styles on romantic relationships. *Journal of Personality and Social Psychology, 59*, 971–980.

Simpson, J. A., Rholes, W. S., & Phillips, D. (1996). Conflict in close relationships: An attachment perspective. *Journal of Personality and Social Psychology, 71*, 899–914.

Smith, E. R., Murphy, J., & Coats, S. (1999). Attachment to groups: Theory and measurement. *Journal of Personality and Social Psychology, 77*, 94–110.

Stanton, J. M., & Weiss, E. M. (2002). *Online panels for social science research: An introduction to the StudyResponse project* (Syracuse University, School of Information Studies, Tech. Rep. No. 13001). Retrieved July 5, 2013, from *www.studyresponse.net/TechRpt13001.pdf.*

Sumer, H. C., & Knight, P. A. (2001). How do people with different attachment styles balance work and family?: A personality perspective on work–family linkage. *Journal of Applied Psychology, 86*, 653–663.

Towler, A. (2005). Charismatic leadership development: Role of parental attachment style and parental psychological control. *Journal of Leadership and Organizational Studies, 11*, 15–25.

Towler, A. J., & Stuhlmacher, A. F. (2013). Attachment styles, relationship satisfaction, and well-being in working women. *Journal of Social Psychology, 153*, 297–298.

Vasquez, K., Durik, A. M., & Hyde, J. S. (2002). Family and work: Implications of adult attachment styles. *Personality and Social Psychology Bulletin, 28*, 874–886.

Wayne, S. J., Shore, L. M., & Linden, R. C. (1997). Perceived organizational support and leader–member exchange: A social exchange perspective. *Academy of Management Journal, 40*, 82–111.

Health and Attachment Processes

Paula R. Pietromonaco
Cassandra C. DeVito
Fiona Ge
Jana Lembke

People with supportive social relationships, more social connections, and greater social integration typically evidence better emotional and physical health than those with unsupportive relationships, fewer social connections, and less social integration (Holt-Lunstad, Smith, & Layton, 2010; Uchino, 2009). Marital relationships, in particular, appear to confer health benefits (Kiecolt-Glaser & Newton, 2001), especially when those relationships are high in quality. Researchers have repeatedly found links between close relationships and health, but much remains to be learned about the processes through which relationships affect health.

Research following from attachment theory can offer insights into how relationships contribute to health, because many aspects of attachment processes (e.g., affect regulation, self-regulation, perceptions of support and support seeking, caregiving) are implicated in health. Accordingly, a growing literature has begun to examine the extent to which individual differences in attachment style are associated with health-related biological indicators, health behaviors, and health and disease outcomes from childhood through adulthood (Maunder & Hunter, 2008; Pietromonaco, DeBuse, & Powers, 2013; Pietromonaco, Uchino, & Dunkel Schetter, 2013). In this chapter, we first discuss the relevance of attachment processes for understanding health-related behaviors and outcomes, and present a theoretical framework for understanding potential connections between attachment and health. We then review research examining linkages between and among attachment and health-related biological responses, health behavior, and health and disease outcomes. Throughout our review, we evaluate how attachment processes across the lifespan—from childhood through adulthood—contribute to health-related outcomes. Finally, we discuss several emerging themes, as well as directions for future research that will enhance our understanding of the mechanisms linking attachment processes and health.

Relevance of Attachment Processes for Health

Research and theory point to several ways in which attachment processes contribute to health-related physiological responses and downstream health and disease outcomes. Attachment processes are inextricably tied to how people regulate distress in the face of threat (Mikulincer & Shaver, 2007; Pietromonaco & Beck, 2015), and these regulatory strategies are likely to have long-term consequences for both emotional and physical health. In normative cases, individuals (infants, children, or adults) who face a threatening event seek out their attachment figures, who then provide comfort and reassurance, thereby allowing distressed individuals to regain a sense of calm. People vary, however, in the kinds of regulatory strategies they apply, depending on what they have come to expect about the responsiveness and reliability of attachment figures (i.e., depending on the content of their working models of attachment; Mikulincer & Shaver, 2007). Individuals with an insecure *anxious* attachment style expect that close others will not be readily available; as a result, they respond to threat by using hyperactivating strategies, including persisting in signaling their emotional distress to their partners and in trying to maintain proximity to partners, and excessively seeking reassurance and support from partners. Individuals with an insecure *avoidant* attachment style typically expect that their attachment figures will be unavailable and unresponsive to their needs. As a result, avoidantly attached individuals often respond to threat by suppressing or minimizing their distress and by not turning to close others for support. In contrast, individuals with a *secure* attachment style expect that their attachment figures will be available and responsive, and they are comfortable turning to their attachment figures when they are in need of support or reassurance. These chronic strategies for regulating negative affect are associated with different emotional health outcomes and may raise or lower risks for physical illness as well. For example, both anxious and avoidant individuals are more likely to show symptoms of depression (Carnelley, Pietromonaco, & Jaffe, 1994; Simpson, Rholes, Campbell, Tran, & Wilson, 2003; Wei, Mallinckrodt, Larson, & Zakalik, 2005), which in turn predict impaired immune functioning and the development of infectious diseases and chronic illnesses such as cancer (Antoni et al., 2006; Miller, 2010).

Another way in which attachment may influence health is via perceptions and provision of support; that is, individual differences in attachment-based affect regulation strategies predict the extent to which individuals rely on and benefit from their partners' efforts to provide support and reassurance, how they perceive their partners' supportive attempts, and how they provide support to partners (Beck, Pietromonaco, DeBuse, Powers, & Sayer, 2013; Carnelley, Pietromonaco, & Jaffe, 1996; Collins & Feeney, 2004; Simpson, Winterheld, Rholes, & Oriña, 2007). Given the importance of social support throughout life for later health outcomes (Robles, Slatcher, Trombello, & McGinn, 2014; Uchino, 2009) and the potential benefits of caregiving (Brown et al., 2009), attachment-related expectations and beliefs constitute an important antecedent condition that is likely to predict the extent to which individuals reap the health benefits of receiving and giving social support.

A final pathway linking attachment and health is that individual differences in attachment style and associated affect regulation strategies are connected to the ability to self-regulate and organize behavior in an effort to achieve goals (for a review, see Mikulincer & Shaver, 2007). For example, in young children, attachment security predicts the ability to regulate behavior on tasks that require them to suppress a dominant response (Kochanska, Philibert, & Barry, 2009) or that require social control (Drake, Belsky, & Fearon, 2014). Similarly, in adults, attachment security has been associated with greater self-control (Tangney, Baumeister, & Boone, 2004), as well as more effective behavioral regulation in a variety of domains (e.g., analyzing a problem, concentrating on a task, task persistence; reported in Mikulincer & Shaver, 2007, pp. 229–230). These findings suggest that insecurely attached individuals will have greater difficulty regulating behaviors related to health—including taking preventive measures such as obtaining regular physical exams and immunizations, eating a healthy diet, and avoiding risky behaviors.

Given the hypothesized ways that attachment-related differences in affect regulation, care seeking and support, and self-regulation influence individuals' later health outcomes, we have developed a model (Figure 11.1) that illustrates how these processes, along with physiological and affective responses and health behaviors, may account for the link between attachment and health. The conceptual framework illustrates that in a relationship between two partners (Partner A and Partner B), each partner's own attachment style shapes his or her affect and self-regulation strategies and relationship behavior, which in turn trigger patterns of health-related physiological responses (e.g., cortisol reactivity to stress, cardiovascular reactivity, immune functioning), affect, and health behavior (e.g., diet, exercise). The framework further suggests that these physiological and affective responses and health behaviors then contribute to the development of health conditions and disease. In addition, the theoretical framework emphasizes

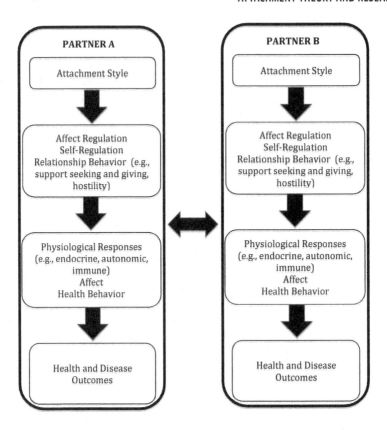

FIGURE 11.1. A theoretical framework for guiding research on attachment and health-related processes and outcomes.

that attachment relationships are dyadic, suggesting that each partner's characteristics, responses, and outcomes can influence the other partner at various points (Pietromonaco, Uchino, et al., 2013). To simplify the model, we have illustrated effects in only one direction (e.g., from attachment to health and disease outcomes), but some effects are likely to be bidirectional (e.g., having a disease may influence attachment security). Although a fair amount of research has examined the connection between attachment and health-related processes and outcomes, few studies have tested the hypothesized mediating links in the model. As an example, little is known about whether the link between attachment insecurity and health conditions such as cardiovascular disease (McWilliams & Bailey, 2010) can be accounted for by the cumulative effects of cortisol reactivity to stress, or health behaviors such as food and exercise patterns, or a combination of these factors. In the following sections, we review evidence indicating that individual differences in attachment style—in both childhood and adulthood—are associated with health-related biological responses, health behavior, and health and disease outcomes. When possible, we discuss evidence relevant to the mediating mechanisms (see Figure 11.1); we return to this issue in the final section, in which we make recommendations for the next generation of studies.

Physiological Mechanisms Linking Attachment and Health

Early adverse attachment experiences can alter the development and functioning of biological regulatory systems, including the hypothalamic–pituitary–adrenal (HPA) axis, the sympathetic–adrenal medullary (SAM) axis, and the immune system, leaving individuals vulnerable to the effects of stress on the body (Felitti et al., 1998; Gunnar & Donzella, 2002; Repetti, Taylor, & Seeman, 2002; Schore, 2001; Shonkoff, Boyce, & McEwen, 2009; Taylor, Way, & Seeman, 2011). Specifically, children who experience harsh circumstances—including neglectful or abusive parents, or environments with high levels of conflict or disorganization—not only evidence difficulty in regulating distress, but also show dysregulation in their physiological stress responses (Repetti et al., 2002; Taylor et al., 2011). Indeed, early childhood adversity and low socioeconomic status (SES) have been linked to higher risk for a variety of chronic health conditions, such as cardiovascular disease, obesity, metabolic syndrome, and cancer (Kelly-Irving et al., 2013; Lehman, Taylor, Kiefe, & Seeman, 2005; Miller & Cole, 2012; Steptoe & Kivimäki, 2013; Tamayo, Christian, & Rathmann, 2010). Thus, as illustrated in Figure 11.1, dysregulation in endocrine, autonomic, and immune responses may provide a pathway through which attachment-related beliefs and expectations developed early in life (e.g., as a result of early adverse experiences) contribute to downstream health and disease outcomes. Similarly, attachment in adulthood also may shape health and disease outcomes through biological response systems, either because of continuity between earlier and later attachment patterns (Fraley & Brumbaugh, 2004), or because attachment in adult relationships also can shape biological stress responses (Pietromonaco, DeBuse, et al., 2013; Pietromonaco, Uchino, et al., 2013). The primary biological indicators that have been examined reflect activity in the HPA axis, SAM axis, and immune system. We selectively review key studies for each of these biological responses.

HPA Responses

A key physiological system subject to the influence of attachment is the HPA axis. Upon activation by a stressor, the HPA axis governs the release of cortisol into the bloodstream. Although this response prepares the body to deal with acute stressors, continued release of cortisol disrupts numerous body processes, including metabolism, immune responses, and autonomic nervous system activity (Pietromonaco, DeBuse, et al., 2013). Indeed, the effect of cortisol on health may be attributed to its inhibitory effect on the immune system, which predisposes individuals to negative health outcomes such as increased susceptibility to infectious disease, flareups of existing allergies or other conditions, and accelerated progression of chronic disease (Miller, Chen, & Zhou, 2007).

Childhood Attachment and HPA Responses

The link between attachment style and health-related biological outcomes emerges very early in life. Support from a large body of research suggests that infants and children raised in a harsh family environment experience mental and physical health problems well into adulthood, and that HPA axis dysregulation is implicated in the link between risky family background and health risks (Taylor, Lerner, Sage, Lehman, & Seeman, 2004). In particular, parental caregiving may influence children's biologically based stress response systems; for example, poorer caregiving by parents (which is associated with children's attachment insecurity) can increase children's baseline cortisol levels, and this dysregulation potentiates lower executive functioning and higher reactivity to stimuli (Blair & Raver, 2012). These outcomes are correlates of poor self-regulation, which places infants and children at risk for serious health problems including heart disease and depression, as well as increases in the prevalence of health-threatening behaviors such as substance abuse and sexual promiscuity (Repetti et al., 2002). In this way, an adverse environment in childhood may have lasting effects on HPA axis functioning, increasing one's propensity for health risks and disease.

Several studies have focused specifically on the link between parent–child attachment and physiological responses. This work has indicated that infants with different attachment classifications exhibit distinctive physiological patterns to stressful stimuli. Infants with a Type D (disorganized/disoriented) attachment classification consistently show significantly higher elevations in cortisol levels and heart rates than infants with other attachment classifications (Hertsgaard, Gunnar, Erickson, & Nachmias, 1995; Spangler & Grossmann, 1993). Similarly, toddlers of mothers who reported more frequently using emotional withdrawal in response to their children (which presumably would increase the likelihood that the children were insecurely attached) were more likely to show higher levels of baseline cortisol (Bugental, Martorell, & Barraza, 2003). Other work has found that attachment moderated the association between behavior inhibition and HPA activity, such that HPA activation was most prominent in fearful or behaviorally inhibited infants who were also insecurely attached (Gunnar, Brodersen, Nachmias, Buss, & Rigatuso, 1996; Nachmias, Gunnar,

Mangelsdorf, Parritz, & Buss, 1996; Spangler & Schieche, 1998). Still other work has examined attachment in early childhood and later patterns of stress reactivity in adolescence among individuals at risk for asthma; in this sample, insecure attachment in early childhood predicted flatter patterns of cortisol reactivity over the course of a standard laboratory stressor, suggesting dysregulated HPA responses (Kelsay, Leung, Mrazek, & Klinnert, 2013). Conversely, attachment security may have a health-protective effect. One study found that attachment security buffered infants from elevations in cortisol when the infants were facing threatening stimuli, such as receiving an immunization (Gunnar et al., 1996). Taken together, the research indicates that childhood attachment insecurity is linked to greater dysregulation in physiological responses to stress. It is possible that these dysregulated physiological patterns, such as the frequency and magnitude of HPA activation, may serve as precursors to childhood health and disease problems.

Adult Attachment and HPA Responses

HPA activation has been shown to affect mental and physical wellness in numerous ways (Jaremka et al., 2013; Miller et al., 2007), but research has only recently addressed whether attachment in adult relationships is connected to physiological stress responses that may predispose individuals to later deleterious health outcomes. One study (Powers, Pietromonaco, Gunlicks, & Sayer, 2006) examined how attachment style in dating couples modulates patterns of cortisol release and recovery in response to an interpersonal stressor: discussing a heated and unresolved area of disagreement with one's partner. Salivary cortisol was assessed at multiple time points before, during, and after each couple's conflict discussion. The findings indicated that patterns of cortisol release and recovery varied as a function of attachment style and gender. For women, higher attachment *avoidance* predicted heightened cortisol responses before and during the discussion, but a rapid recovery after the discussion when they were able to disengage from the stressor. For men, higher attachment *anxiety* predicted a peak in cortisol in anticipation of the stressful discussion and resulted in slower recovery afterward. These findings suggest that different types of attachment insecurity are associated with distinct patterns of HPA axis responses to attachment-related threats such as relationship conflict.

While both attachment avoidance and anxiety appear to support atypical HPA axis activity, anxiously attached individuals are especially vulnerable to exaggerated physiological and affective reactivity to stress, particularly when the stressor is relationship-threatening (Pietromonaco, DeBuse, et al., 2013). For instance, heightened HPA axis activity was observed in anxiously attached individuals during travel separations, reinforcing the notion that an anxious attachment style may enhance sensitivity to threats of decreased partner closeness and availability (Diamond, Hicks, & Otter-Henderson, 2008).

Collectively, these findings suggest that an individual's attachment style is associated with his or her stress responses, especially reactions to attachment-relevant threats. In addition, research suggests that one's *partner's* attachment style may modulate, for better or for worse, one's *own* stress response. For example, when husbands withdrew in response to wives' negativity during a conflict interaction, wives showed increased cortisol reactivity (Kiecolt-Glaser et al., 1996). Additional support for the effect of partners' behaviors on individuals' own physiological stress responses comes from research finding that men with securely attached female partners showed lower cortisol reactivity and faster recovery to relationship conflict than did men with insecure partners (Powers et al., 2006). This finding is thought to be a function of secure individuals' tendency to be more responsive, which may have reduced the physiological stress of men in this study (Powers et al., 2006).

Little research has examined how the interplay between *both* partners' attachment orientations is associated with physiological responses, although developmental models have long recognized the significance of this interplay. Specifically, transactional or goodness-of-fit models (Thomas & Chess, 1977) suggest that the attachment orientations, behavior, and temperament of both infants and their mothers need to be considered in predicting how each dyad member responds (Mangelsdorf, Gunnar, Kestenbaum, Lang, & Andreas, 1990). Recent work in our lab examined how both partners' attachment styles might jointly contribute to their physiological and behavioral responses to a conflict discussion (Beck et al., 2013). In this study of 218 newlywed couples, we found that pairs including a more anxiously attached wife and a more avoidantly attached husband showed a distinctive pattern of cortisol responses in anticipation of and before a discussion of a major area of unresolved conflict in their relationship. Both spouses showed rapid increases in cortisol in anticipation of a conflict discussion, followed by rapid declines. These cortisol patterns were paralleled by less constructive interaction behaviors: More anxiously attached wives had difficulty recognizing their husbands' distress when the husbands were high in avoidance, and more avoidantly attached husbands were less able to express their needs for support and responsiveness when their wives were high in anxiety (Beck et al., 2013). These partner effects suggest that relationship partners dynamically influence each other's physiological activity over time, with potential downstream consequences for psychological well-being and physical health.

SAM Responses

Attachment also may influence health outcomes through the SAM system, which includes the autonomic nervous system (Diamond & Fagundes, 2010). As with HPA axis responses, dysregulated reactivity in the SAM axis is likely to accompany insecure attachment in children and adults, and to affect biological markers with implications for health.

Childhood Attachment and SAM Responses

Researchers have become increasingly interested in the complex interactions among genetic predispositions, childhood experiences, attachment style, and physiological outcomes. For instance, attachment behavior has been hypothesized to modulate infants' genetically based physiological sensitivities to distress, such that secure attachment may protect against SAM hyperactivation in individuals with genetic polymorphisms that put them at risk for dysregulated stress responses (Frigerio et al., 2009).

Along with constitutional factors, experiences early in life (e.g., quality of parental caregiving) shape a child's developing attachment style, and a substantial body of research suggests that adverse experiences may disrupt various physiological systems with the potential for long-term adverse health effects. Research on individuals from risky family backgrounds suggests that continued social challenges in early life—such as parental unavailability or insensitivity—can disrupt a child's SAM system, which over time taxes cardiovascular functioning (Repetti et al., 2002). Another pathway by which attachment style in childhood may predict health risks is via attachment-associated social interaction patterns (attachment → relationship behavior in Figure 11.1) with known health correlates. For example, insecure attachment with caregivers may predispose the development of loneliness, fewer reciprocated friendships, and less social competence in children (Kerns, Klepac, & Cole, 1996), which would appear to increase SAM activation and the risk for coronary heart disease. Taken together, these findings support a model whereby attachment-based influences early in development shape lifelong physical health outcomes via multiple avenues.

Adult Attachment and SAM Responses

The relationship between adult attachment and SAM reactivity may vary as a function of deficient, defensive, or dissociative emotion regulation strategies that have been linked to insecure attachment (Pietromonaco & Beck, 2015). For example, individuals high in attachment avoidance tend to minimize emotional distress and rely on repressive coping in response to emotional and attachment-related tasks, and this strategy has been found to produce heightened and escalating sympathetic nervous system reactivity (Diamond et al., 2008). Indeed, several studies have found that attachment avoidance in adults potentiates hyperactivation in the SAM axis, and that in contrast to the pattern for anxiously attached individuals, this avoidance-related hyperactivation fails to correspond with heightened subjective distress (Diamond & Fagundes, 2010; Diamond et al., 2008). The incongruence between avoidant individuals' physiological activity and their reported distress and negative affect underscores the value of physiological measurements for providing a window into a less conscious aspect of emotional reactions.

Immune Responses

Immune system functioning is another biomarker of health outcomes that can fluctuate depending on the quality of relationship experiences, which are closely associated with attachment style. The literature examining attachment and immune responses is in its infancy, with only a few studies examining these processes in early childhood or adulthood.

Childhood Attachment and Immune Responses

Few studies have directly examined childhood attachment and immune responses, but related research indicates that experiencing adversity in early childhood is associated with immune dysregulation (Fagundes, Glaser, & Kiecolt-Glaser, 2013). One study of a nationally representative sample of U.S. children has shown that children from lower-income families evidenced higher levels of C-reactive protein, an indicator of inflammation (Dowd, Zajacova, & Aiello, 2010), as well as elevated antibody levels of a herpes virus, cytomegalovirus (Dowd, Palermo, & Aiello, 2012).

Adversity early in life appears to shape immune functioning later in life (Miller & Chen, 2010; Slopen, Koenen, & Kubzansky, 2012). In one longitudinal study, individuals who as children had experienced some form of socioeconomic disadvantage or high levels of sexual abuse or physical abuse at a young age were more likely to have higher Epstein–Barr virus antibody titers, which reflect cell-mediated immune functioning (Slopen et al., 2012). The potential role of attachment is suggested by recent work showing that adults from a low-SES background who reported (retrospectively) that their mothers displayed high warmth during childhood evidenced diminished pro-inflammatory responses across several indicators of immune functioning and inflammation, compared to those who reported that their mothers displayed low warmth (Chen, Miller, Kobor, & Cole, 2011). These findings suggest that individuals who were more likely to be securely attached (i.e., those who had mothers higher in warmth) were protected from the adverse effects of low SES. However, the interpretation of these findings is limited because the quality of the mother–child relationships was assessed via participants' self-reports about their mothers' earlier behavior, rather than through direct observation of interactions in the mother–child relationships during childhood. As a result, the findings may reflect that participants who recalled their mothers as low in warmth during childhood differed from those who recalled their mothers as high in warmth in important ways (e.g., depressed mood, quality of current relationship) that may lead to poorer immune functioning.

Adult Attachment and Immune Functioning

The few studies examining attachment in adulthood and immune functioning point to attachment avoidance, anxiety, or both as risk factors for immune system dysregulation, but the findings are not always consistent for men and women. One study found that both husbands' and wives' attachment avoidance predicted a greater inflammatory response to a marital conflict discussion, in addition to more negative and fewer positive behaviors, both of which signal cardiovascular risks (Gouin et al., 2009). Similarly, other work with a small sample of dating couples ($N = 34$ couples) found that women's attachment avoidance predicted slower recovery from a skin barrier wound (which reflects immune functioning) over the course of two potentially stressful discussions on two separate days (a discussion of a personal concern and another about a relationship problem); however, avoidance was unrelated to skin barrier recovery among men (Robles, Brooks, Kane, & Schetter, 2013). Instead, men high in attachment anxiety showed slower skin barrier recovery when the discussion focused on a personal concern. Furthermore, one finding for women ran counter to theoretical predictions: Women high in attachment anxiety showed more rapid skin barrier recovery at both visits. This finding is difficult to explain, given the current scarcity of research in this area (Robles et al., 2013) and in light of other recent work showing that attachment anxiety is linked to poorer immune functioning in both husbands and wives: Husbands and wives who scored higher on a measure of adult attachment anxiety showed lower levels of several types of T-cells (CD3+ T-cells, CD45+ T-cells, CD3+CD4+ helper T-cells, and CD3+CD8+ cytotoxic T-cells), suggesting impaired immune functioning (Jaremka et al., 2013).

Too few studies have been conducted to determine whether attachment avoidance, attachment anxiety, or both are more likely to be connected to immune functioning, and when these effects are likely to vary by gender. The answer may be complex: Attachment anxiety may be associated with some immune markers, whereas avoidance may be associated with others, or the links may vary across different situational contexts (e.g., across quality and type of relationship or type and degree of stress) as well as in relation to the meaning of each context for women versus men. Nevertheless, initial evidence suggests that attachment insecurity in adults is associated with disruptions in immune functioning, and that these disruptions may forecast future health problems. Additional investigations are needed to determine the conditions under which attachment anxiety, avoidance, or both are tied to immune responses, and to provide a clearer picture of the mechanisms underlying such effects.

Health Behavior

Attachment orientations are strongly tied to the strategies people use to regulate their thoughts, feelings, and behavior (see Mikulincer & Shaver, 2007, and Pietromonaco & Beck, 2015); as a result, attachment security or insecurity should predict the extent to which individuals engage in preventive health behaviors or behaviors that increase health risks. Despite the importance of this issue, relatively few studies have examined the extent to which attachment in either childhood or adulthood predicts specific health behaviors. Figure 11.1 illustrates that self-regulation, affect regulation, and relationship processes may be implicated in the link between attachment and health behavior, but this idea has yet to be directly tested.

Childhood Attachment and Health Behavior

Children and adolescents who are insecurely attached to parents show riskier health behavior. For example, insecurely attached children (ages 8–11 years) and adolescents are more likely to evidence eating disorders (Goossens, Braet, Bosmans, & Decaluwé, 2011; O'Shaughnessy & Dallos, 2009). Similarly, children who were insecurely attached at 24 months of age, compared with their securely attached peers, were more likely to be diagnosed with obesity at 4.5 years of age (Anderson & Whitaker, 2011), which also may reflect problematic eating patterns and is a risk factor for various diseases later in life (including heart disease, stroke, and diabetes). Similarly, low maternal sensitivity and children's attachment insecurity (assessed from mother–child interactions at ages 1–3) predicted obesity during early adolescence (12–16 years) (Anderson, Gooze, Lemeshow, & Whitaker, 2012). In addition, insecure attachment has been associated with poorer glycemic control among adolescents with diabetes (Rosenberg & Shields, 2009), suggesting that these adolescents had difficulty adhering to their medical regimen.

Furthermore, adolescents with insecure attachments to their parents are more likely to use alcohol and drugs (Branstetter, Furman, & Cottrell, 2009), smoke cigarettes (Foshee & Bauman, 1994), and engage in risky sexual behavior (Luster & Small, 1994). Research examining African American girls (a group at higher risk for sexually transmitted diseases) has shown that girls who had higher-quality relationships with their mothers (a proxy for secure attachment) were less likely to engage in risky sexual behaviors (e.g., unprotected sex, multiple sexual partners, earlier sexual intercourse) (Crosby et al., 2001; Emerson, Donenberg, & Wilson, 2012; Moore & Chase-Lansdale, 2001), suggesting a protective effect of attachment security.

The mechanisms underlying the link between children's attachment and health behavior have yet to be tested. Children who have poorer-quality relationships with parents also have greater difficulty regulating emotions (Contreras, Kerns, Weimer, Gentzler, & Tomich, 2000), which is likely to interfere with their ability to engage in and persist at behaviors such as resisting attractive but potentially health-damaging foods or following a regular exercise routine. Children who are insecurely attached (especially avoidantly attached) may be reluctant to seek assistance from parents or other adults, and discussions with parents about health-protective behaviors may be difficult (Brody et al., 2006). Alternatively, parents who provide less sensitive and responsive caregiving themselves may be more likely to engage in riskier behaviors and less likely to engage in health-protective behaviors, and therefore transmit similar attitudes and behaviors to their children through modeling.

Adult Attachment and Health Behavior

Limited research indicates that attachment insecurity (anxiety, avoidance, or both) in young adults is associated with using drugs, having a poorer body image, engaging in risky sexual behavior, reporting greater alcohol use, having a poorer diet, and exercising less (Feeney, Peterson, Gallois, & Terry, 2000; Huntsinger & Luecken, 2004). In a similar vein, a recent study of 701 adult women found that attachment anxiety predicted riskier sexual behavior, and that avoidance predicted being more likely to smoke (Ahrens, Ciechanowski, & Katon, 2012).

Other work has demonstrated that individuals with insecure attachment styles are less likely to take preventive health measures. For example, women who are higher in avoidance or anxiety are less likely to report receiving cervical cancer screening and perceive more barriers to screening, even after their sexual experience and levels of neuroticism are taken into account (Hill & Gick, 2013). Avoidantly attached women also are less likely to use seat belts routinely (Ahrens et al., 2012). In addition, evidence from a sample of over 4,000 primary care patients with diabetes indicated that those with dismissing/avoidant attachments (i.e., high in avoidance and low in anxiety) showed less adherence to their treatment plans; they were less likely to follow diet, foot care, medication, exercise, and smoking recommendations (Ciechanowski et al., 2004).

Research in this area would be enhanced by examining attachment and health behavior at a dyadic level, taking into account how relationship partners' attachment orientations and associated relational behavior might shape each partner's health behaviors. Research on relationships and health behavior has increasingly shown that dyadic processes contribute to health behaviors, including weight loss attempts (Novak & Webster, 2011), smoking (Lewis & Butterfield, 2007), and management of one partner's diabetes (August, Rook, Franks, & Stephens, 2013; Stephens et al., 2013). For example, one recent diary study found that on days when spouses provided support and encouragement about following the recommended diet, their partners with Type 2 diabetes were more likely to adhere to their dietary regimen on the following day; however, on days when spouses exerted pressure or coercion, their partners were less likely to adhere to their diet on the following day (Stephens et al., 2013). Incorporating an attachment perspective into dyadic studies of health behavior will be useful for identifying whether individuals with particular attachment styles (e.g., avoidant) or couples with particular attachment pairings (e.g., a more anxious caregiving partner with a more avoidant patient partner) may be especially prone to veer from their diet when partners exert pressure, or whether support is effective for some patients (e.g., securely attached) but less so for others (e.g., avoidantly attached). Future work investigating how individuals' own attachment styles together with their partners' attachment styles shape dyadic efforts to manage and change health behaviors will be important for developing interventions that take into account individual differences, and that can be tailored for different individuals and types of couples.

Physical Health

All of the factors discussed so far may ultimately contribute to physical health and disease risks and outcomes, as illustrated in Figure 11.1. We now discuss the research linking attachment in childhood and adulthood to known health risks and health conditions.

Childhood Attachment and Health Conditions

A number of studies have examined whether health conditions *during childhood* vary as a function of early childhood attachment insecurity (Maunder & Hunter, 2001). One general finding is that insecure attachment to parents is more prevalent among children diagnosed with a clinical condition, compared with healthy controls; for instance, this pattern has been found for premature infants or infants affected by atopic dermatitis (Cassibba, van IJzendoorn, & Coppola, 2012), infants with congenital heart disease (Goldberg, Simmons, Newman, Campbell, & Fowler, 1991), and asthmatic preschool children (Mrazek, Casey, & Anderson, 1987).

Although studies have demonstrated an association between childhood attachment and children's health conditions and outcomes, the direction of this association remains elusive. It is possible that early attachment contributes to childhood health conditions through physiological pathways, such as the HPA axis; an additional possibility is that disease conditions alter parent–child interactions in ways that increase the likelihood that children will become insecurely attached. Few studies have addressed this question; however, one study has shown that children born with congenital heart disease were more likely to be classified as avoidantly attached at 12–18 months of age (based on behavior in the Strange Situation) than healthy controls were (Goldberg et al., 1991). Furthermore, of the children with congenital heart disease, 70% of those classified as securely attached showed improvement in cardiac function from an earlier initial intake interview to the laboratory session in which attachment behavior was observed, whereas only 30% of children classified as insecurely attached showed improvement, even though the two groups did not differ in the initial severity of their illness. This finding suggests that improvement in a child's health condition may alter parent–child interactions in ways increasing the likelihood that the child will show secure attachment behavior; however, prospective data are needed to evaluate the direction of these effects more precisely.

Few studies have examined whether childhood attachment to parents predicts health conditions *in adulthood*. Evidence from studies in which individuals retrospectively reported on their childhood relationships suggests that individuals with poorer-quality family relationships are more likely to have health problems in adulthood (Stewart-Brown, Fletcher, & Wadsworth, 2005). Interpreting findings from studies relying on retrospective reports of childhood attachment is difficult, however, because participants' current states (e.g., current attachment, mood, physical health conditions) could bias their memory for earlier childhood experiences. Other work has used self-report indicators of early attachment disruption that are less likely to be biased by participants' current states. For example, one study examined whether the self-reported death of a biological parent before age 16 predicted adults' health-related physiological responses to stress (Luecken, 1998). This research found that young adults who had lost a parent before age 16 showed higher blood pressure and cortisol levels in response to novel stressful stimuli (watching a video clip depicting loss of a parent or giving an impromptu speech) in comparison to young adults who had not experienced the loss of a parent. If physiological responses such as those observed in this study accumulate over time, they may contribute to the development of adverse health conditions. Similarly, research using childhood SES as an indicator of early childhood environment has found that individuals from lower-SES backgrounds are more likely to develop adult metabolic syndrome; however, this association appears to be stronger among participants who report poorer maternal nurturance (possibly reflecting insecure attachment) and weaker among individuals who report better maternal nurturance (possibly reflecting secure attachment) (Miller, Lachman, et al., 2011).

The best way to examine the role of childhood attachment and future health and disease outcomes in adulthood is to assess attachment in childhood and then follow these individuals into adulthood (Maunder & Hunter, 2001). Although nearly 30 years ago researchers pointed to the importance of taking a developmental perspective to understand how early childhood experiences shape health in later life (e.g., Boyce, 1985), few studies have examined this question by using prospective, longitudinal designs. A recent landmark study, however, used a prospective design to follow individuals from infancy to age 32, providing the most compelling evidence yet for a connection between attachment in childhood and health outcomes in adulthood (Puig, Englund, Simpson, & Collins, 2013). In this study, childhood attachment was assessed when participants were 12 and 18 months of age with an objective measure: the infants' behavior (coded by trained observers) in response to separation and reunion with their mothers in the Strange Situation. Physical health was assessed many years later, when participants were 32 years old. Remarkably, individuals' infant attachment classifications predicted their physical health outcomes in middle adulthood, even after potentially related variables (e.g., life stress, negative emotion, body mass index) were taken into account. Specifically, individuals whose attachments had been classified as anxious-resistant in infancy were more likely to report physical illness as adults 32 years later than were individuals who had been classified as securely attached in infancy. Adults whose attachments had previously been classified as anxious-avoidant or anxious-resistant were more likely to report having an inflammation-related illness at age 32 than their secure peers. In addition, participants classified as insecurely attached at both times (12 months and 18 months) during infancy were more likely to report having a physical illness, inflammation-related illness, and nonspecific symptoms at age 32 than participants classified as insecurely attached at one time or as securely attached at both times during infancy.

The Puig et al. (2013) study also examined whether several factors mediated the link between early attachment and later health outcomes—including variables that our model (Figure 11.1) suggests may be important mechanisms, such as the role of childhood emotion regulation ability, interpersonal competence with peers, and emotional health. None of the variables tested significantly mediated the attachment–health link. As Puig et al. note, however, the small percentage of participants with a physical illness may have made it difficult to detect mediation.

This prospective research suggests that the quality of early parent–child relationships is an important antecedent of later physical health. Additional prospective longitudinal studies are needed for replicating this effect and assessing its generality across samples. The infants in the Puig et al. (2013) study were originally from low-SES backgrounds; such individuals carry a greater risk for adverse health outcomes in adulthood, a process that may occur in part through alterations beginning in childhood in the body's physiological stress response systems (Miller, Lachman, et al., 2011). Thus it will be important for additional prospective studies to determine whether the link between childhood attachment and later health outcomes is intensified by early adverse circumstances (e.g., low SES), or whether a similar link emerges among individuals who have not experienced early childhood adversity. Furthermore, research in this area will be advanced by assessing potential physiological pathways (Miller, Chen, & Parker, 2011), as well as further examining possible behavioral and emotional mechanisms (e.g., learned strategies for regulating emotion) through which early experiences shape downstream health outcomes. This knowledge will be vital for developing early intervention programs to target processes that are implicated in the link between early experience and later health and disease outcomes.

Adult Attachment and Health/Disease Outcomes in Adulthood

A growing literature suggests that adult attachment is associated with physical symptoms (e.g., sleep problems, perceptions of pain) and health and disease risks and conditions (e.g., cardiovascular reactivity, high blood pressure, stroke, heart attack).

Physical Symptoms

Anxiously attached individuals, who show greater affective reactivity (Pietromonaco, Barrett, & Powers, 2006; Pietromonaco & Barrett, 1997), also may be more sensitive to physical distress and pain. Consistent with this idea, individuals characterized by anxious attachment report more physical and somatic symptoms than individuals with other forms of attachment do (Feeney & Ryan, 1994; Kidd & Sheffield, 2005; Ciechanowski, Walker, Katon, & Russo, 2002).

Most of the studies have examined adult attachment and reported physical symptoms at the same point in time, making it difficult to know whether attachment style influences symptom reporting, or whether experiencing unpleasant physical symptoms creates conditions that lead to attachment insecurity. For example, people who are in pain may find it difficult to engage in positive interactions with others, which over time may increase their attachment insecurity.

Studies of experimentally induced pain suggest that attachment anxiety is associated not only with anxiously attached individuals' reports of pain experienced in their daily lives, but also with their reactions to induced pain. Individuals higher in attachment anxiety show more intense reactions to experimentally induced pain, including a lower pain threshold, greater catastrophizing about the pain (e.g., ruminating about it, feeling overwhelmed by it), and greater perceptions of pain (Meredith, Strong, & Feeney, 2006; Wilson & Ruben, 2011), although some work has not found this association (Andrews, Meredith, & Strong, 2011).

The link between attachment avoidance and experimentally induced pain is less clear. Some work has found greater pain tolerance among avoidantly attached individuals exposed to an acute laboratory pain induction

(Andrews et al., 2011; Wilson & Ruben, 2011). Other work, however, has found that both attachment anxiety and avoidance predict pain intensity. In a diary study of women with chronic pain, those high in attachment anxiety reported greater pain intensity and showed more pain catastrophizing on days when they reported more intense pain; more avoidant women also reported greater pain intensity and catastrophizing, but they were less likely to cope by relying on others on days when they showed higher catastrophizing (Kratz, Davis, & Zautra, 2012).

These findings suggest that for women with chronic pain, both attachment anxiety and avoidance are associated with perceptions of pain and coping strategies, especially on days that are more difficult (the pain is more intense, or worries about the pain are high). Findings vary somewhat across studies, possibly because the extent to which either attachment anxiety, avoidance, or both are associated with pain responses may depend on the context (e.g., an acute laboratory stressor or chronic pain), the nature of the sample (e.g., individuals with or without chronic pain, age of sample), and other contextual variables (e.g., the extent to which the pain sufferers feel supported or rejected) (Andrews et al., 2011; MacDonald, 2008). For example, anxiously attached individuals who were reminded of rejection evidenced a lower pain threshold than anxiously attached individuals in a control condition did (MacDonald, 2008), suggesting that social pain may trigger greater sensitivity to physical pain among those with anxious attachments.

Another symptom associated with attachment is difficulty sleeping, which is linked to greater health risks such as contracting the common cold (Cohen, Doyle, Alper, Janicki-Deverts, & Turner, 2009), poorer immune function (Prather et al., 2012), and metabolic and cardiovascular diseases (Grandner, Jackson, Pak, & Gehrman, 2012). Attachment anxiety in adults may be relevant for sleep quality, because an individual's worries about the relationship and partner (e.g., concerns about closeness, rejection) may become salient when the individual attempts to fall asleep (Carmichael & Reis, 2005). In line with this reasoning, one study of married couples found that attachment anxiety predicted difficulties with sleeping for husbands and wives, even after the researchers controlled for individuals' symptoms of depression, which also are linked to sleep problems (Carmichael & Reis, 2005). Similarly, research using a diverse sample of older adults (ages 60–85 years) found that individuals who were preoccupied with attachment (high in anxiety and low in avoidance) were more likely to use medication to help them sleep and more likely to take naps during the daytime, possibly as a side effect of the medications or because they had trouble sleeping at night (Verdecias, Jean-Louis, Zizi, Casimir, & Browne, 2009).

Other work has found a link between anxious attachment and objective sleep quality, but, surprisingly, not subjective sleep quality (Troxel, Cyranowski, Hall, Frank, & Buysse, 2007; Troxel & Germain, 2011). In this work, anxiously attached women with major depression showed poorer sleep quality on objective measures: They showed the lowest percentage of sleep during stages 3 and 4 (deep sleep), especially if they had lost a spouse through divorce, separation, or death (Troxel et al., 2007). Similarly, military veterans with posttraumatic stress disorder who were more anxiously attached showed less sleep in stages 3 and 4 (Troxel & Germain, 2011).

Overall, the findings consistently show that attachment anxiety is associated with sleep disturbances, whereas few studies have shown a similar link between avoidance and sleep disturbances (Maunder, Hunter, & Lancee, 2011). Importantly, the link between relationship functioning and sleep disruptions appears to be bidirectional (Hasler & Troxel, 2010). As a result, individuals who are anxiously attached may experience a vicious cycle in which attachment-related worries lead to poorer sleep quality, and being fatigued may increase the likelihood of problematic interactions with their partners, which can then interfere with subsequent sleep. This idea fits with findings from a diary study showing that more anxiously attached couple members reported greater sleep problems on mornings following days of greater conflict with their partners, and fewer sleep problems on mornings following days of lower conflict (Hicks & Diamond, 2011). In contrast, individuals higher in avoidance showed a weaker association between experiencing conflict on the previous day and sleep problems the next morning than did those low in avoidance, perhaps because highly avoidant individuals are better able to suppress potentially disturbing thoughts about conflict.

Health Risks and Conditions

Cardiovascular reactivity to stress, particularly if cumulative, is a risk factor for later cardiovascular disease (Uchino, Cacioppo, & Kiecolt-Glaser, 1996). Several studies suggest that attachment insecurity is associated with cardiovascular reactivity. For example, individuals who were anxiously or avoidantly attached responded with increased heart rate and blood pressure after separation from their romantic partners during a stress task (Feeney & Kirkpatrick, 1996) or when they imagined themselves in hypothetical scenarios about their romantic partners that evoked anger (Mikulincer, 1998). In addition, adolescents who were more anxiously attached in their relationships with close others showed higher ambulatory diastolic and systolic blood pressure in response to interactions with friends, and those who were more avoidantly attached showed higher diastolic blood pressure in response to interpersonal conflict (Gallo & Matthews, 2006). (Although this study examined adolescents, it is included in this section because the attachment measure did not specifically assess parent–child attachment.) Although these studies point to attachment insecurity as a risk factor for downstream health problems, no studies have yet demonstrated that attachment-related fluctuations in blood pressure predict health and disease outcomes later in life.

Some work has examined whether adult attachment predicts the likelihood of having a health condition. The best evidence comes from cross-sectional data from the National Comorbidity Survey Replication, in which researchers examined the links between adult attachment and a range of health conditions in a large ($N = 5,692$) national probability sample from the United States (McWilliams & Bailey, 2010). In analyses that simultaneously included attachment ratings for security, anxiety, and avoidance and controlled for demographic variables (gender, marital status, race, age, education), attachment avoidance was associated with greater odds of having conditions defined primarily by pain (headaches, arthritis, back and neck problems, other chronic pain). Attachment anxiety was associated with greater odds of having headaches and some forms of chronic pain, as well as more serious conditions such as ulcers, high blood pressure, heart attack, and stroke.

Attachment insecurity also has been associated with risks for depression, anxiety symptoms and disorders, and substance abuse (Carnelley et al., 1994; Mickelson, Kessler, & Shaver, 1997; Simpson et al., 2003). For this reason, it is important that researchers take into account psychological disorders when examining the connection between attachment and physical health conditions. Following this reasoning, in additional analyses of the data from the National Comorbidity Survey Replication, McWilliams and Bailey (2010) controlled for psychiatric disorders (e.g., depression, anxiety) associated with attachment insecurity. These analyses indicated that attachment anxiety remained significantly associated with some forms of chronic pain and with stroke, heart attack, and high blood pressure, over and above any associations with psychiatric conditions. Attachment avoidance, however, was no longer significantly associated with chronic pain conditions after the investigators took into account psychological health, suggesting that some forms of psychopathology (especially depression and anxiety disorders) may account for the link between attachment avoidance and pain-related conditions. These findings are intriguing and invite further research in this understudied area. In particular, prospective longitudinal studies are essential for clarifying the nature of the attachment–health link, as well as for investigating the possible mediating roles of negative affect such as depression and anxiety.

Emerging Themes and Future Directions

Much of the literature linking attachment in childhood and adulthood to health is newly developing. The work so far suggests that attachment insecurity is a risk factor for a variety of health problems, including dys-regulated stress responses, maladaptive health behaviors, physical symp-toms, and serious outcomes such as heart disease and stroke. Nonethe-less, the small number of studies (particularly regarding the links between attachment and immune responses or health behavior) makes it difficult to generalize about connections between specific forms of attachment insecu-rity (i.e., attachment anxiety, avoidance, or both) and particular response patterns. Some of the variation across studies probably results from differ-ences in the context of the situations or stressors (e.g., relationship-related, achievement-related, relevance to the self) as well as gender-related charac-teristics, and we expect that further work allowing for comparisons across a broader range of contexts will clarify the nature of these links. We sug-gest several promising directions for advancing knowledge about the nature of the attachment–health link, and especially the processes through which attachment from infancy through adulthood shapes later health outcomes.

One important avenue for future research is to pinpoint specific mech-anisms that might account for the link between attachment and health-related outcomes. As Figure 11.1 suggests, physiological responses are likely to be mediating pathways through which attachment influences subsequent health outcomes, but there is no direct evidence on this point. Specifically, further work needs to determine the conditions under which physiological responses (e.g., HPA, SAM responses) to acute stressors mediate the link between attachment and longer-term health/disease outcomes. In addition, most research examines one or two physiological markers or systems in isolation; more needs to be known about how the interplay among dif-ferent physiological markers and systems contributes to the attachment–health link (Diamond & Fagundes, 2010). This work will necessarily entail the use of prospective longitudinal designs that examine the link between attachment and physiological responses at earlier time points, and then test whether physiological responses mediate the link between attachment and later physical health outcomes. Similarly, additional work will be required to determine whether other factors in the model—self-regulatory skills, affect regulation strategies, affective responses, and health behaviors—mediate the relationship between attachment and downstream health out-comes.

Attachment insecurity predicts problematic relationship behaviors, including poorer communication, hostility, and poorer care seeking and caregiving (Beck et al., 2013; Collins & Feeney, 2000; Simpson, Rholes, & Phillips, 1996; Beck, Pietromonaco, DeVito, Powers, & Boyle, 2014). And, as shown in Figure 11.1, such relationship behaviors may provide a key pathway connecting attachment style to health-related physiological responses, health behavior, and downstream health outcomes. Although a few studies have explored links between relationship behavior and physiological responses (Gouin et al., 2009; Kiecolt-Glaser et al., 1993, 1996), no research has directly tested the extent to which relationship behaviors account for links between attachment and subsequent health-related outcomes. Identifying the mediating role of relationship behaviors in the attachment–health link will facilitate efforts to develop interventions to promote health. For example, positive interaction styles or having securely attached partners may act as a *buffer* against negative relationship outcomes for insecure individuals (Salvatore, Kuo, Steele, Simpson, & Collins, 2011). In a similar manner, positive interactions with relationship partners may help to protect insecure individuals from later adverse health consequences. For example, engaging in a positive-mindset emotion regulation intervention prior to discussing a conflict with one's partner decreased cardiovascular arousal and negative affect in both the manipulated person *and* his or her partner; interestingly, this effect was especially robust for individuals high in attachment anxiety (Ben-Naim, Hirschberger, Ein-Dor, & Mikulincer, 2013).

The dyadic context is important for understanding the link between attachment and health-related outcomes (Beck et al., 2013; Pietromonaco, Uchino, et al., 2013; Powers et al., 2006). For example, given the theorized mediating role of physiological activity in the attachment–health link, questions about how romantic partners modulate each other's physiology and downstream health demand further exploration. Emerging research on coregulation focuses on how relationship partners influence each other's psychological and physiological responses (Sbarra & Hazan, 2008). For example, wives who displayed negative behavior in a conflict interaction showed heightened cortisol responses when their husbands withdrew (Kiecolt-Glaser et al., 1996), and the interplay between husbands' avoidance and wives' anxiety has been found to predict distinctive cortisol patterns in response to a conflict discussion (Beck et al., 2013), suggesting the importance of dyadic processes in physiological response patterns. Other work indicates that spouses' cortisol levels are associated with each other (Papp, Pendry, Simon, & Adam, 2013; Saxbe & Repetti, 2010), and that spouses' cortisol levels in response to conflict show convergence over the first 3 years of marriage (Laws, Sayer, Pietromonaco, & Powers, 2014). A challenge for future work will be to determine the conditions under which coregulation processes (and other dyadic processes) contribute over time to health-related behaviors and outcomes.

Still other work underscores the value of taking a dyadic approach for understanding how attachment shapes individuals' health behaviors and illness outcomes. For example, some work has demonstrated the value of incorporating both partners into health behavior change programs (Lewis & Butterfield, 2007), and research in this area would benefit from examining how partners' attachment styles and associated relationship processes affect health behavior change. Recent work highlights the role of dyadic processes in predicting patients' outcomes: Anxiously attached patients with Alzheimer's disease reported more physical and psychological symptoms, especially when their spouses/caregivers were also anxiously attached (Monin, Schulz, & Kershaw, 2013).

Another important set of questions concern the extent to which attachment patterns in childhood versus adulthood contribute to health outcomes via the same or different pathways. For example, little is known about the stability of health-related physiological responses from childhood to adulthood. To what extent are stability between childhood and adult attachment, and the physiological correlates of each, able to account for the links between adult attachment and health outcomes? And to what extent does attachment at different points in development uniquely predict such outcomes? In addition, experiences in early childhood may be more likely than those in adulthood to alter underlying physiological stress response systems (e.g., see Schore, 2001). If so, then early experiences may be more potent predictors of later physical health.

Finally, it will be important to place the connection between attachment and health within the larger context of other kinds of relationships, such as those with health care providers. For example, insecurely attached patients often desire close, supportive relationships with their physicians (Noyes et al., 2003) and trust their physicians less (Holwerda et al., 2013). Such perceptions may contribute to patients' disease outcomes. For instance, patients with diabetes and with dismissing/avoidant attachments who reported lower-quality communications with their provider showed poorer metabolic control (Ciechanowski, Katon, Russo, & Walker, 2001). Research incorporating the perspectives of both health care providers and patients, as well as spouses or close others who may be involved in the care process, will inform the development of tailored interventions that take into account which kinds of communication strategies promote health for which patients.

Conclusions

Attachment patterns from childhood through adulthood are associated with a range of health-related outcomes, including physiological stress responses, health behavior, and health and disease conditions. Although research in this area is growing, many questions remain about how attachment patterns translate into later health and disease outcomes. We hope that our model illustrating potential pathways underlying the attachment–health link, as well as our recommendations for future research, will serve as a roadmap to guide the next generation of studies.

Acknowledgment

Preparation of this chapter was facilitated by a grant from the National Cancer Institute of the National Institutes of Health (Grant No. R01CA133908) to Paula R. Pietromonaco.

References

Ahrens, K. R., Ciechanowski, P. S., & Katon, W. (2012). Associations between adult attachment style and health risk behaviors in an adult female primary care population. *Journal of Psychosomatic Research, 72*(5), 364–370.

Anderson, S. E., Gooze, R. A., Lemeshow, S., & Whitaker, R. C. (2012). Quality of early maternal–child relationship and risk of adolescent obesity. *Pediatrics, 129*(1), 132–140.

Anderson, S. E., & Whitaker, R. C. (2011). Attachment security and obesity in US preschool-aged children. *Archives of Pediatrics and Adolescent Medicine, 165*(3), 235–242.

Andrews, N. E., Meredith, P. J., & Strong, J. (2011). Adult attachment and reports of pain in experimentally-induced pain. *European Journal of Pain, 15*(5), 523–530.

Antoni, M. H., Lutgendorf, S. K., Cole, S. W., Dhabhar, F. S., Sephton, S. E., McDonald, P. G., et al. (2006). The influence of bio-behavioural factors on tumour biology: Pathways and mechanisms. *Nature Reviews Cancer, 6*(3), 240–248.

August, K. J., Rook, K. S., Franks, M. M., & Stephens, M. A. P. (2013). Spouses' involvement in their partners' diabetes management: Associations with spouse stress and perceived marital quality. *Journal of Family Psychology, 27*(5), 712–721.

Beck, L. A., Pietromonaco, P. R., DeBuse, C. J., Powers, S. I., & Sayer, A. G. (2013). Spouses' attachment pairings predict neuroendocrine, behavioral, and psychological responses to marital conflict. *Journal of Personality and Social Psychology, 105*(3), 388–424.

Beck, L. A., Pietromonaco, P. R., DeVito, C. C., Powers, S. I., & Boyle, A. M. (2014). Congruence between spouses' perceptions and observers' ratings of responsiveness: The role of attachment avoidance. *Personality and Social Psychology Bulletin, 40*(2), 164–174.

Ben-Naim, S., Hirschberger, G., Ein-Dor, T., & Mikulincer, M. (2013). An experimental study of emotion regulation during relationship conflict interactions: The moderating role of attachment orientations. *Emotion, 13*(3), 506–519.

Blair, C., & Raver, C. C. (2012). Child development in the context of adversity: Experiential canalization of brain and behavior. *American Psychologist, 67*(4), 309–318.

Boyce, W. T. (1985). Social support, family relations, and children. In S. Cohen & S. L. Syme (Eds.), *Social support and health* (pp. 151–173). San Diego, CA: Academic Press.

Branstetter, S. A., Furman, W., & Cottrell, L. (2009). The influence of representations of attachment, maternal–adolescent relationship quality, and maternal monitoring on adolescent substance use: A 2-year longitudinal examination. *Child Development, 80*(5), 1448–1462.

Brody, G. H., Murry, V. M., Gerrard, M., Gibbons, F. X., McNair, L., Brown, A. C., et al. (2006). The Strong African American Families Program: Prevention of youths' high-risk behavior and a test of a model of change. *Journal of Family Psychology, 20*(1), 1–11.

Brown, S. L., Smith, D. M., Schulz, R., Kabeto, M. U., Ubel, P. A., Poulin, M., et al. (2009). Caregiving behavior is associated with decreased mortality risk. *Psychological Science, 20*(4), 488–494.

Bugental, D. B., Martorell, G. A., & Barraza, V. (2003). The hormonal costs of subtle forms of infant maltreatment. *Hormones and Behavior, 43*(1), 237–244.

Carmichael, C. L., & Reis, H. T. (2005). Attachment, sleep quality, and depressed affect. *Health Psychology, 24*(5), 526–531.

Carnelley, K. B., Pietromonaco, P. R., & Jaffe, K. (1994). Depression, working models of others, and relationship functioning. *Journal of Personality and Social Psychology, 66*(1), 127–140.

Carnelley, K. B., Pietromonaco, P. R., & Jaffe, K. (1996). Attachment, caregiving, and relationship functioning in couples: Effects of self and partner. *Personal Relationships, 3*(3), 257–277.

Cassibba, R., van IJzendoorn, M. H., & Coppola, G. (2012). Emotional availability and attachment across generations: Variations in patterns associated with infant health risk status. *Child: Care, Health and Development, 38*(4), 538–544.

Chen, E., Miller, G. E., Kobor, M. S., & Cole, S. W. (2011). Maternal warmth buffers the effects of low early-life socioeconomic status on pro-inflammatory signaling in adulthood. *Molecular Psychiatry, 16*(7), 729–737.

Ciechanowski, P. S., Katon, W. J., Russo, J. E., & Walker, E. A. (2001). The patient–provider relationship: Attachment theory and adherence to treatment in diabetes. *American Journal of Psychiatry, 158*(1), 29–35.

Ciechanowski, P. S., Russo, J., Katon, W., Von Korff, M., Ludman, E., Lin, E., et al. (2004). Influence of patient attachment style on self-care and outcomes in diabetes. *Psychosomatic Medicine, 66*(5), 720–728.

Ciechanowski, P. S., Walker, E. A., Katon, W. J., & Russo, J. E. (2002). Attachment theory: A model for health care utilization and somatization. *Psychosomatic Medicine, 64*(4), 660–667.

Cohen, S., Doyle, W. J., Alper, C. M., Janicki-Deverts, D., & Turner, R. B. (2009). Sleep habits and susceptibility to the common cold. *Archives of Internal Medicine, 169*(1), 62–67.

Collins, N. L., & Feeney, B. C. (2000). A safe haven: An attachment theory perspective on support seeking and caregiving in intimate relationships. *Journal of Personality and Social Psychology, 78*(6), 1053–1073.

Collins, N. L., & Feeney, B. C. (2004). Working models of attachment shape perceptions of social support: Evidence from experimental and observational studies. *Journal of Personality and Social Psychology, 87*(3), 363–383.

Contreras, J. M., Kerns, K. A., Weimer, B. L., Gentzler, A. L., & Tomich, P. L. (2000). Emotion regulation as a mediator of associations between mother–child attachment and peer relationships in middle childhood. *Journal of Family Psychology, 14*(1), 111–124.

Crosby, R., DiClemente, R., Wingood, G., Cobb, B., Harrington, K., Davies, S., et al. (2001). HIV/STD-protective benefits of living with mothers in perceived supportive families: A study of high-risk African American female teens. *Preventive Medicine, 33*(3), 175–178.

Diamond, L. M., & Fagundes, C. P. (2010). Psychobiological research on attachment. *Journal of Social and Personal Relationships, 27*(2), 218–225.

Diamond, L. M., Hicks, A. M., & Otter-Henderson, K. D. (2008). Every time you go away: Changes in affect, behavior, and physiology associated with travel-related separations from romantic partners. *Journal of Personality and Social Psychology, 95*(2), 385–403.

Dowd, J. B., Palermo, T. M., & Aiello, A. E. (2012). Family poverty is associated with cytomegalovirus antibody titers in U.S. children. *Health Psychology, 31*(1), 5–10.

Dowd, J. B., Zajacova, A., & Aiello, A. E. (2010). Predictors of inflammation in U.S. children aged 3–16 years. *American Journal of Preventive Medicine, 39*(4), 314–320.

Drake, K., Belsky, J., & Fearon, R. M. P. (2014). From early attachment to engagement with learning in school: The role of self-regulation and persistence. *Developmental Psychology, 50*(5), 1350–1361.

Emerson, E., Donenberg, G. R., & Wilson, H. W. (2012). Health-protective effects of attachment among African American girls in psychiatric care. *Journal of Family Psychology, 26*(1), 124–132.

Fagundes, C. P., Glaser, R., & Kiecolt-Glaser, J. K. (2013). Stressful early life experiences and immune dysregulation across the lifespan. *Brain, Behavior, and Immunity, 27*, 8–12.

Feeney, B. C., & Kirkpatrick, L. A. (1996). Effects of adult attachment and presence of romantic partners on physiological responses to stress. *Journal of Personality and Social Psychology, 70*(2), 255–270.

Feeney, J. A., Peterson, C., Gallois, C., & Terry, D. (2000). Attachment style as a predictor of sexual attitudes and behavior in late adolescence. *Psychology and Health, 14*(6), 1105–1122.

Feeney, J. A., & Ryan, S. M. (1994). Attachment style and affect regulation: Relationships with health behavior and family experiences of illness in a student sample. *Health Psychology, 13*(4), 334–345.

Felitti, V. J., Anda, R. F., Nordenberg, D., Williamson, D. F., Spitz, A. M., Edwards, V., et al. (1998). Relationship of childhood abuse and household dysfunction to many of the leading causes of death in adults: The Adverse Childhood Experiences (ACE) Study. *American Journal of Preventive Medicine, 14*(4), 245–258.

Foshee, V., & Bauman, K. E. (1994). Parental attachment and adolescent cigarette smoking initiation. *Journal of Adolescent Research, 9*(1), 88–104.

Fraley, R. C., & Brumbaugh, C. C. (2004). A dynamical systems approach to conceptualizing and studying stability and change in attachment security. In W. S. Rholes & J. A. Simpson (Eds.), *Adult attachment: Theory, research, and clinical implications* (pp. 86–132). New York: Guilford Press.

Frigerio, A., Ceppi, E., Rusconi, M., Giorda, R., Raggi, M. E., & Fearon, P. (2009). The role played by the interaction between genetic factors and attachment in the stress response in infancy. *Journal of Child Psychology and Psychiatry, 50*(12), 1513–1522.

Gallo, L. C., & Matthews, K. A. (2006). Adolescents' attachment orientation influences ambulatory blood pressure responses to everyday social interactions. *Psychosomatic Medicine, 68*(2), 253–261.

Goldberg, S., Simmons, R. J., Newman, J., Campbell, K., & Fowler, R. S. (1991). Congenital heart disease parental stress and infant–mother relationships. *Journal of Pediatrics, 119*(4), 661–666.

Goossens, L., Braet, C., Bosmans, G., & Decaluwé, V. (2011). Loss of control over eating in pre-adolescent youth: The role of attachment and self-esteem. *Eating Behaviors, 12*(4), 289–295.

Gouin, J.-P., Glaser, R., Loving, T. J., Malarkey, W. B., Stowell, J., Houts, C., et al. (2009). Attachment avoidance predicts inflammatory responses to marital conflict. *Brain, Behavior, and Immunity, 23*(7), 898–904.

Grandner, M. A., Jackson, N. J., Pak, V. M., & Gehrman, P. R. (2012). Sleep disturbance is associated with cardiovascular and metabolic disorders. *Journal of Sleep Research, 21*(4), 427–433.

Gunnar, M. R., Brodersen, L., Nachmias, M., Buss, K., & Rigatuso, J. (1996). Stress reactivity and attachment security. *Developmental Psychobiology, 29*(3), 191–204.

Gunnar, M. R., & Donzella, B. (2002). Social regulation of the cortisol levels in early human development. *Psychoneuroendocrinology, 27*(1–2), 199–220.

Hasler, B. P., & Troxel, W. M. (2010). Couples' nighttime sleep efficiency and concordance: Evidence for bidirectional associations with daytime relationship functioning. *Psychosomatic Medicine, 72*(8), 794–801.

Hertsgaard, L., Gunnar, M., Erickson, M. F., & Nachmias, M. (1995). Adrenocortical responses to the Strange Situation in infants with disorganized/disoriented attachment relationships. *Child Development, 66*(4), 1100–1106.

Hicks, A. M., & Diamond, L. M. (2011). Don't go to bed angry: Attachment, conflict, and affective and physiological reactivity. *Personal Relationships, 18*(2), 266–284.

Hill, E. M., & Gick, M. L. (2013). Attachment and barriers to cervical screening. *Journal of Health Psychology, 18*(5), 648–657.

Holt-Lunstad, J., Smith, T. B., & Layton, J. B. (2010). Social relationships and mortality risk: A meta-analytic review. *PLoS Medicine, 7*(7), 1–20.

Holwerda, N., Sanderman, R., Pool, G., Hinnen, C., Langendijk, J., A., Bemelman, W. A., et al. (2013). Do patients trust their physician?: The role of attachment style in the patient–physician relationship within one year after a cancer diagnosis. *Acta Oncologica, 52*(1), 110–117.

Huntsinger, E., & Luecken, L. (2004). Attachment relationships and health behavior: The mediational role of self-esteem. *Psychology and Health, 19*(4), 515–526.

Jaremka, L. M., Glaser, R., Loving, T. J., Malarkey, W. B., Stowell, J. R., & Kiecolt-Glaser, J. K. (2013). Attachment anxiety is linked to alterations in cortisol production and cellular immunity. *Psychological Science, 24*(3), 272–279.

Kelly-Irving, M., Lepage, B., Dedieu, D., Lacey, R., Cable, N., Bartley, M., et al. (2013). Childhood adversity as a risk for cancer: Findings from the 1958 British birth cohort study. *BMC Public Health, 13*(1), 1–13.

Kelsay, K., Leung, D. Y. M., Mrazek, D. A., & Klinnert, M. D. (2013). Prospectively assessed early life experiences in relation to cortisol reactivity in adolescents at risk for asthma. *Developmental Psychobiology, 55*(2), 133–144.

Kerns, K. A., Klepac, L., & Cole, A. (1996). Peer relationships and preadolescents' perceptions of security in the child–mother relationship. *Developmental Psychology, 32*(3), 457–466.

Kidd, T., & Sheffield, D. (2005). Attachment style and symptom reporting: Examining the mediating effects of anger and social support. *British Journal of Health Psychology, 10*(4), 531–541.

Kiecolt-Glaser, J. K., Malarkey, W. B., Chee, M., Newton, T., Cacioppo, J. T., Mao, H. Y., et al. (1993). Negative behavior during marital conflict is associated with immunological down-regulation. *Psychosomatic Medicine, 55*(5), 395–409.

Kiecolt-Glaser, J. K., & Newton, T. L. (2001). Marriage and health: His and hers. *Psychological Bulletin, 127*(4), 472–503.

Kiecolt-Glaser, J. K., Newton, T., Cacioppo, J. T., MacCallum, R. C., Glaser, R., & Malarkey, W. B. (1996). Marital conflict and endocrine function: Are men really more physiologically affected than women? *Journal of Consulting and Clinical Psychology, 64*(2), 324–332.

Kochanska, G., Philibert, R. A., & Barry, R. A. (2009). Interplay of genes and early mother–child relationship in the development of self-regulation from toddler to preschool age. *Journal of Child Psychology and Psychiatry, 50*(11), 1331–1338.

Kratz, A. L., Davis, M. C., & Zautra, A. J. (2012). Attachment predicts daily catastrophizing and social coping in women with pain. *Health Psychology, 31*(3), 278–285.

Laws, H., Sayer, A. G., Pietromonaco, P. R., & Powers, S. I. (2014). *Longitudinal changes in spouses' cortisol response patterns: Physiological convergence in newlywed couples.* Manuscript under review.

Lehman, B. J., Taylor, S. E., Kiefe, C. I., & Seeman, T. E. (2005). Relation of childhood socioeconomic status and family environment to adult metabolic functioning in the CARDIA study. *Psychosomatic Medicine, 67*(6), 846–854.

Lewis, M. A., & Butterfield, R. M. (2007). Social control in marital relationships: Effect of one's partner on health behaviors. *Journal of Applied Social Psychology, 37*(2), 298–319.

Luecken, L. J. (1998). Childhood attachment and loss experiences affect adult cardiovascular and cortisol function. *Psychosomatic Medicine, 60*(6), 765–772.

Luster, T., & Small, S. A. (1994). Factors associated with sexual risk-taking behaviors among adolescents. *Journal of Marriage and the Family, 56*(3), 622–632.

MacDonald, G. (2008). Use of pain threshold reports to satisfy social needs. *Pain Research and Management, 13*(4), 309–319.

Mangelsdorf, S., Gunnar, M., Kestenbaum, R., Lang, S., & Andreas, D. (1990). Infant proneness-to-distress temperament, maternal personality, and mother–infant attachment: Associations and goodness of fit. *Child Development, 61*(3), 820–831.

Maunder, R. G., & Hunter, J. J. (2001). Attachment and psychosomatic medicine: Developmental contributions to stress and disease. *Psychosomatic Medicine, 63*(4), 556–567.

Maunder, R. G., & Hunter, J. J. (2008). Attachment relationships as determinants of physical health. *Journal of the American Academy of Psychoanalysis and Dynamic Psychiatry, 36*(1), 11–32.

Maunder, R. G., Hunter, J. J., & Lancee, W. J. (2011). The impact of attachment insecurity and sleep disturbance on symptoms and sick days in hospital-based health-care workers. *Journal of Psychosomatic Research, 70*(1), 11–17.

McWilliams, L., & Bailey, S. (2010). Associations between adult attachment ratings and health conditions: Evidence from the National Comorbidity Survey Replication. *Health Psychology, 29*(4), 446–453.

Meredith, P. J., Strong, J., & Feeney, J. A. (2006). The relationship of adult attachment to emotion, catastrophizing, control, threshold and tolerance, in experimentally-induced pain. *Pain, 120*(1–2), 44–52.

Mickelson, K. D., Kessler, R. C., & Shaver, P. R. (1997). Adult attachment in a nationally representative sample. *Journal of Personality and Social Psychology, 73*, 1092–1106.

Mikulincer, M. (1998). Adult attachment style and individual differences in functional versus dysfunctional experiences of anger. *Journal of Personality and Social Psychology, 74*(2), 513–524.

Mikulincer, M., & Shaver, P. R. (2007). *Attachment in adulthood: Structure, dynamics, and change.* New York: Guilford Press.

Miller, A. H. (2010). Depression and immunity: A role for T cells? *Brain, Behavior, and Immunity, 24*(1), 1–8.

Miller, G. E., & Chen, E. (2010). Harsh family climate in early life presages the emergence of a proinflammatory phenotype in adolescence. *Psychological Science, 21*(6), 848–856.

Miller, G. E., Chen, E., & Parker, K. J. (2011). Psychological stress in childhood and susceptibility to the chronic diseases of aging: Moving toward a model of behavioral and biological mechanisms. *Psychological Bulletin, 137*(6), 959–997.

Miller, G. E., Chen, E., & Zhou, E. S. (2007). If it goes up, must it come down?: Chronic stress and the hypothalamic–pituitary–adrenocortical axis in humans. *Psychological Bulletin, 133*(1), 25–45.

Miller, G. E., & Cole, S. W. (2012). Clustering of depression and inflammation in adolescents previously exposed to childhood adversity. *Biological Psychiatry, 72*(1), 34–40.

Miller, G. E., Lachman, M. E., Chen, E., Gruenewald, T. L., Karlamangla, A. S., & Seeman, T. E. (2011). Pathways to resilience: Maternal nurturance as a buffer against the effects of childhood poverty on metabolic syndrome at midlife. *Psychological Science, 22*(12), 1591–1599.

Monin, J. K., Schulz, R., & Kershaw, T. S. (2013). Caregiving spouses' attachment orientations and the physical and psychological health of individuals with Alzheimer's disease. *Aging and Mental Health, 17*(4), 508–516.

Moore, M. R., & Chase-Lansdale, P. L. (2001). Sexual intercourse and pregnancy among African American girls in high-poverty neighborhoods: The role of family and perceived community environment. *Journal of Marriage and Family, 63*(4), 1146–1157.

Mrazek, D. A., Casey, B., & Anderson, I. (1987). Insecure attachment in severely asthmatic preschool children: Is it a risk factor? *Journal of the American Academy of Child and Adolescent Psychiatry, 26*, 516–520.

Nachmias, M., Gunnar, M., Mangelsdorf, S., Parritz, R. H., & Buss, K. (1996).

Behavioral inhibition and stress reactivity: The moderating role of attachment security. *Child Development, 67*(2), 508–522.

Novak, S. A., & Webster, G. D. (2011). Spousal social control during a weight loss attempt: A daily diary study. *Personal Relationships, 18*(2), 224–241.

Noyes, R., Stuart, S. P., Langbehn, D. R., Happel, R. L., Longley, S. L., Muller, B. A., et al. (2003). Test of an interpersonal model of hypochondriasis. *Psychosomatic Medicine, 65*(2), 292–300.

O'Shaughnessy, R., & Dallos, R. (2009). Attachment research and eating disorders: A review of the literature. *Clinical Child Psychology and Psychiatry, 14*(4), 559–574.

Papp, L. M., Pendry, P., Simon, C. D., & Adam, E. K. (2013). Spouses' cortisol associations and moderators: Testing physiological synchrony and connectedness in everyday life. *Family Process, 52*(2), 284–298.

Pietromonaco, P. R., & Barrett, L. F. (1997). Working models of attachment and daily social interactions. *Journal of Personality and Social Psychology, 73*(6), 1409–1423.

Pietromonaco, P. R., Barrett, L. F., & Powers, S. I. (2006). Adult attachment theory and affective reactivity and regulation. In D. K. Snyder, J. Simpson, & J. N. Hughes (Eds.), *Emotion regulation in couples and families: Pathways to dysfunction and health* (pp. 57–74). Washington, DC: American Psychological Association.

Pietromonaco, P. R., & Beck, L. A. (2015). Attachment processes in adult romantic relationships. In M. Mikulincer, P. R. Shaver, J. A. Simpson, & J. F. Dovidio (Eds.), *APA handbook of personality and social psychology: Vol. 3. Interpersonal relations* (pp. 33–64). Washington, DC: American Psychological Association.

Pietromonaco, P. R., DeBuse, C. J., & Powers, S. I. (2013). Does attachment get under the skin?: Adult romantic attachment and cortisol responses to stress. *Current Directions in Psychological Science, 22*(1), 63–68.

Pietromonaco, P. R., Uchino, B., & Dunkel Schetter, C. (2013). Close relationship processes and health: Implications of attachment theory for health and disease. *Health Psychology, 32*(5), 499–513.

Powers, S. I., Pietromonaco, P. R., Gunlicks, M., & Sayer, A. (2006). Dating couples' attachment styles and patterns of cortisol reactivity and recovery in response to a relationship conflict. *Journal of Personality and Social Psychology, 90*(4), 613–628.

Prather, A. A., Hall, M., Fury, J. M., Ross, D. C., Muldoon, M. F., Cohen, S., & Marsland, A. L. (2012). Sleep and antibody response to hepatitis B vaccination. *Sleep, 35*(8), 1063–1069.

Puig, J., Englund, M. M., Simpson, J. A., & Collins, W. A. (2013). Predicting adult physical illness from infant attachment: A prospective longitudinal study. *Health Psychology, 32*(4), 409–417.

Repetti, R. L., Taylor, S. E., & Seeman, T. E. (2002). Risky families: Family social environments and the mental and physical health of offspring. *Psychological Bulletin, 128*(2), 330–366.

Robles, T. F., Brooks, K. P., Kane, H. S., & Schetter, C. D. (2013). Attachment, skin deep?: Relationships between adult attachment and skin barrier recovery. *International Journal of Psychophysiology, 88*(3), 241–252.

Robles, T. F., Slatcher, R. B., Trombello, J. M., & McGinn, M. M. (2014). Marital quality and health: A meta-analytic review. *Psychological Bulletin, 140*(1), 140–187.

Rosenberg, T., & Shields, C. (2009). The role of parent–adolescent attachment in the glycemic control of adolescents with type 1 diabetes: A pilot study. *Families, Systems and Health: Journal of Collaborative Family HealthCare, 27*(3), 237–248.

Salvatore, J. E., Kuo, S. I.-C., Steele, R. D., Simpson, J. A., & Collins, W. A. (2011). Recovering from conflict in romantic relationships: A developmental perspective. *Psychological Science, 22*(3), 376–383.

Saxbe, D., & Repetti, R. L. (2010). For better or worse?: Coregulation of couples' cortisol levels and mood states. *Journal of Personality and Social Psychology, 98*(1), 92–103.

Sbarra, D. A., & Hazan, C. (2008). Coregulation, dysregulation, self-regulation: An integrative analysis and empirical agenda for understanding adult attachment, separation, loss, and recovery. *Personality and Social Psychology Review, 12*(2), 141–167.

Schore, A. N. (2001). Effects of a secure attachment relationship on right brain development, affect regulation, and infant mental health. *Infant Mental Health Journal, 22*(1–2), 7–66.

Shonkoff, J., Boyce, W., & McEwen, B. (2009). Neuroscience, molecular biology, and the childhood roots of health disparities: Building a new framework for health promotion and disease prevention. *Journal of the American Medical Association, 301*(21), 2252–2259.

Simpson, J. A., Rholes, W. S., Campbell, L., Tran, S., & Wilson, C. L. (2003). Adult attachment, the transition to parenthood, and depressive symptoms. *Journal of Personality and Social Psychology, 84*(6), 1172–1187.

Simpson, J. A., Rholes, W. S., & Phillips, D. (1996). Conflict in close relationships: An attachment perspective. *Journal of Personality and Social Psychology, 71*(5), 899–914.

Simpson, J. A., Winterheld, H. A., Rholes, W. S., & Oriña, M. M. (2007). Working models of attachment and reactions to different forms of caregiving from romantic partners. *Journal of Personality and Social Psychology, 93*(3), 466–477.

Slopen, N., Koenen, K. C., & Kubzansky, L. D. (2012). Childhood adversity and immune and inflammatory biomarkers associated with cardiovascular risk in youth: A systematic review. *Brain, Behavior, and Immunity, 26*(2), 239–250.

Spangler, G., & Grossmann, K. E. (1993). Biobehavioral organization in securely and insecurely attached infants. *Child Development, 64*(5), 1439–1450.

Spangler, G., & Schieche, M. (1998). Emotional and adrenocortical responses of infants to the strange situation: The differential function of emotional expression. *International Journal of Behavioral Development, 22*(4), 681–706.

Stephens, M. A. P., Franks, M. M., Rook, K. S., Iida, M., Hemphill, R. C., & Salem, J. K. (2013). Spouses' attempts to regulate day-to-day dietary adherence among patients with type 2 diabetes. *Health Psychology, 32*(10), 1029–1037.

Steptoe, A., & Kivimäki, M. (2013). Stress and cardiovascular disease: An update on current knowledge. *Annual Review of Public Health, 34*, 337–354.

Stewart-Brown, S., Fletcher, L., & Wadsworth, M. (2005). Parent–child relationships and health problems in adulthood in three UK national birth cohort studies. *European Journal of Public Health*, 15(6), 640–646.

Tamayo, T., Christian, H., & Rathmann, W. (2010). Impact of early psychosocial factors (childhood socioeconomic factors and adversities) on future risk of type 2 diabetes, metabolic disturbances and obesity: A systematic review. *BMC Public Health*, 10, 525–539.

Tangney, J. P., Baumeister, R. F., & Boone, A. L. (2004). High self-control predicts good adjustment, less pathology, better grades, and interpersonal success. *Journal of Personality*, 72(2), 271–322.

Taylor, S. E., Lerner, J. S., Sage, R. M., Lehman, B. J., & Seeman, T. E. (2004). Early environment, emotions, responses to stress, and health. *Journal of Personality*, 72(6), 1365–1393.

Taylor, S. E., Way, B. M., & Seeman, T. E. (2011). Early adversity and adult health outcomes. *Development and Psychopathology*, 23(3), 939–954.

Thomas, A., & Chess, S. (1977). *Temperament and development*. New York: Brunner/Mazel.

Troxel, W. M., Cyranowski, J. M., Hall, M., Frank, E., & Buysse, D. J. (2007). Attachment anxiety, relationship context, and sleep in women with recurrent major depression. *Psychosomatic Medicine*, 69(7), 692–699.

Troxel, W. M., & Germain, A. (2011). Insecure attachment is an independent correlate of objective sleep disturbances in military veterans. *Sleep Medicine*, 12(9), 860–865.

Uchino, B. N. (2009). Understanding the links between social support and physical health: A life-span perspective with emphasis on the separability of perceived and received support. *Perspectives on Psychological Science*, 4(3), 236–255.

Uchino, B. N., Cacioppo, J. T., & Kiecolt-Glaser, J. K. (1996). The relationship between social support and physiological processes: A review with emphasis on underlying mechanisms and implications for health. *Psychological Bulletin*, 119(3), 488–531.

Verdecias, R. N., Jean-Louis, G., Zizi, F., Casimir, G. J., & Browne, R. C. (2009). Attachment styles and sleep measures in a community-based sample of older adults. *Sleep Medicine*, 10(6), 664–667.

Wei, M., Mallinckrodt, B., Larson, L. M., & Zakalik, R. A. (2005). Adult attachment, depressive symptoms, and validation from self versus others. *Journal of Counseling Psychology*, 52(3), 368–377.

Wilson, C. L., & Ruben, M. A. (2011). A pain in her arm: Romantic attachment orientations and the tourniquet task. *Personal Relationships*, 18(2), 242–265.

Attachment and Aged Care

Gery C. Karantzas
Jeffry A. Simpson

Approximately 524 million people are over the age of 65, and by the year 2050, this figure will rise to 1.5 billion (National Institute on Aging [NIA], 2011; World Health Organization [WHO], 2012). Furthermore, about 80% of people within this age group report having at least one chronic health condition (National Center for Chronic Disease Prevention and Health Promotion, 2011). Because of these trends, the aging of the population has introduced new challenges for couples and families regarding the care of ailing older adults. No longer is aged care the primary responsibility of the state or government. Instead, family members (whether these are aging adults' spouses/partners, or grown children and their partners) are increasingly becoming the primary carers of aging adults, as federal and state governments in most parts of the globe struggle to meet the health care demands of their aging societies (Karantzas, Evans, & Foddy, 2010; NIA, 2011; WHO, 2012). In the coming decades, caring for an older adult is likely to become a normal life task for many—and perhaps most—adult children and their spouses. Caring for an older person, however, is a highly stressful and challenging responsibility, even for family members; it involves coming to terms with the eventual decline and ultimate loss of someone who often has been a primary source of love, comfort, and support across a carer's entire life. From this perspective, attachment theory (Bowlby, 1969/1982) provides a particularly useful and powerful framework for understanding the processes of caregiving and care receiving, as well as the mental health outcomes experienced by both carers and care recipients. Because it is a lifespan theory of development, attachment theory also provides a unique framework to comprehend how both attachment and caring processes operate in later life.

We begin the chapter by outlining key concepts and ideas in attachment theory, especially those relevant to understanding attachment during later life within the context of aged care. We then provide an overview of existing research linking attachment theory to aged care, highlighting important and novel issues associated with attachment, aged care, and later-life attachment more generally. We conclude the chapter by posing and discussing questions that are likely to shape future directions for research on aged care and attachment processes.

Attachment Concepts and Their Relevance to Aging and Aged Care

Attachment Theory: A Diathesis–Stress Model

According to Bowlby (1969/1982), the regulation and management of our emotional bonds with those closest to us is governed by the attachment behavioral system. This integrated behavioral system motivates people to seek proximity to their attachment figures in order to gain comfort and a sense of safety when they feel threatened or distressed. Attachment theory, therefore, is not merely a theory of human bonding; it is a theory of emotional and distress regulation (Mikulincer & Shaver, 2007a; Simpson & Rholes, 1994). As such, the theory provides a comprehensive framework for understanding how close relationships shape the way in which families deal with stressors and strains, such as the emotional highs and lows of caring for an aging parent. Consistent with other research linking attachment theory to stressful family situations (e.g., the transition to parenthood; see, e.g., Rholes, Simpson, Campbell, & Grich, 2001; Simpson, Rholes, Campbell, Tran, & Wilson, 2003), attachment theory provides a diathesis–stress approach for understanding how and why certain family members who encounter the stress of caring for an older adult tend to experience greater difficulty in the caregiving role (see also Simpson & Rholes, 2012). This approach can also aid in identifying which older adults are particularly susceptible to experiencing difficulties in accepting care from certain family members and adjusting to their own ailing health and functional decline. Thus the application of attachment theory as a diathesis–stress model allows us to unpack the familial vulnerabilities as well as the contextual factors/stressors that shape the physical and emotional well-being of both carers and care recipients.

Felt Security, Proximity Seeking, and Protective Behavior

According to Bowlby (1969/1982), the primary goal of the attachment system is to maintain a state of *felt security*—a physical and/or psychological state in which a person feels safe and protected. When this state is compromised (by experiencing a stressful event or being exposed to a threatening situation), most individuals try to seek out their attachment figures in order to reestablish felt security (these efforts are termed *proximity seeking*). In childhood, felt security is achieved by engaging in rather direct proximity-seeking behaviors, such as when an upset child maintains close physical distance to his or her parent/guardian (e.g., Ainsworth, Blehar, Waters, & Wall, 1978; Vaughn, Egeland, Sroufe, & Waters, 1979).

Compared to young children, adults do not require direct or frequent physical contact with their parents in order to feel secure and safe in threatening situations. Rather, adults can achieve a sense of comfort and security by simply thinking about (symbolically representing) their parents—specifically, through generating thoughts or memories of closeness, internalized shared values, goals, or common interests with their parents (Cicirelli, 1993). As Koski and Shaver (1997) point out, "availability becomes more abstract and no longer requires constant, immediate physical presence" (p. 29). This symbolic representation of contact can be periodically reinforced by direct communication with parents during visits, or via telephone calls or other forms of contact. These behaviors can be conceptualized as an extension of an infant's original working models of his or her parents. Attachment during adulthood, in other words, does not always require actual physical proximity, because felt security can be achieved by stimulated closeness via thoughts, fantasies, and imagery of parents (Cicirelli, 1991, 1993; Shaver & Mikulincer, 2004). This symbolic aspect of attachment has been supported by Troll and Smith (1976), who found that strong familial attachments between older parents and their adult children are often maintained, regardless of their contact frequency or proximity maintenance. Therefore, positive recollections of a parent as an attachment figure, coupled with phone calls, e-mails, and other nonphysical contact, can sustain the parent as a secure base and safe haven, even when a child becomes an adult.

Cicirelli (1998) suggests that in later life, a powerful attachment threat for an adult child is the current or imminent ill health of a parent. When parents become ill, most adult children will engage in proximity seeking manifested in caregiving actions, which Cicirelli has termed *protective behavior*. Protective behavior is designed to preserve or restore the existence of the threatened attachment figure (Bowlby, 1979, 1980; Cicirelli, 1983, 1985). As the vulnerability of a child's attachment bond with a parent becomes salient due to the onset of age-related illnesses, the adult child may become motivated to protect the parent, especially if the parent continues to be an important source of emotional security. Through caregiving and other forms of helping behavior, the adult child should attempt to delay the eventual loss of the parent for as long as possible. To put this another way, the parent's ill health and potential dependency pose a threat to the longevity of the familial attachment bond, which in turn should activate a drive in an adult child to protect the parent through some form of helping or caregiving behavior (Cicirelli, 1998; Mikulincer & Shaver, 2007a). Cicirelli's concept of protective behavior is intriguing, and it may help to explain the normative functioning of the attachment system when an adult child (and perhaps his or her spouse) deals with the failing health of an older parent (or older partner). However, research has not yet tested Cicirelli's assumptions about caregiving as a manifestation of protective behavior.

Behavioral Systems

Implicit in much of the work linking attachment to aged care is the interplay between different behavioral systems—namely, the attachment behavioral system in relation to the caregiving system. According to Bowlby (1969/1982), the caregiving system is complementary to the attachment system, in that it motivates an individual to offer assistance, comfort, and support when another person is distressed and needs help. As such, the goal of the caregiving system is to respond to another individual's need for felt security by providing sensitive and responsive care (Canterberry & Gillath, 2012; Gillath, Shaver, & Mikulincer, 2005). The caregiving system is activated when an individual detects that another is distressed or needs help, and is deactivated when the care recipient's need is met or his or her sense of security is reestablished (Canterberry & Gillath, 2012; Gillath et al., 2005). To date, a considerable amount of early childhood and adult attachment research has examined the associations between these two behavioral systems. For example, research on adult attachment orientations and the experimental enhancement of people's sense of security by priming attachment security have provided important insights into the dynamic interplay of these two systems (for reviews, see Canterberry & Gillath, 2012; George & Solomon, 2008; Mikulincer & Shaver, 2007a, 2007b).

Recently, Canterberry and Gillath (2012) have proposed a model of caregiving system activation and dynamics that directly maps onto Mikulincer and Shaver's (2003, 2007a) model of attachment system dynamics. The Canterberry and Gillath model provides an organizational framework that articulates the role that certain individual differences play in the functioning of the caregiving system, and how they align with other individual differences associated with the functioning of the attachment system. Specifically, the model posits that people can engage in one of three broad caregiving strategies: (1) sensitive and responsive caregiving, (2) hyperactivating caregiving, or (3) deactivating caregiving. Sensitive and responsive caregiving strategies reflect caregiving that is delivered in an appropriate manner and that meets the care recipient's specific needs. Hyperactivating caregiving strategies entail caregiving behaviors that are intrusive, compulsive, and persistent in nature and are delivered in a way that usually intensifies the care recipient's distress or fails to meet the person's needs. Deactivating strategies refer to caregiving that is distant, minimal, and lacking in emotional content. Sensitive and responsive caregiving tends to be enacted by securely attached individuals. Hyperactivating caregiving strategies are typically enacted by anxiously attached individuals, who rely on hyperactivating attachment strategies to regulate their emotions when they are distressed (i.e., strategies in which distress and proximity-seeking efforts are intensified). Deactivating caregiving strategies are displayed by avoidantly attached individuals, who use deactivating attachment strategies when they become upset (i.e., strategies in which distress is minimized and proximity seeking is inhibited).

Despite the utility of the Canterberry and Gillath (2012) model and research that has attempted to test connections between the attachment and caregiving systems, aged-care research has not systematically investigated the links between attachment and caregiving from a behavioral systems perspective. The aged-care field needs to incorporate behavioral systems approaches and concepts in studies linking attachment principles to the care of older adults. The framing of research and testing of assumptions proposed in the Canterberry and Gillath model and related models (e.g., Feeney & Collins, 2004) is particularly important, given Cicirelli's (1998) conceptualization of attachment theory and protective behavior. For instance, from a behavioral systems perspective, one can argue that protective behavior represents the functioning of the attachment system. That is, wanting to be near and wanting to assist an ailing attachment figure (parent or partner) could be a form of proximity seeking that is motivated by the need to feel more secure when faced with the impending loss of an attachment figure (parent or partner). Alternatively, protective behavior may reflect the functioning of the caregiving system, in which a carer notices the older adult's distress, concern, or calls for help, which then motivates the carer to alleviate the older adult's distress or suffering. These competing but equally plausible explanations of protective behavior constitute merely one example of the utility of integrating behavioral systems approaches to elucidate the pathways linking attachment behavior with caregiving behavior in the context of aged care.

Research Trends in Attachment Research within Aging and Aged Care

One of John Bowlby's most widely quoted statements is his contention that attachment relationships shape individuals across the entire lifespan "from the cradle to the grave" (1979, p. 129). Despite this assertion, the lion's share of research has investigated attachment processes no further than early to middle adulthood. Thus there is a very large gap in our understanding of the nature of attachment bonds in later life (especially between adult children and their older parents) and how these bonds influence attitudes, behaviors, and outcomes in contexts such as aged care. Given this large gap in our understanding, scholars have called for the greater application of attachment theory to the study of aging families for many decades.

Some of the earliest work on attachment theory and its application to later-life familial relationships can be attributed to Troll and Smith (1976). They documented that the strength of what they termed "familial attachment bonds" between young adults and their kin (which included parents and grandparents) was not dependent on the frequency of contact or on whether family members lived close to one another. This research provided initial evidence that attachment bonds are indeed functional and relevant to the lives of individuals within families as they traverse the lifespan. As a consequence of this and subsequent early research on later-life attachment (e.g., Kalish & Knudtson, 1976; Thompson & Walker, 1984), developmentalists and gerontologists began to see greater value in applying attachment theory to how families navigate important later-life transitions, such as caring for ailing older adults (Cicirelli, 1983; Thompson & Walker, 1984).

Despite this early interest, attachment theory and its principles have received little attention in recent aged-care research (see Karantzas, Evans, et al., 2010; Mikulincer & Shaver, 2007a; Van Assche et al., 2013). In fact, until the last decade, only about 10% of all gerontology research has focused on family relationships (Allen, Blieszner, & Roberto, 2000), and even less research has explicitly focused on attachment theory and its potential applications to aged care. Instead, aged-care research has been surprisingly atheoretical, with approximately half of these studies using no theoretical model(s) to frame the research (see Dilworth-Anderson, Williams, & Gibson, 2002).

Of the studies that have attempted to explain familial responsibilities and outcomes of aged care in terms of existing theories or models, most have used principles of distributive and procedural justice, social exchange, transactional models of stress and coping, gender role socialization and culture, filial obligation, and intergenerational solidarity (e.g., Bengtson, 2001; Blieszner & Mancini, 1987; Guberman, Maheu, & Maille, 1992; Knight, Silverstein, McCallum, & Fox, 2000; Miller & Cafasso, 1992; Silverstein & Bengtson, 1997; Silverstein, Gans, & Yang, 2006). Although these perspectives have provided important insights into familial caregiving, they have fallen short of providing clear insights into *how* established familial relationship dynamics shape (1) the assistance given by family members to older adults, and (2) older adults' reactions to both seeking and receiving care.

Taking stock of the limited research on attachment and aged care, we (Karantzas, Karantzas, Simpson, & McCabe, 2014) recently conducted a systematic review of this literature. This research revealed that 149 studies claimed to have investigated attachment variables or processes in the context of aged care. Of these studies, however, only 26% explicitly measured attachment styles or orientations. The remaining studies either drew on attachment theory to frame the research or claimed to measure attachment styles/orientations, but actually did not. Instead, a number of these studies measured concepts related to attachment, such as affection, parental bonding, or perceptions of emotional closeness.

An Overview of Attachment and Aged-Care Research

Attachment, Caregiving, and Carer Outcomes

Of the research on aged care that has explicitly used attachment measures, most investigations have focused on the carers' perspective, particularly adult children of aging parents (rather than the aging persons' spouses) (Karantzas et al., 2014; Van Assche et al., 2013). Furthermore, research linking attachment and aged care has primarily examined (1) how the *strength* of the attachment bond between a carer and a care recipient is related to caregiving/helping behavior, or (2) how *individual differences* in attachment mental representations and behavior are associated with caregiving behavior and carers' outcomes.

In regard to the strength of attachment, research has found that stronger self-reported attachment ties between carers and care recipients are associated with more helping behavior and better carer outcomes in general. For example, Thompson and Walker (1984) found that more mother–daughter caregiving reciprocity was associated with stronger attachment ties. Pohl, Boyd, Liang, and Given (1995) found that stronger daughter–mother attachment was associated with daughters' providing more care to their aging mothers. Similarly, Cicirelli (1983, 1993) found that stronger daughter–mother attachment was associated with daughters' providing more care to their aging mothers and experiencing less burden.

Individual differences in attachment mental representations and attachment behavior provide additional insights about the connections between and among attachment, caregiving, and care outcomes. In a recent study, Chen et al. (2013) found that adult children's secure base mental representations predicted fewer negatively expressed emotions directed at older parents—a finding that was moderated by adult children's perceptions of their care of elderly parents as difficult.

Our own work and that of others has found that attachment insecurity (i.e., attachment anxiety and attachment avoidance) is negatively associated with the *amount* of care adult children provide to older parents who need assistance, and that it is positively associated with carer burden, depression, anxiety, and stress (e.g., Carpenter, 2001; Crispi, Schiaffino, & Berman, 1997; Karantzas, 2012; Karantzas, Evans, et al., 2010; Magai

& Cohen, 1998; Nelis, Clare, & Whitaker, 2012). In contrast, attachment security is positively associated with the amount and quality of care provided by adult children to their aging parents, and negatively associated with the carers' burden and mental health outcomes (e.g., Carpenter, 2001; Cooper, Owens, Katona, & Livingston, 2008; Karantzas, Evans, et al., 2010; Magai & Cohen, 1998; Nelis et al., 2012).

In regard to the *type* of care rendered to older adults, research has found that attachment anxiety is negatively associated with adult children's provision of both emotional and instrumental support (Carpenter, 2001; Kim & Carver, 2007). Studies of attachment avoidance show less consistent findings, with some reporting negative associations and others reporting no link between adult children's attachment avoidance and the provision of either emotional or instrumental support to older parents (e.g., Carpenter, 2001; Kim & Carver, 2007; Pohl et al., 1995). However, attachment avoidance is positively associated with adult children's tendency to place their aging parents in residential care facilities (Markiewicz, Reis, & Gold, 1997). In contrast, attachment security is positively associated with adult children's provision of emotional and instrumental help to their aging parents, along with a tendency to keep their parents in their own homes rather than put them in residential care facilities (Markiewicz et al., 1997).

In the only study to date investigating attachment and the *style* (the manner) in which care is provided, Braun et al. (2012) found that in older couples dealing with cancer, carers' attachment avoidance was negatively associated with the provision of sensitive care, whereas carers' attachment anxiety was associated with the provision of compulsive caregiving. In addition, both attachment anxiety and attachment avoidance were associated with carers' engaging in more controlling care toward their older spouses.

During the last decade, a handful of studies have examined how attachment is related to the future care of older adults. Specifically, attachment security and attachment strength are positively correlated with adult children's preparedness and willingness to provide future care to older adults (Cicirelli, 1983; Sörensen, Webster, & Roggman, 2002). In contrast, attachment insecurity is negatively associated with carers' willingness to plan or their intentions to give care to older adults in the future (Karantzas, Evans, et al., 2010; Sörensen et al., 2002). Our work and that of others has also found that attachment avoidance is strongly associated with adult children's unwillingness to provide future care to older parents (Karantzas, Evans, et al., 2010; Sörensen et al., 2002).

Attachment, Care Receiving/Care Seeking, and Care Recipient Outcomes

Over the last four decades, very little research has investigated how attachment processes shape how older adults seek and receive care and their physical and mental health outcomes. This is true despite the fact that many studies of attachment and aged care appear to have collected data on care recipients' physical and/or emotional well-being.

In our systematic review of the literature (Karantzas et al., 2014), we found only five studies that reported associations between and among attachment, care receipt/care seeking, and health outcomes from the perspective of the care recipients. In relation to attachment strength, Antonucci (1994) found that older women who reported stronger attachment to their daughters received more emotional support from them. In an innovative study, Steele, Phibbs, and Woods (2004) examined how the behavior of older adults with dementia, when reunited with their adult daughters after separation, predicted the daughters' attachment mental states as assessed by the Adult Attachment Interview (AAI; Main, Kaplan, & Cassidy, 1985). Steele et al. found that older mothers' behaviors during these reunions with their daughters were positively correlated with their daughters' coherence of mind as assessed by the AAI, even when the researchers controlled for the severity of the mothers' dementia symptoms. Specifically, mothers' display of secure reunion behavior (i.e., proximity seeking, maintenance of contact, and responsiveness) was associated with their daughters' being securely attached on the AAI. In another study focusing on people with dementia, Nelis et al. (2012) found that for such people, attachment security was related to having a more positive self-concept and fewer symptoms of dementia-related anxiety. In one of the few longitudinal studies on attachment and caregiving in aged care, Perren, Schmid, Herrmann, and Wettstein (2007) found that among older couples dealing with dementia care, the caregivers' attachment avoidance and the care recipients' insecure attachment (i.e., attachment anxiety or attachment avoidance) were associated with increased levels of dementia-related problem behavior in care recipients.

Our own work has also examined attachment and familial caregiving from the care recipients' perspective. In one study of older parents' perceptions of seeking care and its effect on carers, we found that attachment anxiety was positively associated with older parents' current receipt of care, their future willingness to receive care, and their perceptions of carer burden (Karantzas, Evans, et al., 2010). We also found that older parents' attachment anxiety was positively associated with their perceptions of the sense of obligation that adult children should have in providing care to older parents (i.e., filial obligation). In a path-analytic model, we confirmed that the covariation between older parents' views about filial obligation and their attachment orientation predicted older parents' actual seeking of care from their adult children. This suggests that filial obligation may be interconnected with attachment anxiety. If so, older parents who are highly anxious may impose filial responsibilities on their adult children as a means of safeguarding and controlling their relationship with them.

A Word of Caution

Although this brief review of the current literature on attachment and aged care offers some valuable insights, caution must be exercised regarding how much to read into these findings. A recurrent theme in this review and recent others is the significant variability in how attachment is conceptualized and measured in most aged-care research (see Bradley & Cafferty, 2001; Karantzas, Evans, et al., 2010; Van Assche et al., 2013). We address the issue of the conceptualization and assessment of attachment in later life and aged care in the next section. In doing so, we discuss various conceptualizations of attachment and describe particular measures associated with each one. We also discuss the strengths and weaknesses of the various conceptualizations and assessments as they relate to aged care.

Conceptualizing Attachment in Later Life and in Aged Care

One of the greatest concerns regarding the conceptual and measurement variability of attachment is the inability to compare findings across different studies. In most prior research on attachment and aged care, attachment has been conceptualized and assessed in one of three ways: (1) strength of attachment, (2) attachment states of mind, and (3) attachment orientations/ styles. We discuss each of these distinct conceptualizations and assessment perspectives in turn.

Strength of Attachment

Several studies of attachment and aged care have conceptualized attachment in terms of the strength of the "bond" between older parents and their adult children (e.g., Cicirelli, 1995; Thompson & Walker, 1984; Troll & Smith, 1976), with few measures of this type assessing the romantic attachment orientations of older adults. This conceptualization of attachment places little, if any, emphasis on the distinction between attachment individual differences in the form of attachment orientations or styles; rather, strength is measured as a unidimensional construct, with higher scores reflecting a tighter/closer perceived bond between an older adult and an adult child. A common inference associated with these measures is that a higher score indicates a more secure attachment (Cicirelli, 1993; Thompson & Walker, 1984). However, this inference (as we discuss later in this section) is somewhat tenuous, as a "tighter" or "closer" bond does not necessarily reflect a "secure" attachment. Rather, a secure attachment bond is characterized by a relationship in which closeness is balanced with autonomy and independence (Karantzas, Evans, et al., 2010).

Nearly all of these unidimensional measures are self-report in nature, and various questionnaire measures have been developed. Troll and Smith (1976), for example, developed a measure that mixes obligation and aspects of intergenerational solidarity into their assessment of later-life parent–child attachment. Thompson and Walker (1984) developed a 9-item measure of later-life parent–child attachment (with a specific focus on mother–daughter relationships) in which higher scores reflect "greater attachment." Example items include "We're emotionally dependent on one another," "When we anticipate being apart, our relationship intensifies," and "Our best times are with each other." In 1995, Cicirelli developed the 16-item Adult Attachment Scale (AAS) to measure the degree or strength of aging mother–daughter attachment. The measure assesses four normative aspects of attachment discussed in prior attachment research (e.g., Ainsworth, 1985; Bowlby, 1980; Weiss, 1982): feelings of love, feelings of security and comfort, distress upon separation, and joy on reunion. Cicirelli's (1995) measure also contains items that capture the symbolic or "felt security" nature of attachment in adulthood (Ainsworth, 1989; Cicirelli, 1991; Levitt, 1991; Marvin & Stewart, 1990). Items include "The thought of losing my mother is deeply disturbing to me," and "I feel lonely when I don't see my mother often."

Concentric mapping approaches and interviews have also been used to assess the strength of attachment between older adults or between aging parents and their adult children. The most widely used concentric mapping technique is that devised by Antonucci and colleagues as part of their social convoy theory of human relations (e.g., Antonucci, 1986; Antonucci & Akiyama, 1987; Antonucci, Kahn, & Akiyama, 1989). As part of this measure, individuals are asked to imagine themselves at the center of three concentric circles. They are then instructed to list members of their social network according to how close they perceive each network member is to the self by distributing their social ties across the concentric circles. According to Antonucci and colleagues, network members who are placed within the concentric circle closest to the self are regarded as very close emotional ties and are presumed to be attachment figures. Social convoy studies of adult children and older adults have found that adult children tend to report strong attachments to their older parents (both mothers and fathers), and that older adults report their strongest attachments to be with their spouses and adult children (e.g., Antonucci, Akiyama, & Takahashi, 2004).

Barnas, Pollina, and Cummings (1991) developed an attachment interview designed to measure strength of attachment security. In a semistructured protocol, responses to 12 questions are coded for attachment content on two dimensions: the presence of attachment security, and attachment avoidance/resistance. Scores along both dimensions are then summed to range on a continuum from insecurity to security.

Even though several measures have attempted to capture key attachment constructs, the unidimensional nature of many of these measures (coupled with their scoring procedures) casts some doubt over their validity as good indicators of attachment patterns in later life. As cases in point, higher scores on both Thompson and Walker's (1984) measure and Cicirelli's (1995) AAS are presumed to reflect stronger (and more secure) attachment, whereas lower scores are believed to reflect weaker (and more insecure) attachment. However, this scoring procedure is likely to be inappropriate, because both of these measures were specifically designed to assess attachment bonding between older parents and their adult children (especially aging mothers and adult daughters) within the context of aged care. Several items in these measures—such as "We're emotionally dependent on one another," "The thought of losing my mother is deeply disturbing to me," or "I feel lonely when I don't see my mother often"—suggest that a high score may not reflect attachment security, but attachment insecurity. Within the context of family members involved in aged care, the loss of an older adult is inevitable. According to Bowlby (1980) and Fraley and Shaver (1999), individuals who are securely attached typically go through a cognitive reorganization of their working models after the death of an attachment figure, which allows them to come to terms with the loss and eventually reengage in exploratory behavior. In doing so, the reorganization of their working models is likely to commence prior to death, as in the case of familial caregiving during which an older spouse or adult child witnesses an attachment figure endure a protracted illness (see Fraley & Shaver, 1999).

Thus it seems erroneous to interpret high scores on these unidimensional measures as indexing secure attachment. In fact, it seems more appropriate to infer that *moderate* scores on these measures may be more indicative of secure familial attachment, because secure adult children, while distressed about the eventual loss of their parents, should have started reorganizing their attachment working models during the course of their parents' ill health. Therefore, high scores on these measures are probably indicative of an overly anxious form of attachment characterized by clinginess, a high degree of separation protest, and cognitive inflexibility in the reorganization of attachment working models. Moreover, the items on the AAS and Thompson and Walker's measure assess attachment anxiety, with little emphasis on attachment avoidance. In contrast, the Barnas et al. (1991) interview measure conflates scores on attachment security and attachment avoidance. As a result, it is difficult to determine whether scores on this measure reflect either the presence or absence of security or the presence or absence of avoidance. Moreover, with no explicit assessment of attachment anxiety, this measure excludes a fundamental type of attachment insecurity. Finally, while Antonucci and colleagues' social convoy measure is not solely a measure of attachment strength, the suggestion that inner-circle network members are bona fide "attachment figures" is an assertion rather than a fact. Thus, although it may be true that some "very close" network members are actual attachment figures, there is no definitive way of determining whether this is true for the social convoy measure. In sum, even though these unidimensional assessments of attachment have been used to study aging families and aged care, whether and the extent to which these measures validly capture attachment orientations or styles remain uncertain.

Attachment States of Mind

Born from the developmental psychology tradition, other studies investigating later life attachment and/or aged care have used observational and/or interview assessments to tie early parent–child experiences to attachment states of mind later in life. Specifically, there are a handful of studies that have conceptualized attachment from this perspective and have used adult analogues of Ainsworth's Strange Situation (Ainsworth et al., 1978), the Secure Base Script Assessment (see Chen et al., 2013; Waters & Waters, 2006), or the AAI (see Main et al., 1985; Steele et al., 2004). For instance, in an earlier-described study examining familial attachment processes in later life, Steele et al. (2004) conducted AAI assessments of daughters who were caring for older mothers with dementia. They used a modified version of the Strange Situation to observe the reunion behavior between daughters and their mothers. The concordance between these distinct assessments (i.e., the AAI and reunion behavior in an analogue of the Strange Situation) was then examined as a way of explaining variability in the dementia-related behavior of older adults.

In a study using a modified version of the Secure Base Script Assessment, Chen et al. (2013) investigated how adult children's attachment representations were associated with their care of older parents with dementia. As part of the Secure Base Script Assessment, participants are presented with an attachment topic (e.g., a parent's having an accident) along with a series of word prompts. They are then instructed to verbalize a narrative about the topic, using the word prompts as a guide. Participants are free to develop their own distinctive stories around each topic. The narratives are then scored on a 7-point scale, with higher scores reflecting greater secure base content. In the Chen et al. study, adult children's scores on this assessment were then regressed onto their children's perceptions of difficulty when caring for parents with dementia, including the negative emotions expressed toward their own parents.

The assessment of attachment states of mind in the Steele et al. (2004) and Chen et al. (2013) studies are innovative ways of applying established attachment assessments to the contexts of aging and aged care. Importantly, these assessments place strong emphasis on aspects of the internal working models underlying attachment. Therefore, the application of these assessment procedures to the study of aged care is likely to benefit the field of aged care in two ways. First, the use of the AAI, especially when assessing carers, can provide direct evidence of how early attachment representations are related to the care provided by adult children to ailing adults. Second, interview measures such as the AAI can yield attachment classifications that distinguish how different attachment orientations/styles (i.e., secure, anxious, avoidant, and disorganized) affect carers' caregiving behavior as well as their physical and mental health outcomes. Unfortunately, measures that assess the strength of attachment fall short of allowing such inferences to be made.

Assessments such as the Strange Situation yield behavioral observations of attachment behavior that can be used to validate interview and self-report assessments. Furthermore, behavioral assessments such as the Strange Situation allow for the measurement of actual attachment behavior in older adults who are experiencing varying degrees of cognitive impairment. By and large, older adults experiencing cognitive deficits have frequently been excluded from aged-care studies because of their inability to provide reliable data. Validated observational assessments open the opportunity for the care recipients' perspective to be more firmly embedded in aged-care research on attachment.

The Secure Base Script Assessment is designed to elicit a narrative that taps an individual's generalized expectations about the provision of secure base support (Waters & Waters, 2006). According to Waters and Rodrigues-Doolabh (2001), a prototypic secure base script depicts an event sequence in which

> the caregiver: (1) supports the [care recipient's] exploration; (2) remains available and responsive and serves as a resource as necessary; (3) the [care recipient] encounters an obstacle or threat and becomes distressed; (4) either the [care recipient] retreats to the caregiver or the caregiver goes to the [care recipient]; (5) the difficulty is resolved or removed; (6) proximity and/or contact with the caregiver effectively comforts the [care recipient]; (7) the [care recipient] (possibly with the caregiver's assistance) returns to constructive [activity] (or ends [the activity] comfortably and makes a transition to another activity). (p. 1)

As a result, this assessment measures the degree to which an individual's story regarding attachment topics yields a narrative with "extensive secure base content and a strong interpersonal framework" (Waters & Rodrigues-Doolabh, 2001, p. 2). Scores on this measure range from low to high, with higher scores indicative of narratives that encompass greater and more elaborate secure base content. The application of this measure to aged-care research can provide important insights into how carers' expectations about secure base support underpin their own mental representations (i.e., attitudes, expectations, and working models) and behaviors relevant to their role as caregivers.

Despite the benefits of using different types of assessments that target attachment states of mind, it is difficult to make comparisons across these studies, due to the distinct nature of these attachment assessments. AAI classifications, for example, provide information about individual differences in attachment mental states, whereas the Secure Base Script Assessment yields a unidimensional score reflecting the extent of people's secure base script content. Hence these two measures do not necessarily assess the same construct. If aged-care research is going to make good use of these assessment tools, taxometric and scaling procedures will need to demonstrate convergence between assessments of attachment orientations/styles and attachment mental states indexed by measures such as the AAI and the Strange Situation (see Fraley & Spieker, 2003; Roisman, Fraley, & Belsky, 2007). Preliminary evidence regarding links between the Secure Base Script Assessment and individual-difference measures of attachment suggest that individuals who are insecurely attached (i.e., have insecure classifications on the AAI and high scores on self-report measures of attachment anxiety and/or avoidance) score lower on the Secure Base Script Assessment (Coppola, Vaughn, Cassiba, & Costantini, 2006; Dykas, Woodhouse, Cassidy, & Waters, 2006). However, further work needs to determine both the degree of association and the convergence of these measures in later-life familial bonds and the aged-care context.

Attachment Orientations/Styles

The most widely used of the validated attachment measures in aging and aged-care research are self-report assessments of attachment orientations/styles. Generally speaking, these self-report measures have been either categorical assessments or dimensional assessments of attachment. The most commonly used categorical measures are Hazan and Shaver's (1987) three category descriptors (i.e., secure, anxious, and avoidant) and Bartholomew and colleagues' prototype measures of attachment (i.e., secure, preoccupied, dismissing, and fearful, assessed by the Relationship Questionnaire [the RQ; Bartholomew & Horowitz, 1991] or the Relationship Styles Questionnaire [the RSQ; Griffin & Bartholomew, 1994]). The most popular dimensional measures have been the Experiences in Close Relationships (ECR) scale (Brennan, Clark, & Shaver, 1998) and revisions of it (e.g., the ECR-R; Fraley, Waller, & Brennan, 2000), and the Attachment Style Questionnaire (ASQ; Feeney, Noller, & Hanrahan, 1994; Karantzas, Feeney, & Wilkinson, 2010). Both the ECR and the ASQ tap the two primary dimensions underlying attachment orientations/styles—attachment anxiety and attachment avoidance. The ASQ also taps specific facets of attachment insecurity (for reviews, see Feeney et al., 1994; Karantzas, Feeney, et al., 2010; Mikulincer & Shaver, 2007a). Scores derived from these categorical and dimensional assessments have been linked to caregiving behavior outcomes, carer outcomes, and anticipated caregiving behavior (e.g., Braun et al., 2012; Carpenter, 2001; Karantzas, Evans, et al., 2010; Magai & Cohen, 1998; Nelis et al., 2012).

The adoption of these self-report measures in aged-care research has introduced more uniformity in how individual differences in attachment are conceptualized and measured (Bradley & Cafferty, 2001). They have also provided greater psychometric rigor, and these measures are yielding important insights into the links between attachment and aged care. As a result, differential predictions can be made regarding how attachment security and different forms of insecurity are likely to affect the provision of care and the seeking and/or receipt of care.

Given that these measures were designed to measure adult romantic or global attachment orientations/styles, various gerontological researchers have modified or adapted their instructions or reworded the items to focus on attachments between adult children and older adults. Although these adaptations are presumed to be more context-specific and ecologically valid assessments of attachment, research is mixed regarding the extent to which alterations of instructions and items yield assessments that are similar to general attachment representations (see Cameron, Finnegan, & Morry, 2012; Mikulincer & Shaver, 2007a). Given these mixed findings, the use of self-report measures originally designed to assess romantic or general attachment orientations during young and middle adulthood raises questions about the validity of these assessments when they are applied to aged-care contexts, especially when assessments target familial attachments between older parents and their adult children. For instance, items that typically capture attachment insecurity in romantic relationships—such as "I want to merge completely with another person" and "I want to be completely emotionally intimate with others" (i.e., attachment anxiety), and "I am nervous when partners get too close to me" and "I am too busy with other activities to put much time into relationships" (i.e., attachment avoidance)—may not apply very well to how older parents or their adult children perceive their relationships. The use of these self-report measures in aged-care research, in fact, has often yielded low reliability coefficients, indicating poor internal consistency and/or factor structures that do not neatly map onto the dimensions of the original measures (e.g., Carpenter, 2001; Magai et al., 2001). These findings suggest that these revised measures may not capture attachment insecurity in a way that is age-appropriate and/or relationship-appropriate when researchers are investigating bonds between older adults and their adult children.

Therefore, considerable caution needs to be taken when self-report measures are implemented in the aging and aged-care contexts, especially for the purpose of measuring attachment relationships between older parents and their adult children. One way forward may be to develop self-report measures that assess the critical features of attachment security, anxiety, and avoidance, but that contain items worded in a manner that more aptly captures familial attachments in later life. The development of such measures may involve creating new items, rather than just modifying existing ones that are currently used in attachment research to target romantic relationships or earlier stages of the lifespan.

Where to Next?: Future Directions in Attachment and Aged-Care Research

When highlighting particular attachment concepts and ideas earlier in this chapter, we have identified specific aspects of attachment theory and research that require further extension and investigation in the context of aging and aged care. In our overview of attachment research on aging and particularly aged care, we have reviewed the research conducted to date, but have also highlighted which areas need further attention. When discussing how attachment orientations/styles are conceptualized and assessed later in life with respect to aged care, we have identified problems in the area, but have proposed courses of action that can be taken to advance our understanding of attachment processes through the application of existing attachment measures and the development of new measures. In this final section, we reiterate and expand upon some of our earlier themes, and suggest some new and promising directions for future research on aging and aged care.

The concepts of diathesis–stress, protective behavior, and behavioral systems are all highly relevant to aged care research. To date, however, there has been no systematic investigation of these concepts in aged samples. Applying these concepts in systematic, well-designed studies is likely to yield important and novel insights into the impact of certain attachment processes on aged care. For instance, do the vulnerabilities of insecurely attached carers and care recipients lead to different outcomes, depending on the severity or chronicity of distress associated with family caregiving arrangements? Studies identifying the specific types of family caregiving arrangements that put insecurely attached carers and care recipients at the most risk for physical or mental health problems could inform future models of health care and carer support. By identifying the types of familial caregiving situations that most adversely affect insecurely attached families, health care and carer support systems can determine what kinds of caregiving circumstances are likely to require specific forms of professional intervention. Therefore, attachment research into aged care that implements a diathesis–stress approach is not only likely to advance our theoretical understanding of attachment processes in aged care; it is also likely to have important applied value to the aged-care sector.

The concept of protective behavior, coupled with behavioral systems research on the interplay between the attachment and caregiving systems in the context of aged care, also offers exciting opportunities to advance our theoretical understanding of these two behavioral systems. As noted earlier in the chapter, the help given by a carer to a care recipient is likely to reflect attachment system dynamics, according to Cicirelli (1998). In particular, the ill health of an aging parent may spark proximity-seeking behavior in the carer, in the form of rendering comfort and assistance to safeguard the attachment bond between the carer and his or her aging parent (i.e., protective behavior). However, it is equally plausible that the comfort and assistance given by a carer may reflect activation of the caregiving system, in which an aging parent's ill health alerts the carer to the parent's suffering. In this case, the carer may be motivated to provide assistance not to meet the aging parent's attachment needs, but to alleviate the parent's distress or suffering. Thus Cicirelli's (1983) ideas regarding protective behavior may reflect caregiving rather than attachment system functioning. Researchers need to test these plausible competing behavioral system explanations.

A more systematic investigation of the interplay between the attachment and caregiving behavioral systems in the context of aged care also provides an important opportunity to test some critical theoretical assumptions that could significantly advance our understating of attachment and caregiving dynamics. To date, research linking attachment to caregiving has been studied primarily in social support situations in which romantic couples have been exposed to temporary stressors (e.g., Simpson, Rholes, & Nelligan, 1992), or in studies examining prosocial behavior when helping strangers (e.g., Gillath et al., 2005; Mikulincer, Shaver, Gillath, & Nitzberg, 2005). The findings of these studies suggest that securely attached individuals, unlike insecurely attached ones, usually forgo their own attachment needs and instead attend to the needs of their romantic partners or complete strangers. According to Gillath et al. (2005) and Mikulincer and Shaver (2007a), securely attached people have the capacity to self-soothe, as well as the cognitive and affective regulatory ability to delay meeting their own needs until a later time. One assumption underlying this research is that the caregiving system overrides the attachment system in most securely attached people to ensure that assistance is given to another in need (Gillath et al., 2005; Mikulincer et al., 2005).

However, to what extent are these assumptions and explanations true in typical aged-care situations, when the stress of both the carer *and* the care recipient is severe and chronic, and in many instances will result in the permanent loss of the carer's attachment figure? Under these extreme conditions, can we really expect the caregiving system to override or inhibit the functioning of the attachment system? Couldn't it be just as plausible that under these conditions, the strong activation of the attachment system inhibits the functioning of the caregiving system? Alternatively, could the chronic and extreme stress often associated with aged care result in the concurrent activation of the caregiving and attachment systems (i.e., both systems become activated), or the relative activation of the caregiving and attachment systems (i.e., both systems become activated, but one system is activated more than the other)? Finally, could the activation of these two behavioral systems be moderated by attachment strength or individual differences in attachment orientations/styles? The aged-care context offers unique opportunities for significantly advancing our understanding of how the attachment and caregiving behavioral systems jointly operate.

Our own thinking on the interplay between the attachment and caregiving systems in the aged-care context leads us to believe that individual differences may moderate the dynamics of these behavioral systems. We contend that secure people are likely to have attachment and caregiving systems that are fairly balanced in terms of their typical activation and operation. Carers who are secure in their attachment orientation/style should have systems that become activated in situations that warrant their activation, such as when an adult child feels some degree of attachment threat in response to a sudden change in an aging parent's health status. If, however, it becomes clear that the parent requires substantial assistance, the caregiving system of a secure adult child should override the activation of his or her attachment system to render support. Not only are secure people likely to be more attentive to signs of help, but their capacity to regulate their own distress and emotions should allow them to move more easily between meeting their own attachment needs (at least eventually) and meeting the needs of distressed others in ways that satisfy both systems.

Secure care recipients should also experience more balanced activation of the two systems. When they truly need care, secure care recipients ought to seek proximity or attention in order to receive support and ameliorate their distress. However, the type and amount of support that is sought should be commensurate with the chronicity and severity of the threat, and secure care recipients should experience deactivation of the attachment system after appropriate help is received. In relation to the caregiving system, secure care recipients should also be sensitive and responsive to signs of stress or strain in caregivers. When they notice carer distress, for example, secure recipients may provide support to alleviate the carers' strain, such as through words of encouragement, a hug, or a supportive embrace.

Avoidantly attached people should need more stress (either their own or their care recipients') to trigger either behavioral system. When either system becomes operative, the type and amount of care they provide should follow what is already known about their care provision tendencies. Specifically, avoidant individuals should strive to suppress activation of both behavioral systems. As a result, any care they provide is likely to be emotionally distant, underinvolved, and superficial. Thus the amount and type of caregiving (or lack thereof) typical of avoidant caregivers should short-circuit or suppress both behavioral systems simultaneously. Similarly, avoidant care recipients ought to minimize their distress as a means of deactivating the attachment system.

Avoidantly attached care recipients should refrain from actively seeking help from carers, and they may even reject, dismiss, or devalue its importance when support is provided. Avoidant individuals should also be less in tune with the distress and strain of their carers. As a result, they may be less likely to notice signs of distress in their carers, which may ensure that their caregiving system is not triggered.

Anxiously attached people should have attachment and caregiving systems that are more easily and chronically activated. Due to their tendencies to intensify distress, anxious individuals ought to have lower stress thresholds than secure and avoidant individuals (Simpson & Rholes, 1994), so that lower levels of stress in themselves or others are likely to activate either system. When it comes to family caregiving, anxious individuals ought to experience chronic activation of both systems, in which they oscillate between providing compulsive or situationally inappropriate support and seeking attention and validation from their attachment figures, despite their frailty. Furthermore, it may be more difficult for anxious individuals to shut down both systems once they are activated.

When they are receiving care, anxious individuals should experience strong activation of the attachment system. This heightened activation, coupled with their hyperactivating emotional regulation strategies, should lead anxious care recipients to engage in persistent care-seeking behavior, which is rarely fully satisfied by their carers. In fact, the heightened and sustained activation of the attachment system in care recipients may inhibit activation of the caregiving system, even when their carers are experiencing significant distress and burnout.

Further research on individual differences in attachment that takes into account the unique perspectives of a carer and a care recipient is likely to increase our theoretical understanding of the pathways that connect carers' and care recipients' attachment orientations/styles to current family care arrangements. For instance, we still know relatively little about how the amount and type of help that is provided and sought as part of family care arrangements is related to attachment orientations/styles. Even less is known about how individual differences in attachment influence the physical and mental health outcomes of carers and care recipients. Emerging research suggests that attachment insecurity may be differentially associated with caregiving and care-receiving/seeking behavior (Karantzas & Cole, 2011; Karantzas, Evans, et al., 2010; Nelis et al., 2012). Specifically, while research with carers seems to indicate that both forms of attachment insecurity (anxiety and avoidance) are associated with providing less care to aging adults, attachment anxiety may be a particularly important dimension in explaining older adults' seeking and receipt of care (e.g., Karantzas, Evans, et al., 2010; Karantzas et al., 2014).

Future research that adopts a multilevel perspective by examining family caregiving at the dyadic level (i.e., a care recipient and a carer) or the family systems level (i.e., a care recipient nested within a network of family carers) could also provide important explanations for the differential functioning of attachment orientations/styles as they relate to carers and care recipients. This kind of research is likely to have significant clinical implications in aged care as well. For example, developing a better understanding of individual differences in attachment regarding carers and care recipients may help us identify carers and older adults who will not adjust well to certain family care arrangements. Most importantly, an attachment perspective may assist health care professionals (i.e., clinicians, counselors, and social workers) to tailor the counseling of families through understanding the role of attachment in family dynamics, mental health outcomes, and emotional reactions related to caregiving and the planning of future care arrangements. A consideration of attachment issues may therefore improve the efficacy of interventions aimed at reducing family and carer burden, which to date have resulted in only modest improvements for carers (Brodaty & Green, 2002; Cooke, McNally, Mulligan, Harrison, & Newman, 2001; Lopez-Hartmann, Wens, Verhoeven, & Remmen, 2012).

In conclusion, we have highlighted the theoretical and applied value that can be gained by applying attachment theory to the study of later-life family attachment bonds and aged care. To this point, research has been limited; however, the field has an important opportunity to develop significant and groundbreaking investigations that can appreciably enhance our understanding of attachment processes "from the cradle to the grave" (Bowlby, 1979, p. 129). To ensure that the family-based care of older adults is effective and sustainable in the coming decades, and to minimize pressures and stressors on carers and care recipients alike, a better understanding of late-life attachment relationships is vital. Such an understanding will not only provide new ways of supporting and strengthening these critical bonds; it will also facilitate the development of services and supports for family caregivers and care recipients, helping them to cope better with this already difficult stage of life and to enhance family functioning.

References

Ainsworth, M. D. (1985). Attachments across the life-span. *Bulletin of the New York Academy of Medicine, 61,* 792–812.

Ainsworth, M. D. (1989). Attachments beyond infancy. *American Psychologist, 44,* 709–716.

Ainsworth, M. D. S., Blehar, M. C., Waters, E., & Wall, S. (1978). *Patterns of attachment: A psychological study of the Strange Situation.* Hillsdale, NJ: Erlbaum.

Allen, K. R., Blieszner, R., & Roberto, K. A. (2000). Families in the middle and later years: A review and critique of research in the 1990s. *Journal of Marriage and Family, 62,* 911–926.

Antonucci, T. C. (1986). Social support networks: A hierarchical mapping technique. *Generations: Journal of the American Society on Aging, 10,* 10–12.

Antonucci, T. C. (1994). Attachment in adulthood and aging. In M. B. Sperling & W. H. Berman (Eds.), *Attachment in adults: Clinical and developmental perspectives* (pp. 256–272). New York: Guilford Press.

Antonucci, T. C., & Akiyama, H. (1987). Social networks in adult life and a preliminary examination of the convoy model. *Journal of Gerontology, 42,* 519–527.

Antonucci, T. C., Akiyama, H., & Takahashi, K. (2004). Attachment and close relationships across the life span. *Attachment and Human Development, 6,* 353–370.

Antonucci, T. C., Kahn, R., & Akiyama, H. (1989). Psychosocial factors and the response to cancer symptoms. In R. Yancik & J. W. Yates (Eds.), *Cancer in the elderly: Approaches to early detection and treatment* (pp. 40–52). New York: Springer.

Barnas, M. V., Pollina, L., & Cummings, E. (1991). Life-span attachment: Relations between attachment and socioemotional functioning in adult women. *Genetic, Social, and General Psychology Monographs, 117,* 175–202.

Bartholomew, K., & Horowitz, L. M. (1991). Attachment styles among young adults: A test of a four-category model. *Journal of Personality and Social Psychology, 61,* 226–244.

Bengtson, V. L. (2001). Beyond the nuclear family: The increasing importance of multigenerational bonds. *Journal of Marriage and Family, 63,* 1–16.

Blieszner, R., & Mancini, J. A. (1987). Enduring ties: Older adults' parental role and responsibilities. *Family Relations, 36,* 176–180.

Bowlby, J. (1969/1982). *Attachment and loss: Vol. 1. Attachment.* New York: Basic Books.

Bowlby, J. (1979). *The making and breaking of affectional bonds.* London: Tavistock.

Bowlby, J. (1980). *Attachment and loss: Vol. 3. Sadness and depression.* New York: Basic Books.

Bradley, J. M., & Cafferty, T. P. (2001). Attachment among older adults: Current issues and directions for future research. *Attachment and Human Development, 3,* 200–221.

Braun, M., Hales, S., Gilad, L., Mikulincer, M., Rydall, A., & Rodin, G. (2012). Caregiving styles and attachment orientations in couples facing advanced cancer. *Psycho-Oncology, 21,* 935–943.

Brennan, K. A., Clark, C. L., & Shaver, P. R. (1998). Self-report measurement of adult romantic attachment: An integrative overview. In J. A. Simpson & W. S. Rholes (Eds.), *Attachment theory and close relationships* (pp. 46–76). New York: Guilford Press.

Brodaty, H., & Green, A. (2002). Who cares for the carer?: The often forgotten patient. *Clinical Practice: Therapeutic Review, 31,* 1–4.

Cameron, J. J., Finnegan, H., & Morry, M. M. (2012). Orthogonal dreams in an oblique world: A meta-analysis of the association between attachment anxiety and avoidance. *Journal of Research in Personality, 46,* 472–476.

Canterberry, M., & Gillath, O. (2012). Attachment and caregiving. In P. Noller & G. C. Karantzas (Eds.), *The Wiley–Blackwell handbook of couple and family relationships* (pp. 207–219). Chichester, UK: Wiley.

Carpenter, B. D. (2001). Attachment bonds between adult daughters and their older mothers: Associations with contemporary caregiving. *Journals of Gerontology, Series B, 56B,* 257–266.

Chen, C. K., Waters, H. S., Hartman, M., Zimmerman, S., Miklowitz, D. J., & Waters, E. (2013). The secure base script and the task of caring for elderly parents: Implications for attachment theory and clinical practice. *Attachment and Human Development, 15,* 332–348.

Cicirelli, V. G. (1983). Adult children's attachment and helping behaviour to elderly parents: A path model. *Journal of Marriage and the Family, 45,* 815–822.

Cicirelli, V. G. (1985). The role of siblings as family caregivers. In W. J. Sauer & R. T. Cowards, (Eds.), *Social support networks and the care of the elderly* (pp. 93–107). New York: Springer.

Cicirelli, V. G. (1991). *Family caregiving: Autonomous and paternalistic decision making.* Newbury Park, CA: Sage.

Cicirelli, V. G. (1993). Attachment and obligation as daughters' motives for caregiving behavior and subsequent effect on subjective burden. *Psychology and Aging, 8,* 144–155.

Cicirelli, V. G. (1995). A measure of caregiving daughters' attachment to elderly mothers. *Journal of Family Psychology, 9,* 89–94.

Cicirelli, V. G. (1998). A frame of reference for guiding research regarding the relationship between adult attachment and mental health in aging families. In J. Lomranz (Ed.), *Handbook of aging and mental health: An integrative approach* (pp. 341–353). New York: Plenum Press.

Cooke, D. D., McNally, L., Mulligan, K. T., Harrison, M. J. G., & Newman, S. P. (2001). Psychosocial interventions for caregivers of people with dementia: A systematic review. *Aging and Mental Health, 5,* 120–135.

Cooper, C., Owens, C., Katona, C., & Livingston, G. (2008). Attachment style and anxiety in carers of people with Alzheimer's disease: Results from the LASER-AD study. *International Psychogeriatrics, 20,* 494–507.

Coppola, G., Vaughn, B. E., Cassibba, R., & Costantini, A. (2006). The attachment script representation procedure in an Italian sample: Associations with adult attachment interview scales and with maternal sensitivity. *Attachment and Human Development, 8,* 209–219.

Crispi, E. L., Schiaffino, K., & Berman, W. H. (1997). The contribution of attachment to burden in adult children of institutionalized parents with dementia. *The Gerontologist, 37,* 52–60.

Dilworth-Anderson, P., Williams, I. C., & Gibson, B. E. (2002). Issues of race, ethnicity, and culture in caregiving research: A 20-year review (1980–2000). *The Gerontologist, 42,* 237–272.

Dykas, M. J., Woodhouse, S. S., Cassidy, J., & Waters, H. S. (2006). Narrative assessment of attachment representations: Links between secure base scripts and adolescent attachment. *Attachment and Human Development, 8,* 221–240.

Feeney, B. C., & Collins, N. L. (2004). Interpersonal safe haven and secure base caregiving processes in adulthood. In W. S. Rholes & J. A. Simpson (Eds.),

Adult attachment: Theory, research, and clinical implications (pp. 300–338). New York: Guilford Press.

Feeney, J. A., Noller, P., & Hanrahan, M. (1994). Assessing adult attachment. In M. B. Sperling & W. H. Berman (Eds.), *Attachment in adults: Clinical and developmental perspectives* (pp. 128–152). New York: Guilford Press.

Fraley, R. C., & Shaver, P. R. (1999). Loss and bereavement: Attachment theory and recent controversies concerning grief work and the nature of detachment. In J. Cassidy & P. R. Shaver (Eds.), *Handbook of attachment: Theory, research, and clinical applications* (pp. 735–759). New York: Guilford Press.

Fraley, R. C., & Spieker, S. J. (2003). Are infant attachment patterns continuously or categorically distributed?: A taxometric analysis of Strange Situation behavior. *Developmental Psychology, 39,* 387–404.

Fraley, R. C., Waller, N. G., & Brennan, K. A. (2000). An item response theory analysis of self-report measures of adult attachment. *Journal of Personality and Social Psychology, 78,* 350–365.

George, C., & Solomon, J. (2008). The caregiving system: A behavioral systems approach to parenting. In J. Cassidy & P. R. Shaver (Eds.), *Handbook of attachment: Theory, research, and clinical applications* (2nd ed., pp. 833–856). New York: Guilford Press.

Gillath, O., Shaver, P. R., & Mikulincer, M. (2005). An attachment-theoretical approach to compassion and altruism. In P. Gilbert (Ed.), *Compassion: Conceptualizations, research, and use in psychotherapy* (pp. 121–147). London: Brunner-Routledge.

Griffin, D. W., & Bartholomew, K. (1994). The metaphysics of measurement: The case of adult attachment. In K. Bartholomew & D. Perlman (Eds.), *Advances in personal relationships: Vol. 5. Attachment processes in adulthood* (pp. 17–52). London: Jessica Kingsley.

Guberman, N., Maheu, P., & Maille, C. (1992). Women as family caregivers: Why do they care? *The Gerontologist, 32,* 607–617.

Hazan, C., & Shaver, P. R. (1987). Romantic love conceptualized as an attachment process. *Journal of Personality and Social Psychology, 52,* 511–524.

Kalish, R. A., & Knudtson, F. W. (1976). Attachment versus disengagement: A life-span conceptualization. *Human Development, 19,* 171–181.

Karantzas, G. C. (2012). Family caregiving. In P. Noller & G. C. Karantzas (Eds.), *The Wiley–Blackwell handbook of couples and family relationships* (pp. 82–96). Chichester, UK: Wiley.

Karantzas, G. C., & Cole, S. F. (2011). Arthritis and support seeking tendencies: The role of attachment. *Journal of Social and Clinical Psychology, 30,* 404–440.

Karantzas, G. C., Evans, L., & Foddy, M. (2010). The role of attachment in current and future parent caregiving. *Journals of Gerontology, Series B, 65B,* 573–580.

Karantzas, G. C., Feeney, J. A., & Wilkinson, R. B. (2010). Does less mean more?: A confirmatory factor analytic study of the Attachment Style Questionnaire and the Attachment Style Questionnaire—Short Form. *Journal of Social and Personal Relationships, 27,* 749–780.

Karantzas, G. C., Karantzas, K. M., Simpson, J. A., & McCabe, M. (2014). *Examining the associations between attachment and aged care: A systematic review.* Unpublished manuscript.

Kim, Y., & Carver, C. S. (2007). Frequency and difficulty in caregiving among spouses of individuals with cancer: Effects of adult attachment and gender. *Psycho-Oncology, 16,* 714–723.

Knight, B., Silverstein, M., McCallum, T., & Fox, L. (2000). A sociocultural stress and coping model for mental health outcomes among African American caregivers in Southern California. *Journals of Gerontology, Series B, 55B,* 142–150.

Koski, L. R., & Shaver, P. R. (1997). Attachment and relationship satisfaction across the lifespan. In R. J. Sternberg & M. Hojjat (Eds.), *Satisfaction in close relationships* (pp. 26–55). New York: Guilford Press.

Levitt, M. J. (1991). Attachment and close relationships: A life-span perspective. In J. Gewirtz, & W. M. Kurtines (Eds.), *Intersections with attachment* (pp. 183–205). Hillsdale, NJ: Erlbaum.

Lopez-Hartmann, M., Wens, J., Verhoeven, V., & Remmen, R. (2012). The effect of caregiver support interventions for informal caregivers of community-dwelling frail elderly: A systematic review. *International Journal of Integrated Care, 12,* 1–16.

Magai, C., & Cohen, C. I. (1998). Attachment style and emotion regulation in dementia patients and their relation to caregiver burden. *Journals of Gerontology, Series B, 53B,* 147–154.

Magai, C., Cohen, C. I., Milburn, N., Thorpe, B., McPherson, R., & Peralta, D. (2001). Attachment styles in older European American and African American adults. *Journals of Gerontology, Series B, 56B,* 28–35.

Main, M., Kaplan, N., & Cassidy, J. (1985). Security in infancy, childhood, and adulthood: A move to the level of representation. In I. Bretherton & E. Waters (Eds.), Growing points of attachment theory and research. *Monographs of the Society for Research in Child Development, 50*(1–2, Serial No. 209), 66–104.

Markiewicz, D., Reis, M., & Gold, D. P. (1997). An exploration of attachment styles and personality traits in caregiving for dementia patients. *International Journal of Aging and Human Development, 45,* 111–132.

Marvin, R. S., & Stewart, R. B. (1990). A family systems framework for the study of attachment. In M. T. Greenberg, D. Cicchetti, & E. M. Cummings (Eds.), *Attachment in the preschool years: Theory, research, and intervention* (pp. 51–86). Chicago: University of Chicago Press.

Mikulincer, M., & Shaver, P. R. (2003). The attachment behavioral system in adulthood: Activation, psychodynamics, and interpersonal processes. In M. P. Zanna (Ed.), *Advances in experimental social psychology* (Vol. 35, pp. 53–152). San Diego, CA: Academic Press.

Mikulincer, M., & Shaver, P. R. (2007a). *Attachment in adulthood: Structure, dynamics, and change.* New York: Guilford Press.

Mikulincer, M., & Shaver, P. R. (2007b). Boosting attachment security to promote mental health, prosocial values, and inter-group tolerance. *Psychological Inquiry, 18,* 139–156.

Mikulincer, M., Shaver, P. R., Gillath, O., & Nitzberg, R. A. (2005). Attachment, caregiving, and altruism: Boosting attachment security increases compassion and helping. *Journal of Personality and Social Psychology, 89,* 817–839.

Miller, B., & Cafasso, L. (1992). Gender differences in caregiving: Fact or artifact? *The Gerontologist, 32,* 498–507.

National Center for Chronic Disease Prevention and Health Promotion. (2011). *Healthy aging: Helping people to live long and productive lives and enjoy a good quality life*. Atlanta, GA: Centers for Disease Control and Prevention.

National Institute on Aging (NIA). (2011). *Global health and aging* (NIH Publication No. 11-7737). Bethesda, MD: National Institutes of Health.

Nelis, S. M., Clare, L., & Whitaker, C. J. (2012). Attachment representations in people with dementia and their carers: Implications for well-being within the dyad. *Aging and Mental Health, 16,* 845–854.

Perren, S., Schmid, R., Herrmann, S., & Wettstein, A. (2007). The impact of attachment on dementia-related problem behavior and spousal caregivers' well-being. *Attachment and Human Development, 9,* 163–178.

Pohl, J. M., Boyd, C., Liang, J., & Given, C. W. (1995). Analysis of the impact of mother–daughter relationships on the commitment to caregiving. *Nursing Research, 44,* 68–75.

Rholes, W. S., Simpson, J. A., Campbell, L., & Grich, J. (2001). Adult attachment and the transition to parenthood. *Journal of Personality and Social Psychology, 81,* 421–435.

Roisman, G. I., Fraley, R. C., & Belsky, J. (2007). A taxometric study of the Adult Attachment Interview. *Developmental Psychology, 43,* 675–686.

Shaver, P. R., & Mikulincer, M. (2004). What do self-report attachment measures assess? In W. S. Rholes & J. A. Simpson (Eds.), *Adult attachment: Theory, research, and clinical implications* (pp. 17–54). New York: Guilford Press.

Silverstein, M., & Bengtson, V. L. (1997). Intergenerational solidarity and the structure of adult child–parent relationships in American families. *American Journal of Sociology, 103,* 429–460.

Silverstein, M., Gans, D., & Yang, F. M. (2006). Intergenerational support to aging parents: The role of norms and needs. *Journal of Family Issues, 27,* 1068–1084.

Simpson, J. A., & Rholes, W. S. (1994). Stress and secure base relationships in adulthood. In K. Bartholomew & D. Perlman (Eds.), *Advances in personal relationships: Vol. 5. Attachment processes in adulthood* (pp. 181–204). London: Jessica Kingsley.

Simpson, J. A., & Rholes, W. S. (2012). Adult attachment orientations, stress, and romantic relationships. In T. Devine & A. Plante (Eds.), *Advances in experimental social psychology* (Vol. 45, pp. 279–328). New York: Elsevier.

Simpson, J. A., Rholes, W. S., Campbell, L., Tran, S., & Wilson, C. L. (2003). Adult attachment, the transition to parenthood, and depressive symptoms. *Journal of Personality and Social Psychology, 84,* 1172–1187.

Simpson, J. A., Rholes, W. S., & Nelligan, J. S. (1992). Support seeking and support giving within couples in an anxiety-provoking situation: The role of attachment styles. *Journal of Personality and Social Psychology, 62,* 434–446.

Sörensen, S., Webster, J. D., & Roggman, L. A. (2002). Adult attachment and preparing to provide care for older relatives. *Attachment and Human Development, 4,* 84–106.

Steele, H., Phibbs, E., & Woods, R. T. (2004). Coherence of mind in daughter caregivers of mothers with dementia: Links with their mothers' joy and relatedness on reunion in a strange situation. *Attachment and Human Development, 6,* 439–450.

Thompson, L., & Walker, A. J. (1984). Mothers and daughters: Aid patterns and attachment. *Journal of Marriage and the Family, 46*, 313–322.

Troll, E., & Smith, J. (1976). Attachment through the life-span: Some questions about dyadic bonds among adults. *Human Development, 19*, 156–170.

Van Assche, L., Luyten, P., Bruffaerts, R., Persoons, P., van de Ven, L., & Vandenbulcke, M. (2013). Attachment in old age: Theoretical assumptions, empirical findings and implications for clinical practice. *Clinical Psychology Review, 33*, 67–81.

Vaughn, B. E., Egeland, B. R., Sroufe, L. A., & Waters, E. (1979). Individual differences in infant–mother attachment at 12 and 18 months: Stability and change in families under stress. *Child Development, 50*, 971–975.

Waters, H. S., & Rodrigues-Doolabh, L. M. (2001). *Narrative assessment of adult attachment representations: The scoring of Secure Base Script content.* Unpublished manuscript, State University of New York at Stony Brook.

Waters, H. S., & Waters, E. (2006). The attachment working models concept: Among other things, we build script-like representations of secure base experiences. *Attachment and Human Development, 8*, 185–197.

Weiss, R. S. (1982). Attachment in adult life. In C. M. Parkes & J. Stevenson-Hinde (Eds.), *The place of attachment in human behavior* (pp. 171–184). New York: Basic Books.

World Health Organization (WHO). (2012). *Knowledge translation on ageing and health: Policy framework.* Geneva, Switzerland: Author.

13

Psychopathology and Attachment

Tsachi Ein-Dor
Guy Doron

Albert Einstein once stated, "One knows from daily life that one exists for other people—first of all for those upon whose smiles and well-being our own happiness is wholly dependent" (1931, p. 193). In keeping with this view, theory and research have indicated that the roots of mental health and psychopathology may be traced to a person's history of interactions with other people, specifically in times of need (Bowlby, 1980; Sroufe, 2005; Sroufe, Egeland, Carlson, & Collins, 2005). When people, particularly close others, regularly respond sensitively to the person's needs, he or she develops a sense of attachment security that includes acquiring constructive strategies for coping with threats and for regulating negative emotions (see Mikulincer & Shaver, 2007, for an extensive review). But when other people are often unavailable, unreliable, or rejecting of bids for support, the person may become chronically insecure with respect to close relationships. One of the main insecure attachment patterns in adulthood is avoidance, which relates to the extent to which a person distrusts relationship partners' goodwill, strives to maintain independence, and relies on deactivating strategies for dealing with threats and negative emotions (e.g., Fraley & Shaver, 1997). The second main insecure pattern is anxiety, which relates to the extent to which a person worries that others will not be available or helpful in times of need. Anxious individuals exaggerate their sense of vulnerability and insistently call on others for help and care, sometimes to the point of being intrusive (e.g., Feeney & Noller, 1990).

Research has indicated that attachment insecurities (both anxiety and avoidance) are associated with a general vulnerability to mental disorders

(Mikulincer & Shaver, 2012; Sroufe, Duggal, Weinfield, & Carlson, 2000). For example, attachment insecurities are linked with depression (e.g., Catanzaro & Wei, 2010), generalized anxiety disorder (e.g., Marganska, Gallagher, & Miranda, 2013), obsessive–compulsive disorder (e.g., Doron, Moulding, Kyrios, Nedeljkovic, & Mikulincer, 2009), posttraumatic stress disorder (PTSD) (e.g., Ein-Dor, Doron, Solomon, Mikulincer, & Shaver, 2010), eating disorders (e.g., Illing, Tasca, Balfour, & Bissada, 2010), and suicide ideation (e.g., Davaji, Valizadeh, & Nikamal, 2010). Attachment insecurity is also related to many personality disorders (Crawford et al., 2007; Meyer & Pilkonis, 2005). For example, people high on attachment anxiety have higher prevalences of dependent, histrionic, and borderline personality disorders, which often comprise identity confusion, anxiety, emotional liability, cognitive distortions, submissiveness, self-harm, and suspiciousness (the "emotional dysregulation" component of personality disorders; Livesley, 1991). Conversely, avoidant individuals have higher prevalences of schizoid and avoidant personality disorders, which consist of restricted expression of emotions, problems with intimacy, and social avoidance (the "inhibitedness" component of personality problems; Livesley, 1991).

Attachment theory, however, has difficulty simultaneously explaining the mechanisms by which attachment insecurities lead to multiple disorders (i.e., the question of *multifinality*; Cicchetti, 1984; Egeland, Pianta, & Ogawa, 1996), and why one individual with a particular attachment orientation develops one set of symptoms while another with the same attachment vulnerability develops another set of symptoms (i.e., the question of *divergent trajectories*; Nolen-Hoeksema & Watkins, 2011). In addition, attachment research has yet to explore the dyadic processes that play a role in exacerbating or mitigating psychopathology. In this chapter, we unfold a transdiagnostic model of attachment insecurities (in line with Nolen-Hoeksema and Watkins's [2011] heuristic for developing such models; see Figure 13.1 for an outline of the heuristic) that refers to the possible causal processes linking attachment orientation to multiple disorders.

We first review studies of both clinical and nonclinical samples that link attachment dispositions to the two primary dimensions of psychopathology: internalizing (including mood and anxiety disorders, such as major depression, generalized anxiety disorder, panic disorder, and social anxiety disorder [social phobia]; Krueger & Markon, 2006, 2011), and externalizing (including substance use and antisocial disorders; Krueger & Markon, 2006, 2011).

Next, we address the question of multifinality by speculating on the processes (i.e., proximal risk factors) that mediate the linkage between attachment insecurities and multiple disorders, and the question of divergent trajectories by indicating the different contexts (e.g., genetic predisposition, family environment, and cultural environment) that might set one

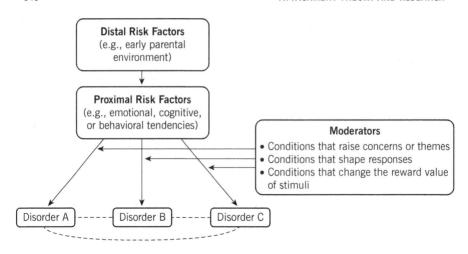

FIGURE 13.1. Nolen-Hoeksema and Watkins's (2011) heuristic for developing transdiagnostic models of psychopathology. Distal risk factors contribute to disorders only through mediating proximal risk factors. Proximal risk factors directly influence symptoms relative to distal risk factors. Distal and proximal risk factors lead to multiple disorders (i.e., multifinality), which are comorbid (indicated by dashed lines). Moderators interact with proximal risk factors to determine which specific disorders individuals will experience (i.e., to determine divergent trajectories).

individual on a trajectory to one set of symptoms, but another individual on a path to a different set of symptoms.

Attachment and Internalizing Disorders

Internalizing refers to a general liability toward negative affect and anxiety disorders. It may be bifurcated into two separable but highly correlated liabilities—*distress* and *fear*. Distress is a liability to major depression, dysthymia (also known as chronic depression), and generalized anxiety disorder, whereas fear is a liability to disorders such as panic disorder, phobias, and PTSD (Krueger & Markon, 2011). In the current review, we focus on anxiety, depression, and PTSD—the three most extensively studied types of internalizing disorders with respect to attachment theory.

Anxiety Disorders

Bowlby (1973) was the first to contend that attachment insecurities can, under specific circumstances, lead to anxiety disorders. When caregivers are unavailable and unsupportive in times of need, the attachment system fails to accomplish its basic function—to protect an individual, alleviate his or her distress and fear, and assure a sense of security. Unsupported individuals begin to internalize perceptions of the world as a dangerous place, full of unexpected threats and perils, devoid of places of assurance and safety. Alongside the internalization of such negative worldviews, these individuals harbor serious doubts about their ability to cope with threats and dangers. The individuals therefore are left to ruminate about their problems, concerns, and feeling of distress, without taking action to make positive changes (Mikulincer & Florian, 1998). These maladaptive cognitive tendencies can exacerbate fearful reactions to threats, as well as heighten the tendency to evade potential anxiety-provoking plights—the clinically familiar fear and avoidance components of most anxiety disorders (American Psychiatric Association, 2013).

Numerous cross-sectional studies have examined the links between attachment dispositions and anxiety symptoms. Results have indicated that a preoccupied state of mind in the Adult Attachment Interview (AAI) (e.g., Adam, Gunnar, & Tanaka, 2004), endorsement of an anxious (categorical) attachment style in close relationships (e.g., Marganska et al., 2013; Muris & Meesters, 2002), or higher ratings of attachment anxiety on self-report scales (e.g., Esbjørn et al., 2013) are all associated with heightened severity of anxiety symptoms. With regard to attachment avoidance, the picture is less consistent: About half of the studies have concluded that people high on attachment avoidance suffer from more anxiety symptoms (Muris & Meesters, 2002; Wei, Heppner, & Mallinckrodt, 2003), whereas other studies have determined that attachment avoidance is not significantly linked with anxiety (e.g., Adam et al., 2004; Costa & Weems, 2005; Sheehan & Noller, 2002). This inconsistency may be resolved, at least to some extent, by carefully examining the positive associations between attachment avoidance and anxiety-related symptoms: Studies using the typology classification of attachment styles have indicated that anxiety symptoms are linked with the fearful aspect rather than the dismissing aspect of attachment avoidance. Thus it seems that the anxious facet of fearful avoidance, which is also shared by people high on attachment anxiety, is associated with vulnerability to anxiety-related symptoms rather than the distancing facet of dismissing avoidance.

Such a conclusion may be biased, however. Epidemiological research has indicated that cross-sectional snapshots mix single-episode and "one-off" cases with recurrent and chronic cases, which are known to differ in the severity and etiology of their conditions. A cross-sectional design also precludes confident conclusions regarding the direction of causality in the link between personality dispositions and psychopathology. Therefore, longitudinal studies are needed to establish the nature of the links between attachment dispositions and anxiety disorders. The Minnesota Study (see

Sroufe et al., 2005, for an extensive review), which set out to explore developmental trajectories of early attachment orientations, revealed that infants classified as anxious-resistant were more likely than their secure counterparts to endorse anxiety disorders at age 17 (Warren, Huston, Egeland, & Sroufe, 1997). This prospective prediction was not apparent among anxious-avoidant infants. In a different study, attachment anxiety, but not avoidance, was also linked with a history of anxiety-related disorders—from emotional dysregulation at age 3.5, through childhood anxiety problems, to anxiety disorders in adolescence (Bosquet & Egeland, 2006).

Depression

Bowlby (1980) posited that attachment insecurities relate to the development of depressive disorders, as well as to that of anxiety. He contended that a loss of a primary attachment figure or a repeated failure to form a secure relationship with a caregiver encourages the formation of pessimistic, hopeless representations of self, other, and world. When an insecure individual encounters subsequent losses, traumatic events, or hardships, his or her abandonment-related cognitions and feelings may trigger symptoms of depression.

To date, more than 100 studies have examined the links between attachment dispositions and the severity of depressive symptoms. For example, studies in special populations with a heightened risk for depression (i.e., low socioeconomic status, stressful life history, and poor health) revealed that people high on either attachment anxiety or avoidance suffer from more depressive symptoms. Specifically, dismissing and preoccupied states of mind according to the AAI, and higher scores on self-report measures of attachment avoidance or anxiety, have been associated with more severe symptoms of depression in samples of psychiatric inpatients (Fowler, Allen, Oldham, & Frueh, 2013); patients with chronic pain (Ciechanowski, Sullivan, Jensen, Romano, & Summers, 2003); patients with diabetes (Ciechanowski, Katon, & Russo, 2005); patients who are HIV-positive (e.g., Hinnen et al., 2012); and outpatients suffering from eating disorders, drug abuse, or major depression (e.g., Eng, Heimberg, Hart, Schneier, & Liebowitz, 2001; Visioli, Senatore, Lepri, & Tondo, 2012).

Studies in nonclinical samples have indicated that a preoccupied state of mind on the AAI (Cole-Detke & Kobak, 1996), endorsement of an anxious (categorical) attachment style in close relationships (e.g., Muris, Meesters, van Melick, & Zwambag, 2001), or higher ratings of attachment anxiety on self-report scales (e.g., Brenning, Soenens, Braet, & Bosmans, 2012; Wei, Mallinckrodt, Larson, & Zakalik, 2005) are associated with heightened severity of depressive symptoms. In keeping with the findings regarding anxiety disorders, the evidence for the link between attachment avoidance and depression is conflicting: About half of the studies have concluded that people high on attachment avoidance (mostly fearful avoidance) suffer from more depressive symptoms (Gamble & Roberts, 2005; Simpson, Rholes, Campbell, Tran, & Wilson, 2003), whereas other studies have determined that attachment avoidance (mostly dismissing avoidance) is not significantly linked with depression (e.g., Adam et al., 2004; Shaver, Schachner, & Mikulincer, 2005). Research on the multiple facets of depression has revealed more about the nature of the avoidance–depression link (Batgos & Leadbeater, 1994; Davila, 2001; Murphy & Bates, 1997; Zuroff & Fitzpatrick, 1995). Attachment avoidance has been found to be associated with achievement-related aspects of depression, such as perfectionism, self-punishment, and self-criticism (also called *introjective* depression; Blatt, 1974), but not with the interpersonal aspects of depression, such as overdependence, lack of autonomy, and neediness (also called *anaclitic* depression; Blatt, 1974).

The developmental trajectory of depression, as assessed in the Minnesota Study, corroborated the conclusions from cross-sectional findings on the link between attachment and depression by indicating that both anxious-avoidant and anxious-resistant attachment styles were related to depression in adolescence (Duggal, Carlson, Sroufe, & Egeland, 2001). Other prospective studies have found that attachment insecurities (anxiety and avoidance) among adults predict subsequent increases in depression over periods of time ranging from 1 month to 2 years (e.g., Hankin, Kassel, & Abela, 2005; Maunder, Lancee, Hunter, Greenberg, & Steinhart, 2005; Whiffen, 2005).

Posttraumatic Stress Disorder

People's reactions to threats and danger comprise elevated distress and arousing emotions. Such experiences may traumatize the persons and leave them at risk for short-term and long-term mental health and adjustment problems (Horowitz, 1982). Commonly, emotional balance is restored shortly after a traumatic event ends. In some cases, however, profound and prolonged mental health sequelae are manifested in the form of PTSD— repeated reexperiencing of the traumatic event (intrusive symptoms such as unwanted and dreaded mental images and dreams), reduced involvement with the external world (trauma-related avoidance), and cognitive–affective hyperarousal (American Psychiatric Association, 2013).

The first systematic attempt to document attachment style differences in the severity of PTSD symptoms concerned reactions of young adults to Iraqi Scud missile attacks on Israel during the 1991 Gulf War (Mikulincer, Florian, & Weller, 1993). Participants with an anxious (categorical) style had more severe PTSD intrusion and avoidance symptoms as compared with their secure counterparts, and participants with an avoidant attachment style reported more severe posttraumatic avoidance symptoms. The effects of attachment dispositions on PTSD symptom severity at the aftermath of war and terror were replicated in several other studies: Attachment anxiety and avoidance heightened PTSD symptoms among Israeli military veterans (Dekel, Solomon, Ginzburg, & Neria, 2004), among former prisoners of war (ex-POWs) in both the United States and Israel (Dieperink, Leskela, Thuras, & Engdahl, 2001; Ein-Dor, Doron, et al., 2010; Mikulincer, Ein-Dor, Solomon, & Shaver, 2011; Solomon, Ginzburg, Mikulincer, Neria, & Ohry, 1998; Zakin, Solomon, & Neria, 2003), among survivors of the 9/11 terrorist attacks in the United States (Fraley, Fazzari, Bonanno, & Dekel, 2006), and among Palestinians who were former political prisoners (Kanninen, Punamaki, & Qouta, 2003). The association between insecure attachment and PTSD symptom severity has also been observed among adults who were sexually or physically abused as children (e.g., Ortigo, Westen, DeFife, & Bradley, 2013; Twaite & Rodriguez-Srednicki, 2004), among patients after cardiac surgery (Parmigiani et al., 2013), among adults living with HIV/AIDS (Gore-Felton et al., 2013), and among people with a diagnosis of psychosis (Picken, Berry, Tarrier, & Barrowclough, 2010).

Recently, the causal role of attachment-related processes in the development of PTSD was examined in research using a prospective design (Mikulincer, Shaver, & Horesh, 2006). This research focused on Israelis' psychological reactions during the 2003 U.S.–Iraq war and examined the effects of dispositional attachment orientations measured before the war on the severity of PTSD-related intrusion and avoidance symptoms during the war (Study 1). Findings indicated that dispositional attachment-related processes shaped daily responses to the trauma of war. Specifically, people high on anxiety or avoidance were found to suffer from more severe war-related PTSD than their more secure counterparts, with anxious people exhibiting more war-related intrusion symptoms and avoidant people showing more war-related avoidance responses.

In addition, research on the link between attachment dispositions and PTSD-related symptoms has indicated that unlike attachment anxiety, which relates to exacerbated PTSD symptoms even under mild stressful conditions, attachment avoidance is linked with PTSD mostly in prolonged or extremely stressful situations (e.g., caring for a child with a life-threatening illness, living in captivity, or experiencing prolonged political violence; Berant, Mikulincer, & Florian, 2001; Ein-Dor, Doron, et al., 2010; Reizer, Ein-Dor, & Possick, 2012; Reizer, Possick, & Ein-Dor, 2010; Wijngaards-de Meij et al., 2007). For example, in a study of the links between attachment dispositions and PTSD among war veterans, the findings indicated that only for ex-POWs, who endured human-engendered, prolonged, and extremely traumatic conditions, was avoidant attachment associated with more severe intrusion and avoidance symptoms of PTSD. Avoidant attachment was not associated with the severity of symptoms among war veterans who were not held in captivity (Ein-Dor, Doron, et al., 2010). It may be that when individuals are challenged over a prolonged period of time under extreme conditions such as captivity, the otherwise relatively effective avoidant strategies of suppressing attachment needs and distress tend to break down, causing attachment-related avoidance to be associated with emotional problems and psychopathology.

Attachment and Externalizing Disorders

Externalizing refers to a general liability to experience substance use and antisocial disorders (Krueger & Markon, 2011). It constitutes disorders that manifest themselves outwardly, and comprises aggressive, impulsive, coercive, and noncompliant reactions. In the current review, we focus on conduct problems.

Conduct Behavior Problems

Bowlby's original interest in attachment processes began with a study of juvenile delinquency, when he followed juvenile thieves and noted that "fourteen of the 44 thieves were distinguished from the remainder by their remarkable lack of affection or warmth of feeling for anyone" (1944, p. 23). He concluded that frustrating and painful experiences with parents, and/or early prolonged, or permanent, separation from a mother, may result in an "affectionless" character marked by distrust and hostility toward parents and a pervasive lack of empathy and compassion toward others. Because excessive animosity and hostility toward parents may be ill adapted, the dysfunctional feelings and frustrations are redirected to other socialization agents, individuals, or institutions without causing guilt, sorrow, or remorse. In this way, insecure attachment can lead to conduct problems and socially deviant or criminal behavior.

Attachment research has documented associations between adolescents' reports of insecure attachment to parents or peers (both anxiety and avoidance) and involvement in delinquent behaviors, such as theft and assault (McElhaney, Immele, Smith, & Allen, 2006; Wade & Brannigan, 1998), approval of norm-violating behavior (Silverberg, Vazsonyi, Schlegel, & Schmidt, 1998), bullying behavior in prison (Ireland & Power, 2004), and antisocial tendencies (e.g., Gwadz, Clatts, Leonard, & Goldsamt, 2004). Other studies have linked only attachment avoidance with conduct problems (e.g., Vungkhanching, Sher, Jackson, & Parra, 2004) or only attachment anxiety with these problems (e.g., McNally, Palfai, Levine, & Moore, 2003). These inconsistencies may be related to differences in measures, samples, and unmeasured variables. Studies using the AAI classifications exhibit the same discrepancy: Whereas some studies have found that conduct problems are associated with an anxious (pre-occupied) state of mind (e.g., Caspers, Cadoret, Langbehn, Yucuis, & Troutman, 2005; McElhaney et al., 2006), others relate these problems to an avoidant (dismissing) state of mind (e.g., Allen, Hauser, & Borman-Spurrell, 1996).

The developmental trajectory of conduct problems with respect to early attachment dispositions has yet to be directly examined. With that being said, poor-quality parenting at infancy (age 42 months), which resulted from maternal attachment avoidance and alienation (Sroufe et al., 2005), was found to be a risk factor for externalizing problems in adulthood in the Minnesota Study (Lorber & Egeland, 2009, 2011).

A Transdiagnostic Model of Attachment Insecurities

As this review has revealed, a vast body of knowledge links attachment dispositions to several types of psychopathology. Recent theory and research in psychiatry and clinical psychology have highlighted the potential value of a transdiagnostic approach to psychiatric disorders, as it holds several theoretical and clinical advantages over disorder-specific models (e.g., Barlow et al., 2011; Mansell, Harvey, Watkins, & Shafran, 2009). In keeping with this view, in the present section we unfold a transdiagnostic model of attachment insecurities that refers to (1) the mechanisms by which attachment dispositions (i.e., the transdiagnostic factors) cause all the different disorders they are associated with (i.e., the mediated pathways underpinning multifinality); and (2) the reasons why a given disposition leads to different disorders in different people or to different disorders within the same person over time (i.e., divergent trajectories). The model is outlined in Figure 13.2.

Mechanisms Linking Attachment Dispositions to Multiple Psychopathological Disorders (Multifinality)

Attachment Anxiety

Research and theory have indicated that people high on attachment anxiety tend to adopt hyperactivating attachment and emotion regulation strategies (i.e., energetic, insistent attempts to obtain care, support, and love from others) as a means of regulating distress and coping with threats (Mikulincer & Shaver, 2003). They are also inclined to exaggerate appraisals of threats (e.g., Mikulincer, Birnbaum, Woddis, & Nachmias, 2000), to have difficulties in suppressing negative thoughts and feelings (e.g., Mikulincer, Dolev, & Shaver, 2004), and to ruminate on distressing thoughts (Mikulincer & Florian, 1998). These tendencies may be the initiating conditions

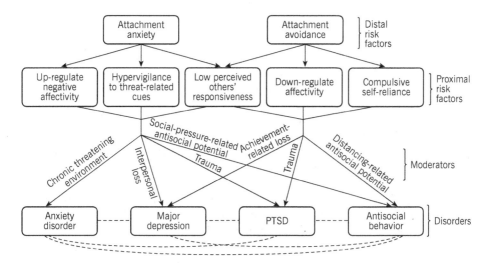

FIGURE 13.2. In this transdiagnostic model, attachment dispositions serve as distal risk factors for multiple psychopathological disorders. Each disposition affects a "dark triad" of proximal risk factors, which mediate the effect of attachment anxiety and avoidance on psychopathology. Specific moderators determine the divergent trajectories that individuals who are high on the proximal risk factors may take.

for a "dark triad" of processes that link attachment anxiety with multiple psychopathological disorders: (1) maladaptive emotion regulation processes, with a tendency to up-regulate negative affectivity; (2) greater vigilance to threat-related cues and heightened empathic accuracy; and (3) a lower level of *perceived others' responsiveness*—that is, seeing others as less responsive and supportive and as less understanding of one's needs (a broader notion than Reis and colleagues' *perceived partner responsiveness*; e.g., Reis, Clark, & Holmes, 2004).

Emotion regulation has been conceptualized as processes through which individuals modulate their emotions to respond appropriately to environmental demands (e.g., Campbell-Sills & Barlow, 2007). Individuals deploy regulatory strategies to modify the magnitude and/or type of their emotional experience or to adjust an emotion-eliciting event itself (e.g., Diamond & Aspinwall, 2003). The attachment system plays an important role in emotion regulation: It is activated by physiological and psychological threats, and causes a threatened individual to seek proximity to others as a means of managing the threat and restoring emotional equilibrium (Mikulincer & Shaver, 2003). Among secure people, these strategies reduce the impact of distressing events, allowing them to experience and acknowledge negative emotions without undue distortion or repression, and to counter negative affectivity. Attachment anxiety interferes with the down-regulation of negative emotions and emboldens intense and persistent distress, which continues even after objective threats subside. As a result, people high on attachment anxiety experience an unmanageable stream of negative thoughts and feelings, which contribute to cognitive disorganization and fuel chronic worries and distress. Attachment anxiety also intensifies fear-related responses to even minimal signs of threats, exaggerates the catastrophic implications of threats, and encourages rumination on threats and their imagined consequences (Ein-Dor, Mikulincer, Doron, & Shaver, 2010).

Difficulties in regulating emotion and exacerbated negative affectivity have been identified as transdiagnostic factors (Aldao, Nolen-Hoeksema, & Schweizer, 2010; Berenbaum, Raghavan, Le, Vernon, & Gomez, 2003; Kring & Sloan, 2010) and have been incorporated into several models of specific psychopathologies, including major depressive disorder (Rottenberg, Gross, & Gotlib, 2005), generalized anxiety disorder (Mennin, Holoway, Fresco, Moore, & Heimberg, 2007) and externalizing disorders (e.g., Sher & Grekin, 2007). Therefore, one potential mediator of the link between attachment anxiety and psychopathology is an up-regulation of negative affectivity.

People high on attachment anxiety do not only intensify negative responses to threats; they have greater vigilance to threat-related cues and are quicker and more accurate in detecting such threats. Specifically, attachment-related anxiety, but not avoidance or security, has recently been associated with a reaction that we (Ein-Dor, Doron, et al., 2010) have called *sentinel behavior*—noticing ambiguous signs of threat, and warning others about the threat (see also Ein-Dor & Orgad, 2012). For example, recent research indicated that people with high scores on attachment anxiety had greater mental access to sentinel-related schemas (Ein-Dor, Mikulincer, & Shaver, 2011a). When compared with their more secure counterparts, individuals high in attachment anxiety recognized sentinel-related sentences more quickly and with greater accuracy than more secure individuals (Study 2). When exposed to an experimentally created threatening situation (a room gradually filling with smoke because of a malfunctioning computer), the most anxious person in a group was the most likely to detect the presence of a threat (Study 6), which contributed to the effectiveness of this person's social group in dealing with the threat (Ein-Dor, Mikulincer, & Shaver, 2011b). Moreover, Ein-Dor and Perry (2014) found that people high in attachment anxiety were more accurate in detecting deceitful statements, and were better poker players; poker is a social game that is partially based on players' ability to detect deception. People high in attachment anxiety were also found to have a greater empathic accuracy in relationship-threatening situations, with respect to their ability to foretell their partners' true thoughts and feelings (e.g., when their partners rated and discussed an attractive person with them; Simpson, Ickes, & Grich, 1999; Simpson et al., 2011). According to Mikulincer and Shaver (2003), these abilities stem from the use of a hyperactivating strategy by people high in attachment anxiety—ruminating about worst-case scenarios and remaining vigilant to signs that close others might not be committed to them.

Attentiveness to threat-related information has been assigned a prominent role in the etiology and maintenance of anxiety and related disorders (e.g., Eysenck, 1992; Mathews & MacLeod, 2002), such as PTSD (Buckley, Blanchard, & Neill, 2000), generalized anxiety disorder (Mogg & Bradley, 2005), and panic disorder and phobias (McNally, 1999). The attentional system of people high on attachment anxiety seems to be distinctively sensitive to and biased in favor of threat-related stimuli in the environment (see Bar-Haim, Lamy, Pergamin, Bakermans-Kranenburg, & van IJzendoorn, 2007, for a recent meta-analysis). This tendency may confer adaptational advantages (Ein-Dor, Mikulincer, et al., 2010), but may also create disadvantages in the form of psychopathology.

Aside from perceiving more threats in the environment and intensively reacting to them, people high on attachment anxiety fear that they may need to face these threats alone: They tend to regard others as less responsive and supportive, and as less understanding to their needs (i.e., they have low perceived others' responsiveness). Research has indicated that perceived social support reflects a personality characteristic rather than the actual helpfulness of others when needed (Sarason et al., 1991). For example, Collins and Feeney (2004) found that people high on attachment anxiety were predisposed to perceive and remember a partner's helpful behavior as less supportive, especially if the behavior was ambiguous, open to subjective construal, and likely to reactivate worries about a partner's availability and supportiveness. Moreover, they often choose unsupportive partners and tend to act in ways that cause partners to act unsupportively, thus confirming and strengthening their doubts about other people's supportiveness (Rholes, Simpson, Campbell, & Grich, 2001).

Perceived availability of social support (and not actual support received) has been found to play an important role in the prediction of specific psychopathologies, including PTSD (e.g., Besser & Neria, 2012), depression (e.g., Grav, Hellzèn, Romild, & Stordal, 2012), and externalizing disorders (e.g., Lifrak, McKay, Rostain, Alterman, & O'Brien, 1997).

We therefore contend that the dark triad of people high on attachment anxiety—hypervigilance to threats, intensified negative affectivity, and low perceived others' responsiveness—may constitute the proximal transdiagnostic risk factors (see Nolen-Hoeksema & Watkins, 2011; also called *intermediate phenotypes*) that mediate the relationships between attachment anxiety and multiple psychopathologies, and that launch anxious individuals on pathways probabilistically related to various psychopathological outcomes.

Attachment Avoidance

Theory and research have indicated that attachment avoidance is organized around deactivating strategies of affect regulation, which involve deemphasizing threats and trying to cope with them alone, without seeking help or support from other people (e.g., Kobak, Cole, Ferenz-Gillies, & Fleming, 1993; Shaver & Mikulincer, 2002). Avoidant people also deny attachment needs and suppress attachment-related thoughts and emotions (Mikulincer & Shaver, 2003). These tendencies may be the initiating conditions for a second "dark triad" of processes—ones that, in this case, link attachment avoidance with multiple psychopathological disorders: (1) maladjusted emotion regulation processes, with a tendency to down-regulate affectivity and employing distancing strategies; (2) compulsive self-reliance; and (3) lower levels of social support and perceived others' responsiveness.

The attachment behavioral system fosters emotion regulation in a socially based way (Coan, 2008; Sroufe et al., 2004): It motivates a person to alleviate his or her distress by seeking actual or symbolic proximity to significant others. People high on attachment avoidance tend to forgo this tendency and to maintain a defensive façade of security and composure, while managing cognitive and emotional avoidance and dealing with threats without seeking help from others (Shaver & Mikulincer, 2002). To independently overcome life's many challenges, they tend to block access to emotions and to cope with stress by ignoring, suppressing, or denying it (e.g., Dozier & Kobak, 1992). These deactivation strategies may be effective in regulating mild levels of stress (e.g., Ein-Dor, Doron, et al., 2010), but they leave suppressed distress unresolved nonetheless. When avoidant persons are faced with prolonged and demanding stressful experiences that require active confrontation of a problem and mobilization of external sources of support, the suppressed distress can impair their ability to deal with inevitable adversities. In these cases, avoidant people may feel inadequate to cope and may undergo a marked decline in functioning (Horowitz, 1982).

Cognitive and emotional avoidance, together with suppression of negative affectivity, have been found to predict a large array of psychopathological disorders: depression and anxiety (Blalock & Joiner, 2000; Holahan, Moos, Holahan, Brennan, & Schutte, 2005), eating disorders (Engler, Crowther, Dalton, & Sanftner, 2006), and conduct problems (Cooper, Wood, Orcutt, & Albino, 2003). For example, Holahan and colleagues (2005) found that cognitive and emotional avoidance predicted increases in depressive symptoms over 10 years in a sample of late-middle-aged adults.

Aside from coping with life's challenges by cognitively and emotionally avoiding the sensation of distress, people high on attachment avoidance are compulsively self-reliant. Bowlby (1978) was the first to note that avoidant people disclaim the need for close interpersonal relationships, distrust these relationships, mock their necessity, and avoid situations where they might be either rejected or relied upon by others. Compulsive self-reliance helps to foster positive appraisals of self and high self-efficacy (Mikulincer & Shaver, 2007), which are essential resources for coping. Bowlby (1988) also noted, however, that no one of any age is completely free from reliance on actual others, and that compulsive self-reliance favors unrealistic positive appraisals of self, not genuine ones. Thus extreme self-criticism is fostered alongside the positive evaluations of self, which may result in psychopathology—especially when an individual repeatedly receives external feedback that he or she is weak, mistaken, or imperfect. Theory and research have indeed indicated that compulsive self-reliance is related to different forms of introjective psychopathology (Blatt, 1974), such as paranoia, obsessive–compulsive disorder, guilt-ridden depression, and phallic narcissism (Blatt & Blass, 1996).

The impact of cognitive, emotional, and behavioral distancing of people high on attachment avoidance on the liability for psychopathology may be further exacerbated in times of genuine need, because avoidant people are low on perceived others' responsiveness (Collins & Feeney, 2004; Ognibene & Collins, 1998). Avoidant people are deficient in interpersonal sensitivity and have problems in maintaining a flexible balance between self-concern and concern for others. These tendencies tend to erode relationship quality and engender relationship instability. Because people high on attachment avoidance are unable or unwilling to care sensitively for others in times of need, they alienate their social network, which in turn fuels a vicious cycle of feelings of rejection, anger, and isolation. According to interpersonal theories of psychopathology (Joiner & Coyne, 1999; Segrin, 2001), these negative relationship experiences and the low levels of perceived others' responsiveness may provide additional pathways to psychological disorders.

We therefore contend that the dark triad of people high in attachment avoidance—cognitive and emotional avoidance, compulsive self-reliance, and low perceived others' responsiveness—may comprise the proximal transdiagnostic risk factors that mediate the relationships between attachment avoidance and multiple psychopathologies.

Moderators of the Effects of Proximal Risk Factors

The moderators in our transdiagnostic model of attachment dispositions determine what particular symptoms proximal transdiagnostic risk factors will lead to in a given individual. Moderators create symptoms by (1) raising concerns or themes that proximal risk factors then act upon, (2) shaping responses through conditioning, or (3) determining the reinforcement value of certain stimuli (Nolen-Hoeksema & Watkins, 2011). In this section of the chapter, we describe the possible moderators that may launch people with different attachment dispositions on pathways to internalizing or externalizing disorders.

The dark triad of people high in attachment anxiety (hypervigilance to threats, intensified negative affectivity, and low perceived others' responsiveness), and that of people high in attachment avoidance (cognitive and emotional avoidance, compulsive self-reliance, and low perceived others' responsiveness), both increase the liability to suffer from internalizing and externalizing disorders. Nevertheless, "most of those with histories of anxious attachment do not have serious behavior problems or qualify for psychiatric diagnoses. Avoidant and resistant patterns of infant attachment are only moderate risks for disturbance" (Sroufe, 2005, p. 360). Therefore, we contend that the dark triad for each type of attachment insecurity should foment psychopathology only when a person is faced with specific moderators.

One possible moderator is an environment that poses chronic mild to moderate threat (e.g., living in a rough neighborhood or facing constant but mild political violence). In such an environment, emotions of fear and anxiety often arise (LeDoux, 2000). The tendency of people high on attachment anxiety to be emotionally overreactive and hyperattentive to threats should exacerbate and maintain these feelings of anxiety and fear. At the same time, their low perceived others' responsiveness should hinder an effective alleviation of these feelings by the aid of supportive others. As a result, the likelihood of developing an anxiety disorder may increase. In contrast, the cognitive and emotional distancing strategies of people high on attachment avoidance may shield them from mild to moderate feelings of anxiety and fear, and therefore may reduce the likelihood of their developing anxiety-based disorders under such threat conditions.

A second moderator may be the experience of loss. At its aftermath, a person may be more likely to develop major depression than an anxiety-related disorder, as loss has been linked with sadness, which in turn is related to depression (Brown & Harris, 1986). The nature of loss, however, may determine the type of depressive symptoms that one may endorse and the likelihood that one will suffer from the disorder. A relationship-related loss, such as the ending of a romantic relationship, may trigger depression among people high on attachment anxiety, because their anxiety relates specifically to separation and abandonment. In such an event, anxious individuals' emotional reactivity and attentional bias should maintain their sad emotions and increase awareness of their loss, potentially leading to anaclitic depression (i.e., interpersonally related depression; Blatt, 1974). Loss related to death of a significant other (e.g., a parent or a spouse), however, may confer more profound consequences and increase the likelihood of developing depressive symptoms among both anxious and avoidant people. This may occur because the distancing defenses of people high on avoidance may collapse under such conditions. Finally, an achievement-related loss such as losing a job (Catalano, Aldrete, Vega, Kolody, & Aguilar-Gaxiola, 2000) may cause introjective depression (Blatt, 1974) among people high on attachment avoidance, but not anxiety, because avoidance is closely tied to excessive self-criticism and compulsive self-reliance.

A third moderator may be the experience of trauma such as rape, assault, car accidents, floods, war, and a host of other natural and human-made disasters. The intensity of the traumatic event and the nature of the trauma-invoking stimulus may determine the liability to suffer from PTSD (and related psychopathology) among people high on anxiety or avoidance. The dark triad of people high on attachment anxiety makes them prone to the psychological ramifications of trauma. Therefore, almost any acute anxiety-provoking event may launch them on a pathway to PTSD. Research has indicated, however, that human-engendered traumatic experiences increase the likelihood, severity, and duration of PTSD more than other kinds of traumatic events (Charuvastra & Cloitre, 2008). Aside from increasing the liability for PTSD among anxious people, human-engendered events may also increase the likelihood of suffering anaclitic depression (comorbid with PTSD), because such events (e.g., rape and captivity) may obliterate any remaining shred of interpersonal trust. A greater sense of uncertainty may also elicit comorbidity of anxiety disorders, because in such events the sense of anxiety is harder to rationalize and the extent of rumination is greater.

A different pattern may be seen among avoidant people. Research on PTSD (Berant et al., 2001; Ein-Dor, Doron, et al., 2010; Reizer et al., 2010, 2012; Wijngaards-de Meij et al., 2007), has shown that people high on attachment avoidance are less likely to suffer from PTSD under mild levels of stress (e.g., natural disasters, car accidents without human casualties). Conversely, when faced with severe levels of stress (e.g., rape, captivity), their psychological defenses may collapse; this may make not only PTSD more likely, but also the comorbidity of introjective depression (because of the loss of the unrealistic positive appraisals of self) and anxiety (because of the inability to maintain the uncontrollable anxiety-related emotions).

A fourth and final moderator may be the types of modeling, observational learning, and reinforcement that increase the likelihood of conduct problems among people high on anxiety or avoidance. Numerous studies have linked childhood conduct disorder and juvenile delinquencies with adult antisocial behavior (for extensive reviews, see Connor, 2002; Hill & Maughan, 2001; Kalb, Farrington, & Loeber, 2001). According to the *integrated cognitive antisocial potential* theory (Farrington, 2005), the key construct underlying offending is antisocial potential—a continuum construct on which people may be ordered from low to high. High antisocial potential may characterize people who are exposed to and influenced by antisocial models, such as criminal parents, delinquent siblings, and delinquent peers (e.g., friends in high-crime schools and neighborhoods). We contend that distancing-related antisocial potential may launch avoidant people on a pathway to adult antisocial behavior because it is more congruent with their perception of and expectations from others. Conversely, social-pressure-related antisocial potential may cast anxious people on such a pathway because the source of their anxiety is separation and abandonment. For example, research has indicated that high-delinquency-rate schools have high levels of distrust between teachers and students, low commitment to the school by students, and unclear and inconsistently enforced rules (Graham, 1988). In such conditions of exposure to distancing-related antisocial models, the dark triad of people high on attachment avoidance may lead them to antisocial behavior. Conversely, social-pressure-related factors such as having antisocial friends (Keenan, Loeber, Zhang, Stouthamer-Loeber, & van Kammen, 1995) or antisocial parents (Lipsey & Derzon, 1998) may cause the dark triad of people high on attachment anxiety to elicit adult antisocial behavior.

Concluding Comments

Numerous studies have linked attachment dispositions (anxiety and avoidance) to multiple psychopathological disorders. In the present chapter, we have unfolded a transdiagnostic model of attachment insecurities to address two open questions in attachment research: (1) What are the potential mechanisms by which attachment dispositions cause all the different disorders they are associated with; and (2) why does a given disposition lead to different disorders in different people, or to different disorders within the same person over time? We have suggested that each attachment orientation has its own "dark triad" of processes that link it to psychopathology, and that by interacting with a specific moderator, these processes launch an individual on a pathway for a particular disorder.

Two key aspects fall outside the scope of the present model and ought to be considered in future transdiagnostic models of attachment dispositions: the moderating effect of genetic predispositions, and the dyadic and interpersonal processes that may affect the liability to psychopathology. Specifically, we contend that particular genetic predispositions may interact with the dark triads of people high on anxiety or avoidance as well as with environmental moderators to predict the likelihood for psychopathology. Of specific interest are the polymorphisms of the receptor genes for oxytocin (OT) and arginine vasopressin (AVP). OT and AVP are mammalian neuropeptides that have been found to be linked not only with development and expression of social behavior and emotion regulation (Bartz,

Zaki, Bolger, & Ochsner, 2011), but also with stress-related behavior and disorders, including anxiety disorders, comorbid depression, and their neuroendocrine concomitants (see Meyer-Lindenberg, Domes, Kirsch, & Heinrichs, 2011, for a review). For example, Thompson, Parker, Hall-mayer, Waugh, and Gotlib (2011) have shown that the AA/AG genotype of the *OTR rs2254298* polymorphism, which has been associated with insecure attachment (Chen, Barth, Johnson, Gotlib, & Johnson, 2011) was also associated with physical, social, and separation anxieties among people with adverse childhood experiences. Therefore, specific OT and AVP polymorphisms may interact with a specific dark triad and environmental moderator to launch an individual on a pathway for a particular psychopathology.

In addition, dyadic processes may play a role in exacerbating or mitigating psychopathology. Specifically, the attachment orientations of a person presenting with psychopathological symptoms may influence his or her spouse's symptom severity. For example, research has indicated that spouses of anxious people may present with greater secondary traumatization and more psychopathology-related symptoms because of the tendency of anxious people to up-regulate their emotional states. Conversely, spouses of avoidant people may paradoxically present with fewer psychopathology symptoms because avoidant people tend to down-regulate their emotional states (e.g., Ein-Dor, Doron, et al., 2010).

Despite these shortcomings, if our model is supported in future studies, it will enable a more comprehensive yet efficient view on the developmental trajectory linking early environmental influences with adult psychopathology.

References

Adam, E. K., Gunnar, M. R., & Tanaka, A. (2004). Adult attachment, parent emotion, and observed parenting behavior: Mediator and moderator models. *Child Development, 75*, 110–122.

Aldao, A., Nolen-Hoeksema, S., & Schweizer, S. (2010). Emotion regulation strategies across psychopathology: A meta-analytic review. *Clinical Psychology Review, 30*, 217–237.

Allen, J. P., Hauser, S. T., & Borman-Spurrell, E. (1996). Attachment theory as a framework for understanding sequelae of severe adolescent psychopathology: An 11-year follow-up study. *Journal of Consulting and Clinical Psychology, 64*, 254–263.

American Psychiatric Association. (2013). *Diagnostic and statistical manual of mental disorders* (5th ed.). Arlington, VA: Author.

Bar-Haim, Y., Lamy, D., Pergamin, L., Bakermans-Kranenburg, M. J., & van IJzendoorn, M. H. (2007). Threat-related attentional bias in anxious and nonanxious individuals: A meta-analytic study. *Psychological Bulletin, 133*, 1–24.

Barlow, D. H., Farchione, T. J., Fairholme, C. P., Ellard, K. K., Boisseau, C. L., Allen, L. B., et al. (2011). *The unified protocol for transdiagnostic treatment of emotional disorders: Therapist guide.* New York: Oxford University Press.

Bartz, J. A., Zaki, J., Bolger, N., & Ochsner, K. N. (2011). Social effects of oxytocin in humans: Context and person matter. *Trends in Cognitive Sciences, 15,* 301–309.

Batgos, J., & Leadbeater, B. J. (1994). Parental attachment, peer relations, and dysphoria in adolescence. In M. B. Sperling & W. H. Berman (Eds.), *Attachment in adults: Clinical and developmental perspectives* (pp. 155–178). New York: Guilford Press.

Berant, E., Mikulincer, M., & Florian, V. (2001). The association of mothers' attachment style and their reactions to the diagnosis of infant's congenital heart disease. *Journal of Social and Clinical Psychology, 20,* 208–232.

Berenbaum, H., Raghavan, C., Le, H. N., Vernon, L. L., & Gomez, J. J. (2003). A taxonomy of emotional disturbances. *Clinical Psychology: Science and Practice, 10,* 206–226.

Besser, A., & Neria, Y. (2012). When home isn't a safe haven: Insecure attachment orientations, perceived social support, and PTSD symptoms among Israeli evacuees under missile threat. *Psychological Trauma: Theory, Research, Practice, and Policy, 4,* 34–46.

Blalock, A., & Joiner, T. (2000). Interaction of cognitive avoidance coping and stress in predicting depression/anxiety. *Cognitive Therapy and Research, 24,* 47–65.

Blatt, S. J. (1974). Levels of object representation in anaclitic and introjective depression. *Psychoanalytic Study of the Child, 24,* 107–157.

Blatt, S. J., & Blass, R. B. (1996). Interpersonal relatedness and self-definition: Two basic dimensions in personality development and psychopathology. In G. G. Noam & K. W. Fischer (Eds.), *Development and vulnerabilities in close relationships* (pp. 309–338). Hillsdale, NJ: Erlbaum.

Bosquet, M., & Egeland, B. (2006). The development and maintenance of anxiety symptoms from infancy through adolescence in a longitudinal sample. *Development and Psychopathology, 18,* 517–550.

Bowlby, J. (1944). Forty-four juvenile thieves: Their character and home-life. *International Journal of Psychoanalysis, 25,* 19–52.

Bowlby, J. (1973). *Attachment and loss: Vol. 2. Separation: Anxiety and anger.* New York: Basic Books.

Bowlby, J. (1978). Attachment theory and its therapeutic implications. In S. C. Feinstein & P. Giovacchini (Eds.), *Adolescent psychiatry: Developmental and clinical studies* (Vol. 6, pp. 5–23). Chicago: University of Chicago Press.

Bowlby, J. (1980). *Attachment and loss: Vol. 3. Sadness and depression.* New York: Basic Books.

Bowlby, J. (1988). *A secure base: Clinical applications of attachment theory.* London: Routledge.

Brenning, K. M., Soenens, B., Braet, C., & Bosmans, G. (2012). Attachment and depressive symptoms in middle childhood and early adolescence: Testing the validity of the emotion regulation model of attachment. *Personal Relationships, 19,* 445–464.

Brown, G. W., & Harris, T. O. (1986). Establishing causal links: The Bedford College studies of depression. In H. Katsching (Ed.), *Life events and psychiatric disorders* (pp. 107–187). Cambridge, UK: Cambridge University Press.

Buckley, T. C., Blanchard, E. B., & Neill, W. T. (2000). Information processing and PTSD: A review of the empirical literature. *Clinical Psychology Review, 20*, 1041–1065.

Campbell-Sills, L., & Barlow, D. H. (2007). Incorporating emotion regulation into conceptualizations and treatments of anxiety and mood disorders. In J. J. Gross (Ed.), *Handbook of emotion regulation* (pp. 542–559). New York: Guilford Press.

Caspers, K. M., Cadoret, R. J., Langbehn, D., Yucuis, R., & Troutman, B. (2005). Contributions of attachment style and perceived social support to lifetime use of illicit substances. *Addictive Behaviors, 30*, 1007–1011.

Catalano, R., Aldrete, E., Vega, W., Kolody, B., & Aguilar-Gaxiola, S. (2000). Job loss and major depression among Mexican Americans. *Social Science Quarterly, 81*, 477–487.

Catanzaro, A., & Wei, M. (2010). Adult attachment, dependence, self-criticism, and depressive symptoms: A test of a mediational model. *Journal of Personality, 78*, 1135–1162.

Charuvastra, A., & Cloitre, M. (2008). Social bonds and posttraumatic stress disorder. *Annual Review of Psychology, 59*, 301–328.

Chen, F. S., Barth, M. E., Johnson, S. L., Gotlib, I. H., & Johnson, S. C. (2011). Oxytocin receptor (OXTR) polymorphisms and attachment in human infants. *Frontiers in Psychology, 2*, 200.

Cicchetti, D. (1984). The emergence of developmental psychopathology. *Child Development, 55*, 1–7.

Ciechanowski, P. S., Katon, W. J., & Russo, J. E. (2005). The association of depression and perceptions of interpersonal relationships in patients with diabetes. *Journal of Psychosomatic Research, 58*, 139–144.

Ciechanowski, P. S., Sullivan, M., Jensen, M., Romano, J., & Summers, H. (2003). The relationship of attachment style to depression, catastrophizing and health care utilization in patients with chronic pain. *Pain, 104*, 627–637.

Coan, J. A. (2008). Toward a neuroscience of attachment. In J. Cassidy & P. R. Shaver (Eds.), *Handbook of attachment: Theory, research, and clinical applications* (2nd ed., pp. 241–265). New York: Guilford Press.

Cole-Detke, H., & Kobak, R. (1996). Attachment processes in eating disorder and depression. *Journal of Consulting and Clinical Psychology, 64*, 282–290.

Collins, N. L., & Feeney, B. C. (2004). Working models of attachment shape perceptions of social support: Evidence from experimental and observational studies. *Journal of Personality and Social Psychology, 87*, 363–383.

Connor, D. F. (2002). *Aggression and antisocial behavior in children and adolescents*. New York: Guilford Press.

Cooper, M. L., Wood, P. K., Orcutt, H. K., & Albino, A. (2003). Personality and predisposition to engage in risky behaviors or problem behaviors during adolescence. *Journal of Personality and Social Psychology, 84*, 390–410.

Costa, N. M., & Weems, C. F. (2005). Maternal and child anxiety: Do attachment beliefs or children's perceptions of maternal control mediate their association? *Social Development, 14*, 574–590.

Crawford, T. N., Livesley, W. J., Jang, K. L., Shaver, P. R., Cohen, P., & Ganiban, J. (2007). Insecure attachment and personality disorder: A twin study of adults. *European Journal of Personality, 21*, 191–208.

Davaji, R. B. O., Valizadeh, S., & Nikamal, M. (2010). The relationship between attachment styles and suicide ideation: The study of Turkmen students, Iran. *Procedia—Social and Behavioral Sciences, 5*, 1190–1194.

Davila, J. (2001). Refining the association between excessive reassurance seeking and depressive symptoms: The role of related interpersonal constructs. *Journal of Social and Clinical Psychology, 20*, 538–559.

Dekel, R., Solomon, Z., Ginzburg, K., & Neria, Y. (2004). Long-term adjustment among Israeli war veterans: The role of attachment style. *Journal of Stress, Anxiety and Coping, 17*, 141–152.

Diamond, L. M., & Aspinwall, L. G. (2003). Emotion regulation across the life span: An integrative perspective emphasizing self-regulation, positive affect, and dyadic processes. *Motivation and Emotion, 27*, 125–156.

Dieperink, M., Leskela, J., Thuras, P., & Engdahl, B. (2001). Attachment style classification and posttraumatic stress disorder in former prisoners of war. *American Journal of Orthopsychiatry, 71*, 374–378.

Doron, G., Moulding, R., Kyrios, M., Nedeljkovic, M., & Mikulincer, M. (2009). Adult attachment insecurities are related to obsessive compulsive phenomena. *Journal of Social and Clinical Psychology, 28*, 1022–1049.

Dozier, M., & Kobak, R. (1992). Psychophysiology in attachment interviews: Converging evidence for deactivating strategies. *Child Development, 63*, 1473–1480.

Duggal, S., Carlson, E. A., Sroufe, L. A., & Egeland, B. (2001). Depressive symptomatology in childhood and adolescence. *Development and Psychopathology, 13*, 143–164.

Egeland, B., Pianta, R., & Ogawa, J. (1996). Early behavior problems: Pathways to mental disorders in adolescence. *Development and Psychopathology, 8*, 735–749.

Ein-Dor, T., Doron, G., Solomon, Z., Mikulincer, M., & Shaver, P. R. (2010). Together in pain: Attachment-related dyadic processes and posttraumatic stress disorder. *Journal of Counseling Psychology, 57*(3), 317–327.

Ein-Dor, T., Mikulincer, M., Doron, G., & Shaver, P. R. (2010). The attachment paradox: How can so many of us (the insecure ones) have no adaptive advantages? *Perspectives on Psychological Science, 5*, 123–141.

Ein-Dor, T., Mikulincer, M., & Shaver, P. R. (2011a). Attachment insecurities and the processing of threat-related information: Studying the schemas involved in insecure people's coping strategies. *Journal of Personality and Social Psychology, 101*, 78–93.

Ein-Dor, T., Mikulincer, M., & Shaver, P. R. (2011b). Effective reaction to danger: Attachment insecurities predict behavioral reactions to an experimentally induced threat above and beyond general personality traits. *Social Psychological and Personality Science, 2*, 467–473.

Ein-Dor, T., & Orgad, T. (2012). Scared saviors: Evidence that people high in attachment anxiety are more effective in alerting others to threat. *European Journal of Social Psychology, 42*, 667–671.

Ein-Dor, T., & Perry, A. (2014). Full house of fears: Evidence that people high in attachment anxiety are more accurate in detecting deceit. *Journal of Personality, 82*(2), 83–92.

Einstein, A. (1931). The world as I see it. *Forum and Century, 84,* 193–194.

Eng, W., Heimberg, R. G., Hart, T. A., Schneier, F. R., & Liebowitz, M. R. (2001). Attachment styles in individuals with social anxiety disorder: The relationship among adult attachment styles, social anxiety, and depression. *Emotion, 1,* 365–380.

Engler, P. A., Crowther, J. H., Dalton, G., & Sanftner, J. L. (2006). Predicting eating disorder group membership: An examination and extension of the sociocultural model. *Behavior Therapy, 37,* 69–79.

Esbjørn, B. H., Pedersen, S. H., Daniel, S. I. F., Hald, H. H., Holm, J. M., & Steele, H. (2013). Anxiety levels in clinically referred children and their parents: Examining the unique influence of self-reported attachment styles and interview-based reflective functioning in mothers and fathers. *British Journal of Clinical Psychology, 52*(4), 394–407.

Eysenck, M. W. (1992). *Anxiety: The cognitive perspective.* Hove, UK: Psychology Press.

Farrington, D. P. (2005). Childhood origins of antisocial behavior. *Clinical Psychology and Psychotherapy, 12,* 177–190.

Feeney, J. A., & Noller, P. (1990). Attachment style as a predictor of adult romantic relationships. *Journal of Personality and Social Psychology, 58,* 281–291.

Fowler, J. C., Allen, J. G., Oldham, J. M., & Frueh, B. C. (2013). Exposure to interpersonal trauma, attachment insecurity, and depression severity. *Journal of Affective Disorders, 149,* 313–318.

Fraley, R. C., Fazzari, D. A., Bonanno, G. A., & Dekel, S. (2006). Attachment and psychological adaptation in high exposure survivors of the September 11th attack on the World Trade Center. *Personality and Social Psychology Bulletin, 32,* 538–551.

Fraley, R. C., & Shaver, P. R. (1997). Adult attachment and the suppression of unwanted thoughts. *Journal of Personality and Social Psychology, 73,* 1080–1091.

Gamble, S. A., & Roberts, J. E. (2005). Adolescents' perceptions of primary caregivers and cognitive style: The roles of attachment security and gender. *Cognitive Therapy and Research, 29,* 123–141.

Gore-Felton, C., Ginzburg, K., Chartier, M., Gardner, W., Agnew-Blais, J., McGarvey, E., et al. (2013). Attachment style and coping in relation to posttraumatic stress disorder symptoms among adults living with HIV/AIDS. *Journal of Behavioral Medicine, 36,* 51–60.

Graham, J. (1988). *Schools, disruptive behaviour and delinquency.* London: Her Majesty's Stationery Office.

Grav, S., Hellzèn, O., Romild, U., & Stordal, E. (2012). Association between social support and depression in the general population: The HUNT study, a cross-sectional survey. *Journal of Clinical Nursing, 21,* 111–120.

Gwadz, M. V., Clatts, M. C., Leonard, N. R., & Goldsamt, L. (2004). Attachment style, childhood adversity, and behavioral risk among young men who have sex with men. *Journal of Adolescent Health, 34,* 402–413.

Hankin, B. L., Kassel, J. D., & Abela, J. R. Z. (2005). Adult attachment dimensions and specificity of emotional distress symptoms: Prospective investigations of cognitive risk and interpersonal stress generation as mediating mechanisms. *Personality and Social Psychology Bulletin, 31,* 136–151.

Hill, J., & Maughan, B. (Eds.). (2001). *Conduct disorders in childhood and adolescence.* Cambridge, UK: Cambridge University Press.

Hinnen, C., Schreuder, I., Jong, E., van Duijn, M., Dahmen, R., & van Gorp, E. C. M. (2012). The contribution of adult attachment and perceived social support to depressive symptoms in patients with HIV. *AIDS Care, 24,* 1535–1542.

Holahan, C. J., Moos, R. S., Holahan, C. K., Brennan, P. L., & Schutte, K. K. (2005). Stress generation, avoidance coping, and depressive symptoms: A 10-year model. *Journal of Consulting and Clinical Psychology, 73,* 658–666.

Horowitz, M. J. (1982). Psychological processes induced by illness, injury, and loss. In T. Millon, C. Green, & R. Meagher (Eds.), *Handbook of clinical health psychology* (pp. 53–68). New York: Plenum Press.

Illing, V., Tasca, G. A., Balfour, L., & Bissada, H. (2010). Attachment insecurity predicts eating disorder symptoms and treatment outcomes in a clinical sample of women. *Journal of Nervous and Mental Disease, 198,* 653–659.

Ireland, J. L., & Power, C. L. (2004). Attachment, emotional loneliness, and bullying behaviour: A study of adult and young offenders. *Aggressive Behavior, 30,* 298–312.

Joiner, T., & Coyne, J. C. (1999). *The interactional nature of depression: Advances in interpersonal approaches.* Washington, DC: American Psychological Association.

Kalb, L. M., Farrington, D. P., & Loeber, R. (2001). Leading longitudinal studies on delinquency, substance use, sexual behavior, and mental health problems with childhood samples. In R. Loeber & D. P. Farrington (Eds.), *Child delinquents: Development, intervention, and service needs* (pp. 415–423). Thousand Oaks, CA: Sage.

Kanninen, K., Punamaki, R. L., & Qouta, S. (2003). Personality and trauma: Adult attachment and posttraumatic distress among former political prisoners. *Peace and Conflict: Journal of Peace Psychology, 9,* 97–126.

Keenan, K., Loeber, R., Zhang, Q., Stouthamer-Loeber, M., & van Kammen, W. B. (1995). The influence of deviant peers on the development of boys' disruptive and delinquent behavior: A temporal analysis. *Development and Psychopathology, 7,* 715–726.

Kobak, R., Cole, H., Ferenz-Gillies, R., & Fleming, W. (1993). Attachment and emotional regulation during mother–teen problem solving: A control theory analysis. *Child Development, 64,* 231–245.

Kring, A. M., & Sloan, D. M. (Eds.). (2010). *Emotion regulation and psychopathology: A transdiagnostic approach to etiology and treatment.* New York: Guilford Press.

Krueger, R. F., & Markon, K. E. (2006). Reinterpreting comorbidity: A model-based approach to understanding and classifying psychopathology. *Annual Review of Clinical Psychology and Aging, 2,* 111–133.

Krueger, R. F., & Markon, K. E. (2011). A dimensional-spectrum model of psychopathology: Progress and opportunities. *Archives of General Psychiatry, 68,* 10–11.

LeDoux, J. E. (2000). Emotion circuits in the brain. *Annual Review of Neuroscience, 23,* 155–184.

Lifrak, P. D., McKay, J. R., Rostain, A., Alterman, A. I., & O'Brien, C. P. (1997). Relationship of perceived competencies, perceived social support, and gender to substance use in young adolescents. *Journal of the American Academy of Child and Adolescent Psychiatry, 36*, 933–940.

Lipsey, M. W., & Derzon, J. H. (1998). Predictors of violent or serious delinquency in adolescence and early adulthood: A synthesis of longitudinal research. In R. Loeber & D. P. Farrington (Eds.), *Serious and violent juvenile offenders: Risk factors and successful interventions* (pp. 86–105). Thousand Oaks, CA: Sage.

Livesley, W. J. (1991). Classifying personality disorders: Ideal types, prototypes, or dimensions? *Journal of Personality Disorders, 5*, 52–59.

Lorber, M. F., & Egeland, B. (2009). Infancy parenting and externalizing psychopathology from childhood through adulthood: Developmental trends. *Developmental Psychology, 45*, 909–912.

Lorber, M. F., & Egeland, B. (2011). Parenting and infant difficulty: Testing a mutual exacerbation hypothesis to predict early onset conduct problems. *Child Development, 82*, 2006–2020.

Mansell, W., Harvey, A., Watkins, E., & Shafran, R. (2009). Conceptual foundations of the transdiagnostic approach to CBT. *Journal of Cognitive Psychotherapy, 23*, 6–19.

Marganska, A., Gallagher, M., & Miranda, R. (2013). Adult attachment, emotion dysregulation, and symptoms of depression and generalized anxiety disorder. *American Journal of Orthopsychiatry, 83*, 131–141.

Mathews, A., & MacLeod, C. (2002). Induced processing biases have causal effects on anxiety. *Cognition and Emotion, 16*, 331–354.

Maunder, R. G., Lancee, W. J., Hunter, J. J., Greenberg, G. R., & Steinhart, A. H. (2005). Attachment insecurity moderates the relationship between disease activity and depressive symptoms in ulcerative colitis. *Inflammatory Bowel Diseases, 11*, 919–926.

McElhaney, K. B., Immele, A., Smith, F. D., & Allen, J. P. (2006). Attachment organization as a moderator of the link between friendship quality and adolescent delinquency. *Attachment and Human Development, 8*, 33–46.

McNally, A. M., Palfai, T. P., Levine, R. V., & Moore, B. M. (2003). Attachment dimensions and drinking-related problems among young adults: The meditational role of coping motives. *Addictive Behaviors, 28*, 1115–1127.

McNally, R. J. (1999). Panic and phobias. In T. Dalgleish & M. J. Power (Eds.), *Handbook of cognition and emotion* (pp. 479–496). Chichester, UK: Wiley.

Mennin, D. S., Holoway, R. M., Fresco, D. M., Moore, M. T., & Heimberg, R. G. (2007). Delineating components of emotion and its dysregulation in anxiety and mood psychopathology. *Behavior Therapy, 38*, 284–302.

Meyer, B., & Pilkonis, P. A. (2005). An attachment model of personality disorders. In M. F. Lenzenweger & J. F. Clarkin (Eds.), *Major theories of personality disorder* (2nd ed., pp. 231–281). New York: Guilford Press.

Meyer-Lindenberg, A., Domes, G., Kirsch, P., & Heinrichs, M. (2011). Oxytocin and vasopressin in the human brain: Social neuropeptides for translational medicine. *Nature Reviews Neuroscience, 12*, 524–538.

Mikulincer, M., Birnbaum, G., Woddis, D., & Nachmias, O. (2000). Stress and accessibility of proximity-related thoughts: Exploring the normative and intraindividual components of attachment theory. *Journal of Personality and Social Psychology, 78,* 509–523.

Mikulincer, M., Dolev, T., & Shaver, P. R. (2004). Attachment-related strategies during thought-suppression: Ironic rebounds and vulnerable self-representations. *Journal of Personality and Social Psychology, 87,* 940–956.

Mikulincer, M., Ein-Dor, T., Solomon, Z., & Shaver, P. R. (2011). Trajectories of attachment insecurities over a 17-year period: A latent growth curve analysis of the impact of war captivity and posttraumatic stress disorder. *Journal of Social and Clinical Psychology, 30,* 960–984.

Mikulincer, M., & Florian, V. (1998). The relationship between adult attachment styles and emotional and cognitive reactions to stressful events. In J. A. Simpson & W. S. Rholes (Eds.), *Attachment theory and close relationships* (pp. 143–165). New York: Guilford Press.

Mikulincer, M., Florian, V., & Weller, A. (1993). Attachment styles, coping strategies, and posttraumatic psychological distress: The impact of the Gulf War in Israel. *Journal of Personality and Social Psychology, 64,* 817–826.

Mikulincer, M., & Shaver, P. R. (2003). The attachment behavioral system in adulthood: Activation, psychodynamics, and interpersonal processes. In M. P. Zanna (Ed.), *Advances in experimental social psychology* (Vol. 35, pp. 52–153). San Diego, CA: Academic Press.

Mikulincer, M., & Shaver, P. R. (2007). *Attachment in adulthood: Structure, dynamics, and change.* New York: Guilford Press.

Mikulincer, M., & Shaver, P. R. (2012). An attachment perspective on psychopathology. *World Psychiatry, 11,* 11–15.

Mikulincer, M., Shaver, P. R., & Horesh, N. (2006). Attachment bases of emotion regulation and posttraumatic adjustment. In D. K. Snyder, J. A. Simpson, & J. N. Hughes (Eds.), *Emotion regulation in families: Pathways to dysfunction and health* (pp. 77–99). Washington, DC: American Psychological Association.

Mogg, K., & Bradley, B. P. (2005). Attentional bias in generalized anxiety disorder versus depressive disorder. *Cognitive Therapy and Research, 29,* 29–45.

Muris, P., & Meesters, C. (2002). Attachment, behavioral inhibition, and anxiety disorders symptoms in normal adolescents. *Journal of Psychopathology and Behavioral Assessment, 24,* 97–105.

Muris, P., Meesters, C., van Melick, M., & Zwambag, L. (2001). Self-reported attachment style, attachment quality, and symptoms of anxiety and depression in young adolescents. *Personality and Individual Differences, 30,* 809–818.

Murphy, B., & Bates, G. W. (1997). Adult attachment style and vulnerability to depression. *Personality and Individual Differences, 22,* 835–844.

Nolen-Hoeksema, S., & Watkins, E. R. (2011). A heuristic for developing transdiagnostic models of psychopathology: Explaining multifinality and divergent trajectories. *Perspectives on Psychological Science, 6,* 589–609.

Ognibene, T. C., & Collins, N. L. (1998). Adult attachment styles, perceived social support and coping strategies. *Journal of Social and Personal Relationships, 15*(3), 323–345.

Ortigo, K. M., Westen, D., DeFife, J. A., & Bradley, B. (2013). Attachment, social cognition, and posttraumatic stress symptoms in a traumatized, urban population: Evidence for the mediating role of object relations. *Journal of Traumatic Stress, 26,* 361–368.

Parmigiani, G., Tarsitani, L., De Santis, V., Mistretta, M., Zampetti, G., Roselli, V., et al. (2013). Attachment style and posttraumatic stress disorder after cardiac surgery. *European Psychiatry, 28*(Suppl. 1), 1.

Picken, A. L., Berry, K., Tarrier, N., & Barrowclough, C. (2010). Traumatic events, posttraumatic stress disorder, attachment style, and working alliance in a sample of people with psychosis. *Journal of Nervous and Mental Disease, 198,* 775–778.

Reis, H. T., Clark, M. S., & Holmes, J. G. (2004). Perceived partner responsiveness as an organizing construct in the study of intimacy and closeness. In D. J. Mashek & A. Aron (Eds.), *Handbook of closeness and intimacy* (pp. 201–225). Mahwah, NJ: Erlbaum.

Reizer, A., Ein-Dor, T., & Possick, H. (2012). Living at risk: Dyadic examination of the links among environmental stress attachment orientations and marital support provision. *Journal of Social and Personal Relationships, 29,* 694–712.

Reizer, A., Possick, H., & Ein-Dor, T. (2010). Environmental threat influences psychological distress and marital satisfaction among avoidantly attached individuals. *Personal Relationships, 17,* 585–598.

Rholes, W. S., Simpson, J. A., Campbell, L., & Grich, J. (2001). Adult attachment and the transition to parenthood. *Journal of Personality and Social Psychology, 81,* 421–435.

Rottenberg, J., Gross, J. J., & Gotlib, I. H. (2005). Emotion context insensitivity in major depressive disorder. *Journal of Abnormal Psychology, 114,* 627–639.

Sarason, B. R., Pierce, G. R., Shearin, E. N., Sarason, I. G., Waltz, J. A., & Poppe, L. (1991). Perceived social support and working models of self and actual others. *Journal of Personality and Social Psychology, 60,* 273–287.

Segrin, C. (2001). Social skills and negative life events: Testing the deficit stress generation hypothesis. *Current Psychology: Developmental, Learning, Personality, Social, 20,* 19–35.

Shaver, P. R., & Mikulincer, M. (2002). Attachment-related psychodynamics. *Attachment and Human Development, 4,* 133–161.

Shaver, P. R., Schachner, D. A., & Mikulincer, M. (2005). Attachment style, excessive reassurance seeking, relationship processes, and depression. *Personality and Social Psychology Bulletin, 31,* 343–359.

Sheehan, G., & Noller, P. (2002). Adolescents' perceptions of differential parenting: Links with attachment style and adolescent adjustment. *Personal Relationships, 9,* 173–190.

Sher, K. J., & Grekin, E. R. (2007). Alcohol and affect regulation. In J. J. Gross (Ed.), *Handbook of emotion regulation* (pp. 560–580). New York: Guilford Press.

Silverberg, S. B., Vazsonyi, A. T., Schlegel, A. E., & Schmidt, S. (1998). Adolescent apprentices in Germany: Adult attachment, job expectations, and delinquency. *Journal of Adolescent Research, 13,* 254–271.

Simpson, J. A., Ickes, W., & Grich, J. (1999). When accuracy hurts: Reactions of anxious-ambivalent dating partners to a relationship-threatening situation. *Journal of Personality and Social Psychology, 76,* 754–769.

Simpson, J. A., Kim, J. S., Fillo, J., Ickes, W., Rholes, W. S., Orina, M. M., & Winterheld, H. A. (2011). Attachment and the management of empathic accuracy in relationship-threatening situations. *Personality and Social Psychology Bulletin, 37*, 242–254.

Simpson, J. A., Rholes, W. S., Campbell, L., Tran, S., & Wilson, C. L. (2003). Adult attachment, the transition to parenthood, and depressive symptoms. *Journal of Personality and Social Psychology, 84*, 1172–1187.

Solomon, Z., Ginzburg, K., Mikulincer, M., Neria, Y., & Ohry, A. (1998). Coping with war captivity: The role of attachment style. *European Journal of Personality, 12*, 271–285.

Sroufe, L. A. (2005). Attachment and development: A prospective, longitudinal study from birth to adulthood. *Attachment and Human Development, 7*, 349–367.

Sroufe, L. A., Duggal, S., Weinfield, N., & Carlson, E. A. (2000). Relationships, development, and psychopathology. In A. J. Sameroff, M. Lewis, & S. M. Miller (Eds.), *Handbook of developmental psychopathology* (2nd ed., pp. 75–91). New York: Kluwer Academic/Plenum.

Sroufe, L. A., Egeland, B., Carlson, E. A., & Collins, A. (2005). *The development of the person: The Minnesota Study of Risk and Adaptation from Birth to Adulthood.* New York: Guilford Press.

Thompson, R. J., Parker, K. J., Hallmayer, J. F., Waugh, C. E., & Gotlib, I. H. (2011). Oxytocin receptor gene polymorphism (rs2254298) interacts with familial risk for psychopathology to predict symptoms of depression and anxiety in adolescent girls. *Psychoneuroendocrinology, 36*, 144–147.

Twaite, J. A., & Rodriguez-Srednicki, O. (2004). Childhood sexual and physical abuse and adult vulnerability to PTSD: The mediating effects of attachment and dissociation. *Journal of Child Sexual Abuse, 13*, 17–38.

Visioli, C., Senatore, R., Lepri, B., & Tondo, L. (2012). Low quality in early attachment bondings as possible predictor of adult depressive disorder. *Journal of Psychopathology, 18*, 273–280.

Vungkhanching, M., Sher, K. J., Jackson, K. M., & Parra, G. R. (2004). Relation of attachment style to family history of alcoholism and alcohol use disorders in early adulthood. *Drug and Alcohol Dependence, 75*, 47–53.

Wade, T. J., & Brannigan, A. (1998). The genesis of adolescent risk-taking: Pathways through family, school and peers. *Canadian Journal of Sociology, 23*, 1–20.

Warren, S. L., Huston, L., Egeland, B., & Sroufe, L. A. (1997). Childhood anxiety disorders and attachment. *Journal of the American Academy of Child and Adolescent Psychiatry, 36*, 637–644.

Wei, M., Heppner, P. P., & Mallinckrodt, B. (2003). Perceived coping as a mediator between attachment and psychological distress: A structural equation modeling approach. *Journal of Counseling Psychology, 50*, 438–447.

Wei, M., Mallinckrodt, B., Larson, L. M., & Zakalik, R. A. (2005). Attachment, depressive symptoms, and validation from self versus others. *Journal of Counseling Psychology, 52*, 368–377.

Whiffen, V. E. (2005). The role of partner characteristics in attachment insecurity and depressive symptoms. *Personal Relationships, 12*, 407–423.

Wijngaards-de Meij, L., Stroebe, M., Schut, H., Stroebe, W., van den Bout, J., van der Heijden, P. G. M., et al. (2007). Patterns of attachment and parents' adjustment to the death of their child. *Personality and Social Psychology Bulletin, 33,* 537–548.

Zakin, G., Solomon, Z., & Neria, Y. (2003). Hardiness, attachment style, and long-term distress among Israeli ex-POWs and combat veterans. *Personality and Individual Differences, 34,* 819–829.

Zuroff, D. C., & Fitzpatrick, D. K. (1995). Depressive personality styles: Implications for adult attachment. *Personality and Individual Differences, 18,* 253–265.

14

Attachment-Related Preventive Interventions

Mary Dozier
Caroline K. P. Roben

Young children are dependent upon their parents for help in regulating attachment, emotions, behaviors, and physiology. When parents themselves experience harsh, adverse conditions and/or have histories of problematic relationships, it is often difficult for them to provide the care children need to flourish. The consideration of clinical phenomena and interventions was central to the development of attachment theory (Bowlby, 1944, 1969/1982). Nonetheless, only relatively recently have attachment-based interventions for parents of young children been developed and tested through experimental design. This chapter focuses upon early attachment-based interventions for parents of infants and young children. Enhancing parenting for infants and young children, especially among parents who are faced with adversity that compromises caregiving, should be a rich and productive avenue for change. Indeed, a number of interventions appear to have important effects on parenting and on child outcomes.

In this chapter, we first review several key principles of attachment, and describe themes specifically relevant to early intervention. We then describe several promising preventive interventions for at-risk children based upon these principles; in particular, we provide an in-depth description of the intervention developed in our lab. We conclude with directions for future research.

Key Foundational Principles

Attachment Theory Is Based on Ethology and Evolutionary Theory

Attachment theory was strongly influenced by ethology (Bowlby, 1969/ 1982). Defining attachment theory as quite distinct from contemporary psychoanalytic and social learning theories, Bowlby drew from the work of evolutionary biologists Lorenz (1935) and Tinbergen (1951), who described behavior such as imprinting among goslings. Bowlby (1969/1982) recognized analogous behaviors among human infants that serve functions in maintaining proximity to caregivers and maximizing chances of survival. In Bowlby's view, such behaviors—especially crying, smiling, clinging, and following—all represent early evolutionarily prepared behaviors displayed by young infants toward their caregivers. He called these evolutionally prepared behaviors the attachment behavioral system.

Humans Are an Altricial Species

Young infants are almost fully dependent upon their caregivers. At birth, infants are dependent upon caregivers for help in regulating body temperature and neuroendocrine functioning, and they become reliant on parents for help in regulating emotions, security, and safety, among other things. Under favorable conditions, parents serve as coregulators for their infants and young children. Although young children gradually take over regulatory functions themselves over time, as described below, there is a protracted period of dependence upon parents as coregulators.

Without an Available Caregiver, There Are Consequences

Availability of caregivers represents an experience-expectant condition. That is, in terms of our evolutionary history, infants would not have survived without caregivers. Therefore, human infants did not need strategies for coping with the lack of caregivers. Not surprisingly, then, significant consequences often result when children lack consistent and adequate caregivers, as Bowlby's (1944) seminal research on the early home lives of 44 thieves demonstrated. Subsequent research has found that children growing up in institutional settings without adequate caregiving show deficits in physical growth, cognitive development, executive functioning, and attachment-related behaviors (Drury et al., 2012; Johnson, Bruce, Tarullo, & Gunnar, 2011; Loman et al., 2013; Nelson et al., 2007; Zeanah, Smyke, Koga, & Carlson, 2005).

Attachment Promotes Physical Proximity

The attachment system evolved to keep infants in close proximity to parents under potentially threatening conditions, thus enhancing their likelihood for survival. By the time infants are capable of moving away from their parents, the attachment system has developed fully, leading children to seek out proximity under threat (Bowlby, 1969/1982). The caregiving system functions in complementary ways to the attachment system, serving to promote parents' protection of their young under conditions of threat (George & Solomon, 1999; Insel, 2000). Although parents differ in how they respond to infants' distress, most nonetheless behave in ways to protect their young from danger.

An Attachment Figure Helps a Child Develop Self-Regulation

A sensitive parent (or other caregiver) serves to help a child regulate physiology, behavior, and emotions, and gradually helps the child take over those regulatory functions him- or herself. As noted above, the parent is therefore a coregulator for the child (Sroufe, 1996), engaging in mutual regulatory experiences that serve as building blocks for the child's developing self-regulation (Kopp, 1982). Without adequate parental input (as in the case of neglect), or with problematic input (as in the case of abuse), parents fail to serve effectively as coregulators. Children who lack appropriate input have difficulty taking over regulatory capabilities themselves, and may have deficits in the ability to regulate physiology, behavior, and emotions (Blair & Raver, 2012; Calkins & Leerkes, 2011; Cicchetti & Toth, 2005).

Key Themes Relevant to Intervention

Parents Are the Focus of the Intervention

Although older children and adolescents may themselves be the focus of intervention, parents are nearly always the focus of intervention involving infants and very young children. Indeed, parenting behaviors, and perhaps aspects of the relationship between parent and child, are seen as important to target, rather than the infant him- or herself. Parents are the most influential aspects of infants' environments, serving as protectors, coregulators, and care providers during most waking hours. In particular, interventions often target helping parents improve their effectiveness as coregulators.

Intervene Early to Change Parental Behavior

Intervening early with at-risk children and their parents can have cascading, lasting effects on developmental trajectories. Infancy and toddlerhood are important times of neurodevelopmental integration of functioning (Johnson & Munakata, 2005), including the neurobiological, social, emotional, and cognitive domains (Gunnar & Quevedo, 2007; Kopp, 1982; Perez & Gauvain, 2007). The vast neurobiological and behavioral changes taking place in early infancy are dependent on repeated and frequent interactions with caregivers (Trevarthen & Aitken, 2001). During this period of rapid development, a child's developing brain and behaviors are especially sensitive to environmental risk; therefore, infancy is an ideal time for intervention (Ramey & Ramey, 1998; Shore, 1997).

Intervene in Families' Homes

Interventions have differed with regard to the emphasis placed on where interventions occur. Some interventions are implemented in offices, whereas others take place in families' homes. We consider it advantageous to intervene in homes, because parents are learning and practicing skills in the context in which they will be using them. The likelihood that behaviors will generalize is increased when these are practiced in the environment in which they will be needed.

Intervene in Critical Parental Behaviors

From an attachment perspective, there are several key characteristics that distinguish sensitive, responsive parenting: nurturance, contingent responsiveness (or synchrony), delight, and nonfrightening behavior. Attachment-related interventions often target these critical parent behaviors, as well as deal with issues related to parental trauma and parents' own caregiving history.

Nurturance

First, young children need nurturing care, and this is especially true for children who have experienced early adversity. Although children from low-risk environments can usually organize attachment around the availability of non-nurturing caregivers, high-risk children have greater difficulty doing so (Cyr, Euser, Bakermans-Kranenburg, & van IJzendoorn, 2010; Dozier, Stovall, Albus, & Bates, 2001). Therefore, an objective of most attachment-based interventions is to help parents behave in nurturing ways when their children are distressed.

Synchrony or Contingent Responsiveness

Children need a responsive environment if they are to develop adequate regulatory capabilities. Children who have experienced early adversity are especially susceptible to problems in regulating their behavior and physiology. When parents follow children's lead and are well attuned to children's signals, they are providing a responsive interpersonal environment (e.g., Beebe et al., 2010; Feldman, 2007; Tronick & Cohn, 1989). As with nurturing care, many attachment-based interventions target this aspect of sensitivity in interventions. Beebe and Lachmann (1984) and Feldman (2007) refer to this quality as *synchrony*, emphasizing the importance of parental attunement to children's signals. Shonkoff et al. (2012) emphasize the "serve and return" nature of successful interactions, with an emphasis on a parent's response to a child-initiated interaction. Other related terms are *following the child's lead* and *contingent responsiveness*.

Parental Delight

Ainsworth, Blehar, Waters, and Wall (1978) emphasized the importance of parents' feeling and showing delight toward their infants. Bernard and Dozier (2011) found that foster parents who indicated that they felt more committed to their foster children showed more delight behaviorally than parents who indicated that they felt less committed. When parents display positive affect to their children, children are more likely to display positive affect themselves (e.g., Forbes, Cohn, Allen, & Lewinsohn, 2004; Tronick, 1989). In contrast, when children's parents (such as parents who are depressed) display emotions characterized as either flat or withdrawn, children are more likely to have dysregulated emotions and behaviors (e.g., Beardslee, Bemporad, Keller, & Klerman, 1983; Cohn & Tronick, 1989; Field, 1984). Delight is explicitly addressed in some interventions.

Nonfrightening Behavior

When parents behave in frightening ways, children have difficulty organizing their attachment behaviors (Schuengel, Bakermans-Kranenburg, & van IJzendoorn, 1999); indeed, such children develop disorganized attachments at high rates (Carlson, Cicchetti, Barnett, & Braunwald, 1989). Children with disorganized attachments have difficulty regulating behavior and physiology (Bernard & Dozier, 2010; Hertsgaard, Gunnar, Erickson, & Nachmias, 1995). Main and Hesse (1990) have suggested that when parents behave in frightening ways, children experience "fright without solution" (p. 163) because they are frightened of the persons from whom they need to seek reassurance. This issue is addressed directly by some interventions.

Parental Trauma and Caregiving History

Parents' history of trauma or inadequate caregiving can affect their ability to respond sensitively to their children. More specifically, parents with their own history of unresolved trauma are at increased risk for behaving in frightening and intrusive ways with their children (Hesse & Main, 1999; Lyons-Ruth & Block, 1996; Schuengel et al., 1999). Interventions that target parental trauma or parents' history of inadequate caregiving directly include Child–Parent Psychotherapy (CPP) and the Circle of Security; Attachment and Biobehavioral Catch-up (ABC) targets these less directly. These three interventions and several others are described below.

Attachment-Based Preventive Interventions

Several attachment-based interventions that have been developed over the last several decades are based on these principles. Some have supporting evidence through randomized clinical trials or pre- to postintervention data. We first provide a detailed overview of ABC, which was developed in our lab, and then go on to describe several other attachment-based interventions. We do not cover the wider range of programs that aim to enhance parental sensitivity more generally.

Attachment and Biobehavioral Catch-up

Overview of the Intervention

ABC is a short-term preventive intervention for high-risk infants and parents. ABC targets four issues, as suggested by attachment and stress neurobiology theory and findings (Bernard, Butzin-Dozier, Rittenhouse, & Dozier, 2010). First, nurturing behavior under conditions of child distress is critical for children who have experienced adversity (Dozier et al., 2001); second, children need parents to behave in contingent, responsive ways when they are not distressed (Bernard et al., 2010: Raver, 1996); third, frightening behavior is problematic for children at all times (Schuengel et al., 1999); and fourth, children need parents to delight in them (Bernard & Dozier, 2011). ABC is specifically designed for infants who have experienced early adversity, and it has been assessed in randomized clinical trials among several populations, including neglecting birth parents, foster parents, and parents adopting internationally.

Description of the Intervention

The ABC intervention is a 10-session program that is conducted in families' homes by a "parent coach" with parents and children present. We consider it critical that the intervention take place in the environment in which parents live their lives, increasing the likelihood that parents will generalize the skills acquired. Sessions are video-recorded for the purposes of providing supervision and video feedback to parents. Sessions include manual-guided discussion of intervention content, review of parent homework, activities that allow parents to practice targeted behavior, and video feedback. Although the intervention is manualized, parent coaches' "in-the-moment" comments, described in more detail below, are considered the most critical aspect of the program.

The ABC intervention has been used with both foster parents and maltreating birth parents referred by child protective services as part of a foster care diversion program. The intervention is best suited to parents of children who are between about 6 and 24 months of age. Although it is possible to intervene with infants between the ages of birth and 6 months, the intervention is likely to be more powerful with children older than 6 months, because there are more opportunities for practice on intervention targets. When the intervention is conducted with newborns and young infants, frequent napping and fewer spontaneous behaviors (vocalizing, reaching for objects, etc.) provide parents with relatively few opportunities to practice targeted behaviors. We are currently testing the efficacy of an intervention for children older than 24 months, which includes attention to helping parents help their children to develop self-regulatory strategies under challenging conditions.

"In-the-Moment" Comments

Parent coaches use "in-the-moment" comments to provide feedback to parents regarding their behaviors that relate to intervention targets. These comments focus attention on parents' opportunities for behaving in nurturing and synchronous ways during the sessions, and help them recognize and practice the key targeted behaviors. Parent coaches are expected to make in-the-moment comments at least once per minute. Parent coaches are expected to pause or interrupt themselves during discussions of manual content to bring the focus of the session back to the parent–child interaction. Manual content is expected to be secondary to in-the-moment comments.

In-the-moment comments can address one or more of three possible components: describing the parent's behavior (e.g., "He bumped his head, and you said, 'Oh, sweetie, are you OK?'"); relating the behavior to an intervention target (e.g., "That's such a good example of your providing her with nurturance"); and/or relating the behavior to long-term outcomes (e.g., "That's the kind of thing that will let him know you'll be there when he needs you"). The first of these three components, describing the behavior, helps the parent clearly identify the behavior that is addressed. Without a clear description, parents are sometimes confused about exactly what the parent coach is focusing upon. Anecdotally, when parent coaches fail to provide clear descriptions, we have seen parents increase behaviors other than those intended. The second of these components, relating the behavior to an intervention target, helps the parent see links between the more general concept and specific behaviors. In other words, it makes the discussion of a general construct (e.g., following the child's lead, nurturance) more specific and concrete, which helps the parent associate his or her own current actions with the manual content being discussed. The third of these components, relating the behavior to a child outcome, provides examples of how the parent's behavior affects child outcomes. The target for parent coaches is an average of one component per comment. Although it is possible (and sometimes desirable) to make comments that include all three components, it can be overwhelming for all comments to include three components.

In the first several intervention sessions, parent coaches are expected to make comments that point out only those times when nurturance, following the child's lead, or delight are observed (even if this means missing many opportunities for making comments when parents fail to nurture or follow the lead). After the first several sessions, when parent coaches have developed sufficient rapport with the parents, they are expected to begin to make comments that point out times when parents have neglected to nurture or follow the lead. These comments can be made gently and in a scaffolding way: "This is one of those times when he might need you to pick him up," or "Are you following or leading right now?"

We have developed a system of coding parent coaches' in the moment comments. Any parental behavior that is relevant to an intervention target is a trigger for a comment. These behaviors include nurturing (or nonnurturing) behavior, synchronous (or nonsynchronous) behavior, delight, and nonfrightening (or frightening) behavior. Parent coaches' behaviors are coded with regard to whether they commented on each relevant parental behavior, along with the number of components included in each comment (description, identification of intervention target, link with child outcome). An automated spreadsheet calculates rates of on-target commenting, average number of components included in comments, and a number of other variables.

Parent coaches are also trained to code their own sessions. A trained coder provides feedback on the reliability of coding and suggests alternative strategies for comments. We have been able to use carefully trained and supervised undergraduate students in this role. The students work with parent coaches to reach predetermined levels of proficiency by the end of a year of supervision. In order to be certified as implementing ABC with fidelity, coaches are expected to reliably make one comment every minute (or miss fewer than 50% of the opportunities available to make a comment); to be on target with their comments at least 80% of the time (e.g., to comment on nurturance when the parent behavior is nurturance instead of a different type of behavior); and to have an average of at least one component (description of the behavior, labeling the target, or providing an outcome) for every comment. An experienced clinician (PhD) also provides clinical supervision.

Randomized clinical trials have found ABC to be effective in improving attachment (Bernard et al., 2012), normalizing diurnal cortisol levels postintervention (Bernard, Dozier, Bick, & Gordon, 2014) and several years after intervention completion (Bernard, Hostinar, & Dozier, in press), reducing child negative affect during a challenging activity (Lind, Bernard, Ross, & Dozier, 2014) and improving executive functioning at age 4 (Lewis-Morrarty, Dozier, Bernard, Terraciano, & Moore, 2012) as compared to a control intervention. Caregivers of children enrolled in ABC have also been shown to have higher levels of sensitivity (Bick & Dozier, 2013) and a more normative ERP response to emotional faces relative to neutral faces when compared to caregivers in the control intervention (Bernard, Simons, & Dozier, 2014).

Child–Parent Psychotherapy

Alicia Lieberman and colleagues at the University of California, San Francisco, developed CPP. CPP grew from the Infant–Parent Psychotherapy intervention developed by Selma Fraiberg (Fraiberg, 1980; Fraiberg, Adelson, & Shapiro, 1975), which considered how parents' "ghosts in the nursery," or challenging attachment experiences, affect parenting. Lieberman adapted CPP to be broader than Infant–Parent Psychotherapy and manualized it (Lieberman, Ghosh Ippen, & Van Horn, 2006). The intervention is designed for parents and their young children who have experienced challenging early attachment experiences, including trauma. The intervention focuses on helping parents become aware of their issues that interfere with sensitivity to their children's needs. The intervention works to help parents provide supportive, safe relationships so that children can cope effectively with trauma, and can develop secure, organized attachments. Among infants, the focus is almost exclusively on parents helping their young children cope, but the intervention increasingly includes children as partners as they become older. Delivered in weekly sessions over about a year, this relatively intensive intervention is intended to help parents gain understanding of their children's challenges in a safe, playful context. The intervention is delivered in the home in some cases and in a clinic-based setting in others.

Through randomized clinical trials, CPP has been shown to reduce disorganized attachment (Cicchetti, Rogosch, & Toth, 2006), reduce negative self-representations (Toth, Maughan, Manly, Spagnola, & Cicchetti, 2002), and reduce posttraumatic stress disorder symptoms among children (Lieberman et al., 2006).

Circle of Security

The Circle of Security (Hoffman, Marvin, Cooper, & Powell, 2006) was developed by three clinicians in Spokane, Washington: Kent Hoffman, Glen Cooper, and Bert Powell. For a number of years, Hoffman, Cooper, and Powell worked with Robert Marvin from the University of Virginia;

more recently, they have worked with Jude Cassidy from the University of Maryland. Two versions of the Circle of Security have been developed—a longer version that requires close work with the model developers to implement, and a briefer, more recent version that is DVD-based and can be implemented independently following training. Both versions of the intervention use a conceptual model of relationship challenges to focus parents' and interventionists' attention. Attachment issues are considered to represent a "circle of security," with parents providing a safe haven when children are distressed, and a secure base when children feel prepared to explore the world. Children are expected to develop confidence in their parents' availability and develop stronger self-esteem when they find that they can venture out into the world supported by their parents, and that they can return to their parents for support when needed.

Parents are asked to think about when their own issues interfere more: when they need to respond to a child's needs for reassurance, or when they need to allow the child to move away to explore. In the longer version, attachment quality is assessed at preintervention to guide and inform the intervention approach, and at postintervention to assess change. In an attempt to reduce the time and resources needed for the longer version, an eight-session parent reflection protocol was developed that uses DVD footage created by the model's founders, rather than individualized video reviews. Groups of parents are encouraged to discuss their own strengths and struggles in parenting in relation to the video clips of other parents and children, and to reflect on parenting behaviors that could serve to maintain attachment problems.

The longer version has been tested in several pre- to postintervention blinded studies, and has been shown to enhance attachment security (Hoffman et al., 2006; Cassidy et al., 2010). At this point, randomized clinical trials have not been reported in the literature, but such trials are under way for both the longer and DVD versions of the model.

Video-Feedback Intervention to Promote Positive Parenting

Juffer, Bakermans-Kranenburg, and van IJzendoorn (2008) developed a brief intervention, the Video-feedback Intervention to promote Positive Parenting (VIPP), to enhance parental sensitivity and thus child attachment security. The intervention uses video feedback to focus mothers' attention on their children's signals, with the goal of enhancing sensitivity and empathy. Video feedback focuses on four themes: exploration versus attachment behavior; giving voice to the child; the chain of events occurring when the parent promptly responds to the child; and the importance of sharing emotions. The interventionist video-records portions of each session while being as unobtrusive as possible, and prepares brief videos for presentation in the subsequent session. Like ABC, VIPP emphasizes parent strengths as observed in specific parental behaviors. (It is very different from ABC, however, because the interventionist remains unobtrusive during filming.) VIPP has been shown to be effective in enhancing parental sensitivity and in enhancing child attachment among a number of different populations (e.g., Juffer et al., 2008; Stein et al., 2006).

Steps Toward Effective Enjoyable Parenting

Byron Egeland and Martha Farrell Erickson developed STEEP in 1986. STEEP was developed directly from an attachment-theoretical perspective, with considerations of the critical factors affecting the development of secure attachments. Using STEEP, interventionists work with parents before their first child is born and throughout the first year of the child's life. This rather intensive and broad-based intervention focuses on helping parents respond sensitively to children's needs, and encouraging them to reflect upon their own attachment issues. STEEP has been found to have positive effects on parental sensitivity, but not on parental state of mind with regard to attachment (Erickson, Korfmacher, & Egeland, 1992; Korfmacher, Adam, Ogawa, & Egeland, 1997).

Interaction Guidance

Susan McDonough developed Interaction Guidance as a brief model using video feedback to enhance parents' awareness of infants' signals and responses, so that children could develop trusting, secure relationships (McDonough, 2004). Targeting parent–infant dyads resistant to other treatments, this model emphasizes the importance of parents' representations of the world more generally, and of their infants more specifically, as the mechanisms of change in parent sensitivity/child attachment. Interventionists are expected to be very positive in their approach to parents, particularly in making suggestions of alternative explanations for children's behaviors.

Robert-Tissot et al. (1996) compared Interaction Guidance with psychodynamic therapy in a randomized clinical trial. Reductions in symptoms and improvements in mothers' self-esteem were seen for both groups, with no significant differences between the groups. In a small matched-comparison-group study, Benoit, Madigan, Lecce, Shea, and Goldberg (2001) found lower levels of maternal atypical behaviors following the intervention among mothers receiving Interaction Guidance than among mothers receiving a feeding-focused intervention.

Minding the Baby

Lois Sadler, Arietta Slade, and others at the Yale Child Study Center developed the Minding the Baby intervention. The focus of Minding the Baby is on promoting reflective parenting by helping give voice to both an infant's and a mother's experiences as a means of enhancing parental sensitivity. The mother is helped to develop the capacity to contemplate these experiences and develop positive feelings for the child, even when faced with challenging emotions. Minding the Baby is an interdisciplinary approach, with a social worker and nurse practitioner working together to enhance secure attachment, health, mental health, self-efficacy, and reflective parenting through intensive home visitation. Preliminary unpublished findings in a sample composed largely of teen mothers suggest that mothers who received the Minding the Baby intervention had babies with higher rates of secure attachment (and lower rates of disorganized attachment) than the rates for babies of mothers in the control condition (*http://medicine.yale.edu/childstudy/mtb/research/currentfindings.aspx*). In addition, mothers in the Minding the Baby intervention reported fewer problem behaviors among their infants than control mothers did. It is important to note, though, that these findings are preliminary.

Promoting First Relationships

Jean Kelly and colleagues at the University of Washington developed Promoting First Relationships with goals similar to those of the other interventions described here (Kelly, Zuckerman, & Rosenblatt, 2008). As the Circle of Security and several other interventions do, Promoting First Relationships uses video recordings of parent–child interactions to help bring parents' attention to times when they behave in nurturing and responsive ways, and times when they fail to do so. Parents are helped to reflect upon their own and their children's behaviors thoughtfully.

The intervention has been assessed through several randomized clinical trials, with varying results. Short-term effects have been seen on parents' sensitivity and knowledge of appropriate parenting behaviors, parents' perceptions of child competence, and observations of child emotion regulation (Spieker, Oxford, Kelly, Nelson, & Fleming, 2012). Effects beyond this initial follow-up period have been nonsignificant, with the exception of differences in sleep problems favoring the Promoting First Relationships group (Spieker et al., 2012). Differences in cortisol production have suggested the possibility of intervention effects as well (Nelson & Spieker, 2013).

New and Promising Directions for Future Research

Dissemination and Implementation

The dissemination of attachment-based preventive interventions is an important issue as researchers work to bring their interventions to scale. The study of dissemination and implementation science (e.g., Southham-Gerow,

Rodriguez, Chorpita, & Daleiden, 2012) highlights many of the critical issues that need to be addressed in moving interventions to larger service systems. Notable challenges arise as interventions move from laboratory to community settings.

Critical to the process of dissemination and implementation is identifying the mechanisms of an intervention's action. When the intervention's mechanisms are identified, local adaptations to the model can be made, with care taken that these adaptations do not interfere with the mechanisms. Fidelity measures can then be developed that carefully assess whether the critical aspects of the interventions are being implemented with fidelity (Carroll, 2012; Landsverk, 2013).

Dissemination of ABC as an Example of the Process

Our lab has begun the process of dissemination and implementation of the ABC intervention. We have proposed in the moment comments as the most critical active ingredient of the intervention. We have found that frequency of in the moment comments is associated with parental synchrony in subsequent sessions and in postintervention assessments (Meade, Dozier, & Bernard, 2014).

Establishing clearly what skill or skills are crucial to an intervention's implementation is an important step, but ensuring that interventionists learn and use the skills is a vital next step. In the early years of ABC, we found that parent coaches often found it difficult to make in-the-moment comments even when supervision focused upon this aspect of the model. We have taken several steps to enhance the likelihood of success and increase our ability to disseminate the model with fidelity.

First, we have developed a screening tool that assesses potential parent coaches' ability to make in the moment comments. They first watch examples of effective in-the-moment comments, and are then asked to generate such comments themselves after watching videos in which the parent coach did not make comments. This screening tool predicts at a very high level later success in making in the moment comments in sessions (Meade, Roben, & Dozier, 2013).

Second, our training and supervision strategies focus on making such comments. In the moment commenting and the coding system are introduced on the first of 2–3 days of training, with extensive practice in the system provided in the rest of the training. Parent coaches receive two types of weekly supervision over the course of a year—one focusing more generally on case conceptualization (i.e., parental strengths with regard to nurturance, following the child's lead, delight, and avoiding frightening behaviors), and one focusing exclusively on in the moment commenting. Each week they code a randomly assigned 5-minute clip of a session, and then meet with their supervisor for consultation on the reliability of their coding and strategies for improving the quantity and quality of comments. Preliminary evidence from eight parent coaches at one training site suggests that adding the coding feedback to regular small-group supervision increased the coaches' rate of commenting across subsequent months (Dozier, Meade, Wallin, & Bernard, 2013).

Finally, we have established clear, quantified criteria that specify how frequently we expect to see in the moment comments and the average number of components expected. Parent coach trainees can therefore gauge their progress toward these criteria. When they meet criteria, they are certified as ABC parent coaches. Since the institution of this system, 80–90% of the parent coaches who have trained in the system have met the criteria and been certified.

Pre- to postintervention assessments provide support for the intervention's effectiveness in changing parental sensitivity in the community (Meade, Dozier, Weston-Lee, & Haggerty, 2014). A randomized clinical trial of ABC is being conducted at another site, but data are not yet available.

Conclusion

A number of attachment-based preventive interventions for parents of young children have been developed in the last several decades. Some of these interventions focus primarily on the parents' own attachment issues that may interfere with caregiving, and others focus primarily on parenting behaviors themselves. In all interventions, goals involve enhancing parental sensitivity and responsiveness, as well as reducing frightening behavior. A growing evidence base supports both of these approaches to enhancing parental sensitivity and responsiveness, with effects seen on children's attachment and self-regulation. This work is exciting in demonstrating the openness of the caregiving and attachment systems to change.

References

Ainsworth, M. D. S., Blehar, M., Waters, E., & Wall, S. (1978). *Patterns of attachment*. Hillsdale, NJ: Erlbaum.

Beardslee, W. R., Bemporad, J., Keller, M. B., & Klerman, G. L. (1983). Children of parents with major affective disorder: A review. *American Journal of Psychiatry, 140*, 825–832.

Beebe, B., Jaffe, J., Markese, S., Buck, K., Chen, H., Cohen, P., et al. (2010). The origins of 12-month attachment: A microanalysis of 4-month mother–infant interaction. *Attachment and Human Development, 12*, 3–141.

Beebe, B., & Lachmann, F. M. (1984). Representation and internalization in infancy: Three principles of salience. *Psychoanalytic Psychology, 11*, 127–165.

Benoit, D., Madigan, S., Lecce, S., Shea, B., & Goldberg, S. (2001). Atypical maternal behavior toward feeding-disordered infants before and after intervention. *Infant Mental Health Journal, 22*, 611–626.

Bernard, K., Butzin-Dozier, Z., Rittenhouse, J., & Dozier, M. (2010). Young children living with neglecting birth parents show more blunted daytime patterns of cortisol production than children in foster care and comparison children. *Archives of Pediatrics and Adolescent Medicine, 164*, 438–443.

Bernard, K., & Dozier, M. (2010). Examining infants' cortisol responses to laboratory tasks among children varying in attachment disorganization: Stress reactivity or return to baseline? *Developmental Psychology, 46*, 1771–1778.

Bernard, K., & Dozier, M. (2011). This is my baby: Foster parents' feelings of commitment and displays of delight. *Infant Mental Health Journal, 32*, 251–262.

Bernard, K., Dozier, M., Bick, J., & Gordon, K. A. (2014). Normalizing blunted diurnal cortisol rhythms among children at risk for neglect: The effects of an early intervention. *Development and Psychopathology.* Advance online publication.

Bernard, K., Dozier, M., Bick, J., Lewis-Morrarty, E., Lindhiem, O., & Carlson, E. (2012). Enhancing attachment organization among maltreated infants: Results of a randomized clinical trial. *Child Development, 83*, 623–636.

Bernard, K., Hostinar, C., & Dozier, M. (in press). Intervention effects on diurnal cortisol rhythms of CPS-referred infants persist into early childhood: Preschool follow-up results of a randomized clinical trial. *JAMA Pediatrics.*

Bernard, K., Simons, R., & Dozier, M. (2014). *Effects of an attachment-based intervention on high-risk mothers' event related potentials to children's emotions.* Manuscript submitted for publication.

Bick, J., & Dozier, M. (2013). The effectiveness of an attachment-based intervention in promoting foster mothers' sensitivity toward foster infants. *Infant Mental Health Journal, 34*, 95–103.

Blair, C., & Raver, C. C. (2012). Child development in the context of adversity: Experiential canalization of brain and behavior. *American Psychologist, 67*, 309–318.

Bowlby, J. (1944). Forty-four juvenile thieves: Their character and home-life. *International Journal of Psychoanalysis, 25*, 19–52.

Bowlby J. (1969/1982). *Attachment and loss: Vol. 1. Attachment.* New York: Basic Books.

Calkins, S. D., & Leerkes, E. M. (2011). Early attachment processes and the development of emotional self-regulation. In K. D. Vohs & R. F. Baumeister (Eds.), *Handbook of self-regulation: Research, theory, and applications* (2nd ed., pp. 355–373). New York: Guilford Press.

Carlson, V., Cicchetti, D., Barnett, D., & Braunwald, K. (1989). Disorganized/disoriented attachment relationships in maltreated infants. *Developmental Psychology, 25*, 525–531.

Carroll, K. (2012). Evidence-based practices: How far we've come, and how much further we've got to go. *Addiction, 107*, 1031–1033.

Cassidy, J., Ziv, Y., Stupica, B., Sherman, L., Butler, H., Karfgin, A., et al. (2010). Enhancing maternal sensitivity and attachment security in the infants of women in a jail-diversion program. *Attachment and Human Development, 12,* 333–353.

Cicchetti, D., Rogosch, F. A., & Toth, S. L. (2006). Fostering secure attachments in infants in maltreating families through preventive interventions. *Development and Psychopathology, 18,* 623–649.

Cicchetti, D., & Toth, S. L. (2005). Child maltreatment. *Annual Review of Clinical Psychology, 1,* 409–438.

Cohn, J. F., & Tronick, E. Z. (1989). Specificity of infants' response to mothers' affective behavior. *Journal of the American Academy of Child and Adolescent Psychiatry, 28,* 242–248.

Cyr, C., Euser, E. M., Bakermans-Kranenburg, M. J., & van IJzendoorn, M. H. (2010). Attachment security and disorganization in maltreating and high-risk families: A series of meta-analyses. *Development and Psychopathology, 22,* 87–108.

Dozier, M., Meade, E., Wallin, A. R., & Bernard, K. (2013). *Implementing an evidence-based intervention for high-risk parents in the community: The importance of model fidelity.* Paper presented at the biennial meeting of the Society for Research on Child Development, Seattle, WA.

Dozier, M., Stovall, K. C., Albus, K. E., & Bates, B. (2001). Attachment for infants in foster care: The role of caregiver state of mind. *Child Development, 72,* 1467–1477.

Drury, S. S., Theall, K., Gleason, M. M., Smyke, A. T., De Vivo, I., Wong, J. Y. Y., et al. (2012). Telomere length and early severe social deprivation: Linking early adversity and cellular aging. *Molecular Psychiatry, 17*(7), 719–727.

Erickson, M. F., Korfmacher, J., & Egeland, B. R. (1992). Attachments past and present: Implications for therapeutic intervention with mother–infant dyads. *Development and Psychopathology, 4,* 495–507.

Feldman, R. (2007). Parent–infant synchrony and the construction of shared timing: Physiological precursors, developmental outcomes, and risk conditions. *Journal of Child Psychology and Psychiatry, 48,* 329–354.

Field, T. (1984). Early interactions between infants and their postpartum depressed mothers. *Infant Behavior and Development, 7,* 527–532.

Forbes, E. E., Cohn, J. F., Allen, N. B., & Lewinsohn, P. M. (2004). Infant affect during parent-infant interaction at 3 and 6 months: Differences between mothers and fathers and influence of parent history of depression. *Infancy, 5,* 61–84.

Fraiberg, S. (1980). *Clinical studies in infant mental health.* New York: Basic Books.

Fraiberg, S., Adelson, E., & Shapiro, V. (1975). Ghosts in the nursery: A psychoanalytic approach to the problems of impaired infant–mother relationships. *Journal of the American Academy of Child Psychiatry, 14,* 387–421.

George, C., & Solomon, J. (1999). Attachment and caregiving: The caregiving behavioral system. In J. Cassidy & P. R. Shaver (Eds.), *Handbook of attachment: Theory, research, and clinical applications* (pp. 649–670). New York: Guilford Press.

Gunnar, M., & Quevedo, K. (2007). The neurobiology of stress and development. *Annual Review of Psychology, 58,* 145–173.

Hertsgaard, L., Gunnar, M., Erickson, M. R., & Nachmias, M. (1995). Adreno-cortical responses to the Strange Situation in infants with disorganized/disori-ented attachment relationships. *Child Development, 66,* 1100–1106.

Hesse, E., & Main, M. (1999). Second-generation effects of unresolved trauma in nonmaltreating parents: Dissociated, frightened, and threatening parental behavior. *Psychoanalytic Inquiry, 19,* 481–540.

Hoffman, K. T., Marvin, R. S., Cooper, G., & Powell, B. (2006). Changing tod-dlers' and preschoolers' attachment classifications: The Circle of Security intervention. *Journal of Consulting and Clinical Psychology, 74,* 1017–1026.

Insel, T. R. (2000) Toward a neurobiology of attachment. *Review of General Psy-chology, 4,* 176–185.

Johnson, A. E., Bruce, J., Tarullo, A. R., & Gunnar, M. R. (2011). Growth delay as an index of allostatic load in young children: Predictions to disinhibited social approach and diurnal cortisol activity. *Development and Psychopathology, 23,* 859–871.

Johnson, M. H., & Munakata, Y. (2005). Processes of change in brain and cogni-tive development. *Trends in Cognitive Sciences, 9,* 152–188.

Juffer, F., Bakermans-Kranenburg, M. J., & van IJzendoorn, M. H. (2008). *Pro-moting positive parenting: An attachment-based intervention.* New York: Erlbaum.

Kelly, J. F., Zuckerman, T., & Rosenblatt, S. (2008). Promoting first relationships: A relationship-focused early intervention approach. *Infants and Young Chil-dren, 21,* 285–295.

Kopp, C. B. (1982). Antecedents of self-regulation: A developmental perspective. *Developmental Psychology, 18,* 199–214.

Korfmacher, J., Adam, E., Ogawa, J., & Egeland, B. (1997). Adult attachment: Implications for the therapeutic process in a home visitation intervention. *Applied Developmental Science, 1,* 43–52.

Landsverk, J. (2013). Reflections on treatment integrity in a dissemination and implementation framework. *Clinical Psychology: Science and Practice, 20,* 114–119.

Lewis-Morrarty, E., Dozier, M., Bernard, K., Terraciano, S., & Moore, S. (2012). Cognitive flexibility and theory of mind outcomes among foster children: Pre-school follow-up results of a randomized clinical trial. *Journal of Adolescent Health, 52,* S17–S22.

Lieberman, A. F., Ghosh Ippen, C., & Van Horn, P. (2006). Child–Parent Psycho-therapy: 6-month follow-up of a randomized controlled trial. *Journal of the American Academy of Child and Adolescent Psychiatry, 45,* 913–918.

Lind, T., Bernard, K., Ross, E., & Dozier, M. (2014). Intervention effects on nega-tive affect of CPS-referred children: Results of a randomized clinical trial. *Child Abuse and Neglect, 9,* 1459–1467.

Loman, M. M., Johnson, A. E., Westerlund, A., Pollak, S. D., Nelson, C. A., & Gunnar, M. R. (2013). The effect of early deprivation on executive attention in middle childhood. *Journal of Child Psychology and Psychiatry, 54,* 37–45.

Lorenz, L. (1935). Der Kumpan in der Umwelt des Vogels. *Journal of Ornithology, 83,* 137–213.

Lyons-Ruth, K., & Block, D. (1996). The disturbed caregiving system: Relations among childhood trauma, maternal caregiving, and infant affect and attachment. *Infant Mental Health Journal, 17,* 257–275.

Main, M., & Hesse, E. (1990). Parents' unresolved traumatic experiences are related to infant disorganized attachment status: Is frightened and/or frightening parental behavior the linking mechanism? In M. T. Greenberg, D. Cicchetti, & E. Cummings (Eds.), *Attachment in the preschool years: Theory, research, and intervention* (pp. 161–182). Chicago: University of Chicago Press.

McDonough, S. C. (2004). Interaction guidance. In A. J. Sameroff, S. C. McDonough, & K. L. Rosenblum (Eds.), *Treating parent–infant relationship problems: Strategies for intervention* (pp. 79–96). New York: Guilford Press.

Meade, E. B., Dozier, M., & Bernard, K. (2014). Using video feedback as a tool in training parent coaches: Promising results from a single-case design. *Attachment and Human Development, 16,* 356–370.

Meade, E., Dozier, M., Weston-Lee, P., & Haggerty, D. (2014). *Effectiveness of community implementation of Attachment and Biobehavioral Catch-up.* Manuscript submitted for review.

Meade, E., Roben, C. K. P., & Dozier, M. (2013). *Screening interventionists for a parent training program.* Unpublished manuscript, University of Delaware.

Nelson, C. A., Zeanah, C. H., Fox, N. A., Marshall, P. J., Smyke, A. T., & Guthrie, D. (2007). Cognitive recovery in socially deprived young children: The Bucharest Early Intervention Project. *Science, 318,* 1937–1940.

Nelson, E. M., & Spieker, S. J. (2013). Intervention effects on morning and stimulated cortisol responses among toddlers in foster care. *Infant Mental Health Journal, 34,* 211–221.

Perez, S. M., & Gauvain, M. (2007). The sociocultural context of transitions in early socioemotional development. In C. A. Brownell & C. B. Kopp (Eds.), *Socioemotional development in the toddler years: Transitions and transformations* (pp. 396–419). New York: Guilford Press.

Ramey, C. T., & Ramey, S. L. (1998). Early intervention and early experience. *American Psychologist, 53,* 109–120.

Raver, C. C. (1996). Relations between social contingency in mother–child interactions and 2-year-olds' social competence. *Developmental Psychology, 32,* 850–859.

Robert-Tissot, C., Cramer, B., Stern, D. N., Serpa, S. R., Bachmann, J. P., Palacio-Espasa, F., et al. (1996). Outcome evaluation in brief mother–infant psychotherapies: Report on 75 cases. *Infant Mental Health Journal, 17*(2), 97–114.

Schuengel, C., Bakermans-Kranenburg, M. J., & van IJzendoorn, M. H. (1999). Frightening maternal behavior linking unresolved loss and disorganized infant attachment. *Journal of Consulting and Clinical Psychology, 67,* 54–63.

Shonkoff, J. P., Garner, A. S., & The Committee on Psychosocial Aspects of Child and Family Health, Committee on Early Childhood, Adoption, and Dependent Care, and Section on Developmental and Behavioral Pediatrics. (2012). The lifelong effects of early childhood adversity and toxic stress. *Pediatrics, 129,* e232–e242.

Shore, R. (1997). *Rethinking the brain: New insights into early development.* New York: Families and Work Institute.

Southham-Gerow, M. A., Rodriguez, A., Chorpita, B. F., & Daleiden, E. L. (2012).

Dissemination and implementation of evidence based treatments for youth: Challenges and recommendations. *Professional Psychology: Research and Practice, 43,* 527–534.

Spieker, S. J., Oxford, M. L., Kelly, J. F., Nelson, E. M., & Fleming, C. B. (2012). Promoting first relationships: Randomized trial of a relationship-based intervention for toddlers in child welfare. *Child Maltreatment, 17,* 271–286.

Sroufe, L. A. (1996). *Emotional development.* New York: Cambridge University Press.

Stein, A., Woolley, H., Senior, R., Hertzmann, L., Lovel, M., Lee, J., et al. (2006). Treating disturbances in the relationship between mothers with bulimic eating disorders and their infants: A randomized, controlled trial of video feedback. *American Journal of Psychiatry, 163,* 899–906.

Tinbergen, N. (1951). *The study of instinct.* Oxford, UK: Oxford University Press.

Toth, S. L., Maughan, A., Manly, J. T., Spagnola, M., & Cicchetti, D. (2002). The relative efficacy of two interventions in altering maltreated preschool children's representational models: Implications for attachment theory. *Development and Psychopathology, 14,* 877–908.

Trevarthen, C., & Aitken, K. (2001). Intersubjectivity: Research, theory, and clinical applications. *Journal of Child Psychology and Psychiatry, 42,* 3–48.

Tronick, E. Z. (1989). Emotions and emotional communication in infants. *American Psychologist, 44,* 112–119.

Tronick, E. Z., & Cohn, J. F. (1989). Infant–mother face-to-face interaction: Age and gender differences in coordination and the occurrence of miscoordination. *Child Development, 60,* 85–92.

Zeanah, C. H., Smyke, A. T., Koga, S. F., & Carlson, E. (2005). Attachment in institutionalized and community children in Romania. *Child Development, 76,* 1015–1028.

Attachment

A Guide to a New Era of Couple Interventions

Susan M. Johnson
Marie-France Lafontaine
Tracy L. Dalgleish

Attachment theory, now recognized as "one of the broadest, most profound, and most creative lines of research" in psychology (Cassidy & Shaver, 2008, p. xi), has permeated the fields of developmental, personality, and social psychology and has arguably changed the culture of parenting in the Western world. Attachment theory is perhaps the prime example of an empirically supported theory of human functioning that systematically integrates what Bowlby (1973, p. 180) called the "inner ring" of emotional processing in the individual with the "outer ring" of patterned interactions in social relationships, outlining how each reciprocally influences the other. This integration would seem to give it obvious relevance for clinical psychology and the tasks of the psychotherapist. Nevertheless, clinical psychologists have been slow to appreciate its significance. Over 25 years ago, Bowlby himself noted that he was "disappointed that clinicians have been so slow to test the theory's uses" (1988, pp. ix–x). The most notable exceptions appear to be the work of more analytically oriented clinicians who use approaches such as mentalizing, derived from attachment theorist Mary Main's (1991) notion of *metacognitive monitoring* (Fonagy et al., 1995; Wallin, 2007), and accelerated experiential dynamic psychotherapy (Fosha, 2000). Both models are used to address individual dysfunction.

In the field of couple therapy, however, attachment theory and science have become increasingly central—forming the basis of one of the only two extant empirically validated couple therapies, emotionally focused therapy (EFT; Johnson, 2004), while beginning to influence the conceptualization of relationship distress in the other, the cognitive-behavioral model of couple therapy (Cobb & Bradbury, 2003). Attachment is also the basis for a new and promising relationship enhancement program based on EFT, the Hold Me Tight: Conversations for Connection program (Johnson, 2010), which is presently being evaluated. This chapter focuses on how attachment science is taking couple therapy and our ability to shape loving relationships, as exemplified by EFT, in new and immensely promising directions; how clinical findings can clarify theoretical issues associated with changing attachment; and how attachment affects other aspects of a relationship, namely sex and caregiving. The chapter does not focus on systematically describing EFT, since such descriptions are already available in numerous texts in the attachment and couple therapy literature (Johnson, 2009a, 2009b). It is sufficient here to summarize EFT as a model where a therapist constantly helps partners to expand their inner emotional awareness, especially of their deeper, softer emotions, and to send new signals to each other that evoke new and more positive responses from each other. These positive responses are then organized into a new "dance" of secure bonding. This dance redefines the partners' relationship and offers them all the benefits that accrue from a stable sense of felt connection with an irreplaceable other.

As a modality, couple therapy is more and more in demand with the public; moreover, the quality of couple relationships is now recognized as a key variable in mental and physical health in general, and in problems such as depression and heart attack in particular (Johnson, 2004; Hawkley, Masi, Berry, & Cacioppo, 2006). However, couple therapy is also a field that has long been accused of being a set of relatively superficial interventions in search of an encompassing theory of relationship and relationship change. Many commentators have suggested that the key defining aspects of love relationships, such as emotional comfort and nurturing, have been conspicuously absent from models of couple therapy, and that many interventions, such as those that focus on teaching sequences of communication and listening skills, are not typical of happy relationships and are not powerful enough to change key relationship-defining interactions outside the therapist's office (Mackay, 1996: Gottman, Coan, Carriere, & Swanson, 1998). In the same vein, Acevedo and Aron (2009)—after completing a recent brain scan study showing that physiological responses to a partner in a certain proportion of recent and long-term lovers were identical, and concluding that romantic love is not ephemeral but can last across time—have now directly challenged couple therapists to begin to focus on shaping the responses that make up what we call love. The key issue in meeting such a challenge is that the creation of a couple therapy that targets the organizing elements of a love relationship, and is powerful enough to have an impact on vital factors such as intimacy, trust, emotional connection, compassion, sexual desire, and tenderness, requires a systematic, pragmatic theory of love and loving. The field of adult attachment, as developed over the last two decades (Mikulincer & Shaver, 2007), offers exactly such a theory. In light of the points made above, it seems to be more and more apparent that the attachment perspective is creating the beginnings of what may be called a revolution in the way couple problems are conceptualized and couple interventions are implemented (Johnson, 2013).

This revolution is exemplified in EFT—a model that now, more than any other approach, exemplifies the ideal in terms of empirical validation as laid out by the American Psychological Association (Sexton et al., 2011), in terms of numerous studies on outcome and the process of change, positive follow-up studies, generalization studies with different populations such as trauma survivors, and studies of the process of learning this model (Lebow, Chambers, Christensen, & Johnson, 2012). It is apparent that attachment theory and science are clarifying the core problem to be addressed in relationship distress, and offer, for the first time, clearly defined criteria for successful treatment and relationship health.

A New Direction: A Secure Base for the Practice of Couple Therapy

First, the essence of any short-term psychotherapy is to find a pertinent focus for intervention. Attachment offers clinicians a clearly detailed map to the emotional territory of a love relationship. It provides an explanatory framework that elucidates the strong emotions and motivations organizing a partner's responses in love relationships, and that explains the powerful impact one partner has on another. As a therapist watches members of a couple move in ubiquitous negative patterns, such as blame/demand followed by defend/withdraw, there are many problematic elements to focus on and many ways to understand what he or she sees. Attachment leads the therapist past individually focused explanations ("She has a personality disorder"), skill deficit issues ("He needs assertiveness training"), content issues ("They need help negotiating their differing parenting styles"), one-dimensional frames ("He needs to learn to reappraise her 'nagging' as concern"), and mythological explanations ("They are not soul mates, so they should separate"). The clear lens of attachment gives precedence to the need for a felt sense of connection with another, and frames emotional isolation in terms of deprivation and starvation; it allows the therapist to see negative responses as desperate attempts to connect with a partner or to stave off the threat of imminent rejection and abandonment. The problem, in attachment terms, is essentially a pervading sense of emotional disconnection and ineffective attempts to remedy this. The central questions in a distressed relationship, often never explicitly stated, are "Are you there for me; am I important to you; and will you come when I call?" Relationship conflict is then seen as separation distress that is continually perpetuated by the negative ways in which a couple deals with attachment signals. As Bowlby himself suggested, through the lens of attachment every apparently dysfunctional response to a partner makes sense, and so the multilevel, often confusing drama of distress is laid bare and becomes amenable to intervention. Partners criticize to evoke responses from each other, but end up pushing each other away; or they shut down and withdraw to avoid rejection, and end up shutting each other out and elicit fears of abandonment. Attachment theory allows therapist to grasp the essential nature of relationship distress on both individual and interactional levels in a manner that clients find salient and compelling and creates a path for the curtailment of negative cycles of interaction and the creation of positive bonding interactions.

The attachment perspective also offers a coherent picture of a healthy, stable relationship that provides a direction for therapy and keeps the therapist on track in the process of change. EFT is conducted in three stages. Stage 1, *deescalation*, involves offering the members of a couple a new understanding of how they influence each other and what they need from each other; the therapist helps them to identify negative patterns of interaction that constantly elicit disconnection, distance, and despair. Once partners can help each other out of such cycles, the relationship becomes a secure base from which to explore the path to deeper connection and Stage 2, *restructuring the bond*. Here partners are guided into a process of becoming more open and responsive to each other, to the point where they can ask for comfort in regard to their attachment fears and clearly state their attachment needs in a manner that invites responsiveness. Stage 3, the last stage, is *consolidation*, where the partners form a coherent narrative of how they changed their relationship and how they can continue to enhance their bond. Process studies of key attachment interactions in Stage 2 inform therapists of the shifts in emotional processing and interactional responses that are necessary and sufficient to create lasting change. The goal in EFT is not simply to lessen negativity and offer a couple some new resources. It is specifically to shape the emotional synchrony typical of positive bonded relationships in the session, and to offer the couple a corrective emotional experience of secure connection. Clarity as to the nature of love and bonding allows for the identification of pivotal moments in therapy—moments where focused, systematic intervention can help partners create not just a more generally positive dance, but one that will answer their primary needs for connection and care, as well as building ongoing commitment and satisfaction.

It is also important to note that this goal, which is admittedly more ambitious than interventions aimed at simply reducing relationship hostility and distress, makes relationship interventions supremely relevant to the welfare of individual partners and so extends the scope of couple therapy as a modality. It is pertinent to consider just a few of the benefits that are associated with more secure attachment. These include being able to retain emotional balance in the fact of stress and threat, rather than becoming flooded with anxiety or anger; tune into one's own emotions and so identify needs; offer consonant, coherent messages to others about fears and needs that evoke responsiveness; trustingly take in care and return to physiological homeostasis; tolerate ambiguous or negative responses from another with less defensiveness and reactivity; turn into the world with the confidence to explore and learn; and respond to another with empathy and sensitive care in a way that constantly renews bonds (Johnson, 2011). A basic tenet of attachment theory is that secure bonds make people stronger and more able to adapt to difficult circumstances. The possibility then arises that couple therapy becomes a potent arena for the growth of more functional individuals that can continue to grow and also to support each other over a lifetime of transitions, uncertainties, and dangers. More secure attachments also have great healing power and can be mobilized in an attachment-oriented therapy as part of any integrated treatment to move individuals from dysfunctional states into improved mental health. EFT has been shown to be easily adapted to couples facing problems such as depression and posttraumatic stress disorder, and to have a positive impact on individual symptomatology (Dalton, Greenman, Classen, & Johnson, 2013; Denton, Wittenborn, & Golden, 2012; MacIntosh & Johnson, 2008).

Attachment-Oriented Innovations in Couple Therapy

There are many ways that an EFT session, guided by attachment theory, differs from other models and from standard practice in the field. First, while many models speak of building a collaborative alliance with clients, in EFT there is a particular emphasis on the therapist's being emotionally present, responsive, and transparent with clients, much as a good attachment figure would be. The most seminal figures in the development of EFT, Carl Rogers (1961) and John Bowlby (1969/1982), both believed in clients' innate desire to grow toward health and advocated empathic responsiveness, and in accepting the validity of clients' present responses and formulations of their reality. A safe environment with an explicitly supportive therapist, then, fosters the exploration of this reality. An EFT therapist will begin by validating a client's anger and placing it in an attachment frame of desperation triggered by perceived abandonment, rather than by pointing out how anger can be dysfunctional and offering corrective directives. The therapist assumes that it is necessary to provide a secure base if new risks are to be taken and difficult emotions explored. In EFT research (Johnson & Talitman, 1997), the quality of the alliance has been found to account for 20% of the variance in therapy outcome. This appears to be a reflection not only of the bond between therapist and clients and agreement about goals, but particularly the perceived relevance of the tasks (such as sharing softer emotions and needs with a partner) structured by the therapist. This speaks to clients' perceptions of the exquisite relevance of the attachment frame, which literally "makes sense" of their struggle and fosters engagement in the therapy process. Attachment offers a unique and very specific version of the therapeutic alliance to the field of psychotherapy.

Second, an attachment framework gives precedence to emotion, offers a map to the emotional territory of love relationships, and also systematically depathologizes attachment anxieties and longings. These three elements, we suggest, all offer new directions to the field. Bowlby always made it very clear that emotion is the core aspect of attachment relationships; however, many models of couple therapy, viewing emotion as the problem, have simply dismissed or, at best, simply labeled and then bypassed it. This is understandable when a therapist has no clear, logical map of the extreme emotions that accompany love relationships. Attachment theory, however, offers such a map. An EFT session resounds with the six basic universal emotions identified by Ekman (2003): anger, which in the case of couple therapy is reactive anger at the partners' perceived unresponsiveness (Bowlby, 1973, called this the anger of despair rather than the anger of hope); surprise and joy, as when a partner responds to an attachment call; sadness, at a partner's pain or for one's own loneliness; shame, when models of self as unworthy and unlovable come to the fore; and fear, which in couple therapy is the fear of abandonment and rejection. Panksepp (2003) refers to this fear as a "primal panic" that arises when contact with a muchneeded loved one is lost and the brain registers this loss as a danger cue. Such a formulation fits with recent findings from brain scan studies that social pain such as rejection is processed in the same part of the brain and in the same way as physical pain (Eisenberger, Lieberman, Matthew, & Williams, 2003), the ultimate danger signal. The attachment perspective outlines key aspects of emotion as it arises in therapy sessions—namely, the compelling need for felt connection with a dependable other that makes sense of intense emotional responses, the triggers for these emotions, the catastrophic meanings associated with them, and the ways they move partners in their interactional dance. Partners and therapists who have no grasp of this perspective often misinterpret or pathologize these emotions, viewing silent fear and shame as indifference, or desperate anger as mental illness or malice rather than an attempt to coerce an unresponsive attachment figure into engagement and responsiveness. The EFT therapist, however, can make coherent sense of, validate, and so help clients effectively regulate such emotions, moving them from numbing out and avoidance or the hyperarousal of attachment anxiety into more emotional balance and more flexible responsiveness. From an attachment perspective, the pathologizing of dependence needs, longings, and anxieties is a significant issue in the field of mental health and in the couple therapy modality in particular, where concepts such as enmeshment and lack of differentiation or individuation are very often offered as explanations for relationship problems (Johnson, 2008b). To change these kinds of conceptualizations into one that values effective dependence, where close connection supports a positive, coherent, and autonomous sense of self, is indeed to take the field in a new direction.

Third, attachment offers the couple therapy field clarity about what is necessary and sufficient to create a corrective emotional experience of connection that is able to redefine a relationship as a stable and satisfying bond. Recent studies (described later in this chapter) have shown that EFT increases attachment security, and that this increase in security is associated with specific processes and events in Stage 2 of EFT (Burgess Moser et al., in press; Burgess Moser, Johnson, Dalgleish, Tasca, & Wiebe, 2014). These results are similar to those from other studies of the process of change in EFT (Dalgleish, Johnson, Burgess Moser, Wiebe, & Tasca, 2014; Greenman & Johnson, 2013), which found that events where the more hostile partner "softened" and asked for needs to be met in a vulnerable fashion, so that partners became mutually accessible and responsive to each other's attachment needs and fears, were associated with positive changes in satisfaction and significant increases in variables such as trust and intimacy. This research also outlines the specific therapist interventions that appear to set up these pivotal moments of change. It is still a relatively rare achievement in the field of psychotherapy to systematically document outcomes, to be able to specify how change occurs, to show that this process is consonant with the theoretical formulations of the model of intervention, and to link moments of change to specific interventions by the therapist. The possibilities for the refinement of intervention, consistently effective practice, and therapist training are clear. We believe the fact that this has been achieved in EFT research and practice speaks to the salience of attachment theory.

Clinical studies on violations of connection or attachment injuries again illustrate the power of attachment—first, to define and clarify clinical issues and impasses so that focused targeted intervention is possible; and second, to provide a compass in the change process to the point that pivotal moments and conditions of change can be specified. The study of injurious events in couple relationships began with the recognition that some partners could not and would not take the risk of opening up and reaching for their lovers to ask for attachment needs to be met, even if these partners became explicitly more accessible. The observation of this impasse as it occurred in video recordings of Stage 2 of EFT led to the formulation of these events as relationship traumas where partners had violated the expectations of an attachment relationship, abandoning or betraying the injured and now untrusting partners at key moments of vulnerability. At times these events may have seemed small or obscure until their attachment meaning and specific emotional significance became clear. Once these ideas were clearly formulated, it was possible to build a model to resolve these injuries and to test its effectiveness (Makinen & Johnson, 2006), and then to examine the process of change and therapist interventions that fostered forgiveness and reconciliation (Zuccarini, Johnson, Dalgleish, & Makinen, 2013). The kinds of injuries studied arouse from key moments of disconnection associated with affairs, health crises, miscarriages, deaths of parents or friends, or significant career losses. These injuries were then exacerbated over time by the couples' inability to discuss and resolve them, and the injuring partners' continued lack of responsiveness in regard to these events.

In the recent study of the process of resolution referred to above, when couples who successfully resolved their injuries were compared to couples who were unable to obtain resolution, members of resolved couples were found to have engaged more deeply in their emotional experiences in key sessions of therapy, to have been more deliberate and reflective in their processing of these experiences, and to have risked more affiliative behaviors when asked by the therapist to communicate directly to each other. Process measures were also used to identify the key steps of resolution and forgiveness as outlined in EFT and to validate that successful couples indeed completed the steps outlined by the theoretical model. At key steps, the therapists of couples who resolved their injury used more reflections of primary emotions, asked more evocative questions to unpack emotions, and heightened emotional experience more often. These therapists also set up powerful enactments focused on attachment-related emotions and needs, and guided partners into increased engagement and responsiveness. This kind of clinical practice and research, guided by the wisdom of adult attachment theory, offers a systematic clinical blueprint that can be used to resolve key impasses in couple therapy and open the door—even for very wounded partners—to renewed relationship satisfaction and connection. Although changes in attachment security were not systematically measured in this study, by the end of therapy resolved couples demonstrated the cognitive flexibility, greater empathy, and trust that are associated with more secure attachment. Resolved, forgiving couples also showed more affiliative responses on the Structural Analysis of Social Behavior (Benjamin, 1981). Such responses have been found to be associated with greater attachment security (Neumann & Tress, 2007).

It is interesting to note that as clinical studies using attachment theory and relationship-oriented neuroscience become more integrated, cross-fertilization is possible. Attachment studies may be able to contribute to ongoing work on understanding and identifying emotions. For example, longing is not identified as one of the basic emotions; however, metaphors such "emotional starvation" and "hunger" are part of the attachment perspective and constantly arise in the practice of EFT. Clinical studies may also be able to expand traditional formulations of attachment theory—for example, by encouraging more emphasis on the emotion regulation aspects of attachment and the consequences of habitual emotion dysregulation, rather than focusing exclusively on cognitive working models as the basic mechanism of long-term stability in attachment patterns. Recent studies on the emotional suppression typical of an avoidant attachment style, for example, suggest that the physiological effort involved in such suppression results in more tension and arousal, which can lead to flooding and sudden rage, and also increases the tension experienced by interactional partners (Gross, 2001). This kind of research allows attachment clinicians and theorists to formulate specific ways in which insecure attachment styles become perpetuated in new relationships.

A recent example of the kind of fertile integration referred to above is the inclusion of a brain scan study (Johnson et al., 2013) as part of a clinical trial focused on demonstrating that EFT is able to increase secure attachment (Burgess Moser et al., in press). Before and after receiving EFT with their partners, insecure and relationally distressed women were placed one by one in a functional magnetic resonance imaging (fMRI) scanner and shown a signal that they knew 20% of the time would result in their receiving an electric shock on their ankles. A woman was shown this signal either while alone in the scanner, with a stranger holding her hand, and with her partner holding her hand. Both before and after EFT, lying alone in the fMRI machine resulted in extreme brain activation when the signal was received, and in reports of significant pain due to the shock. In both pre- and post-EFT conditions, contact with a stranger seemed to reduce brain activation and reported pain. Before EFT, contact with the partner was less effective in reducing activation and pain than was holding the stranger's hand; however, after EFT, this partner contact was associated with a large reduction in brain activation when the threat signal was received, as well as a significant reduction in reported pain. It is also interesting to note that this lack of activation after EFT was observed in the prefrontal cortex (the seat of emotional control), not simply in areas associated with emotional arousal such as the amygdala. This study offers new levels of evidence for one of the most basic tenets of attachment theory—that contact with a loved one who is judged to be dependable and responsive results in more physiological equilibrium in the face of threat, as well as lessened sensitivity or reactivity to pain. Perhaps even more interesting, these results imply that contact comfort influences the perception and encoding of threat itself, rather than simply increasing coping efforts and activity. As Bowlby suggested, it seems that safe connection with a loved one makes the world safer.

The Stability of Attachment: Does EFT Change Attachment Orientations?

Attachment theory posits that accessibility and responsiveness are the building blocks of secure attachment bonds between partners (Bowlby, 1969/1982). The goal of EFT is to create more secure bonding events in therapy sessions by exploring and expressing partners' emotional needs and fears, and by shaping increased emotional accessibility and responsiveness between partners. The question of whether these events indeed revise and modify working models of attachment and long-term emotional regulation strategies has only recently been directly addressed and is discussed below.

This section briefly explores the stability of attachment, change in attachment orientations in the context of psychotherapy, and the specific changes that occur in attachment orientations over the course of EFT. We present findings from two recent studies in our EFT Research Lab (Burgess Moser et al., 2014, in press), which support the notion that EFT is targeting and changing attachment orientations. As EFT researchers and therapists, we see change in attachment orientations as occurring through several pathways: new ways of regulating attachment longings and fears; the shaping of new behaviors, especially in ways of asking for attachment needs to be met; the priming of revised representational models of the present partner; and the delineation of expanded models of self as vulnerable but effective and competent in shaping interactions with loved ones.

Many researchers and theoreticians in the field of attachment theory have testified to the stability of attachment orientations. They suggest that models of attachment formed in childhood display stability throughout adulthood, acting as constant prototypes guiding interpersonal functioning (Fraley, 2002; Fraley, Vicary, Brumbaugh, & Roisman, 2011). They also point out that this is consistent with Bowlby's (1969/1982) early hypothesis that internal working models of attachment contain key information about the self, others, and relationships—information that influences perceptions and expectations, and so guides interpersonal functioning throughout the lifespan. However, others have focused more on the view that childhood attachment patterns can change and can be modified in adulthood by new kinds of interactions with loved ones. Indeed, Bowlby (1969/1982) suggests that to be optimally functional, internal working models must assimilate new information and be amenable to revision. He states (1969, p. 82), "To be useful . . . attachment models must be kept up to date."

Research demonstrates that attachment patterns do in fact change across the lifespan, and that attachment orientations may differ across relationships (Baldwin, Keelan, Fehr, Enns, & Koh-Rangarajoo, 1996; Davila & Cobb, 2004; Caron, Lafontaine, Bureau, Levesque, & Johnson, 2012; Davila, Karney, & Bradbury, 1999). Changes in attachment orientations may be results of situational events and changes in life stress, modifications of relationship status (e.g., entering marriage or parenthood), personality variables, or a combination of these factors (Crowell, Treboux, & Waters, 2002; Davila et al., 1999; Simpson, Rholes, Campbell, & Wilson, 2003). Kirkpatrick and Hazan (1994) found that attachment orientations changed in 30% of individuals over a 4-year period. Although Crowell, Treboux, and Waters (2002) found 78% of spouses to be unchanged in their attachment orientation categories from 3 months before marriage to 18 months after marriage, some spouses did experience changes in their attachment orientations. It is generally presumed that changes to working models begin with new experiences in specific relationships that shift perceptions, biases, and expectations. These shifts then generalize and modify more general relational models. Researchers also suggest that the stability of attachment orientations is dependent on the type of attachment a person possesses. Individuals with higher levels of attachment anxiety are more likely to experience changes in security levels than those with secure and avoidant attachment orientations are (Davila & Cobb, 2003, 2004). It makes sense that once a secure representation is created within a relationship, it tends to be more resistant to distortion when hurtful incidents and relationship difficulties occur, and so to become self-perpetuating—and also that partners with avoidant attachment orientations tend to be less open to new experiences and information, and so less likely to revise their working models.

For the clinician, the key question is whether therapeutic intervention can prime the revision of working models and shape new interpersonal responses. The therapeutic relationship can potentially provide new, emotionally laden experiences of connection that contribute to positive changes in attachment orientation (Bowlby, 1969/1982). The impact of individual and group psychotherapy on attachment orientations indicates that insecurity is amenable to change. In individual psychotherapy, some research suggests that 20–40% of clients move from insecure to more secure attachment after participating in time-limited psychotherapy (Travis, Binder, Bliwise, & Horne-Moyer, 2001) and longer-term psychodynamic therapy (Diamond, Stovall-McCloush, Clarkin, & Levy, 2003; Fonagy et al., 1995). Similar results have been found in group psychotherapy, where attachment anxiety decreases for women with binge-eating disorder who participated in either a cognitive-behavioral or an interpersonal psychodynamic group (Tasca, Balfour, Ritchie, & Bissada, 2007). These results suggest that therapeutic relationships may help clients to move toward attachment security over time. Therapists can act to facilitate clients' formulation and expression of attachment needs, as well as to respond in a manner that disconfirms the expectations created by previous absent or nonresponsive caregivers.

Although positive changes in attachment security have been demonstrated in individual psychotherapy, little to no research has examined changes in attachment security in couple therapy, even though this is the modality where working models may be most accessible and patterns of attachment responses most salient and open to potential modification.

As previously discussed, EFT systematically modifies negative patterns of disconnection and nonresponsiveness, and shapes the elements of more secure interactional cycles and deeper levels of engagement where partners identify and express their attachment longings and needs. Detailed clinical observation over many years has shown that new patterns of mutual accessibility and responsiveness then restructure habitual attachment-oriented interactions and relationship-specific models of attachment. Recently, our research team at the University of Ottawa and the International Centre for Excellence in Emotionally Focused Therapy (ICEEFT; *www.iceeft.com*) more rigorously examined changes in attachment strategies and models over the course of EFT (Burgess Moser et al., 2014, in press).

We recruited 32 moderately distressed and insecurely attached couples. Partners were asked to respond to the relationship-specific version of the Experiences in Close Relationships (ECR) scale (Brennan, Clark, & Shaver, 1998; Mikulincer & Shaver, 2007), and to engage in a conflict resolution task that allowed us to observe and code the manner in which partners tended to seek and provide attachment-based support (the Secure Base Scoring System, or SBSS; Crowell, Treboux, Gao, et al., 2002). Fourteen therapists, each of whom had over 5 years of EFT training, then provided couples with approximately 21 sessions of EFT. Couples also completed the Dyadic Adjustment Scale (DAS; Spanier, 1976) and the ECR—Short Form (ECR-S; Wei, Russell, Mallinckrodt, & Vogel, 2007) after every therapy session. We implemented hierarchical linear modeling (HLM; Singer & Willett, 2003) to examine session-by-session changes in relationship satisfaction and attachment security over the course of therapy.

On the observational measure of attachment (i.e., the SBSS), we found that couples significantly increased their secure base use and secure base provision from pre- to posttherapy (Burgess Moser et al., in press). According to the SBSS (Crowell, Treboux, Gao, et al., 2002), attachment security is defined as the ability to clearly identify and express attachment needs, while also being able to identify and respond to a partner's cries for support and connection. The results of our study suggest that over the course of EFT, members of couples learn to access the attachment longings and needs underlying their negative interaction cycles, and to express these to their partners in a manner that is more open and affiliative. The more congruent expression of these needs then elicits increased responsiveness from the partners. EFT focuses not only on helping members access their own needs, but on guiding them to respond to their partners' calls for care and support in an effective manner. Bowlby (1969/1982) proposed that in addition to preexisting individual attachment orientations, the habitual interaction patterns that develop between adult partners are key in the development and maintenance of attachment security. Both partners need to be able to express their needs clearly and from a place of emotional vulnerability, while at the same time responding to each other to be able to create a secure bond. These results support the notion that EFT is creating unconscious changes in attachment security that show up in explicit responses in seeking and providing support in love relationships.

Our team also examined changes in self-reported attachment security over the course of EFT, using the relationship-specific version of the ECR (administered pre- and posttherapy) and the ECR-S (administered after each therapy session). First, we found that as partners' relationship-specific attachment anxiety and attachment avoidance decreased, relationship satisfaction increased (Burgess Moser et al., in press). This is consonant with the theoretical underpinnings of EFT, suggesting that attachment theory is on target in terms of guiding therapists' interventions that are effective in improving relationship satisfaction. On the ECR-S, we found that reported attachment avoidance significantly decreased over the course of EFT. This suggests that the interventions in EFT are specifically helping avoidant partners to develop more adaptive models and perspectives when interacting with their loved ones. Instead of using deactivation strategies (such as viewing their partners as dangerous and preferring to shut down attachment needs), these individuals are learning to view connection with their partners as a resource, and they begin to depend on them and be more open to sharing fears and needs with their significant others. These results highlight the importance of therapists' helping individuals with higher levels of attachment avoidance (typical of more withdrawn partners) at the start of therapy to turn to their partner rather than inward, and so to develop more adaptive coping mechanisms. These results are contrary to previous research, which suggests that individuals with avoidant attachment may be more difficult to engage in therapy as a result of their deactivating coping strategies (Meyer, Pilkonis, Proietti, Heape, & Egan, 2001; Horowitz, Rosenberg, & Bartholomew, 1993). Rather, EFT and therapists' use of key interventions seem to help such partners modify their internal working models, which paint others as unsafe and minimize attachment needs. Based on these results, therapists should take pains to ensure that withdrawn clients are engaged at the beginning of therapy and are given help to begin to be open to new perceptions of and revised behaviors from their partners.

When we looked at attachment anxiety over the course of EFT, our study at first found no significant change for partners (Burgess Moser et al., in press). However, in a second study, Burgess Moser et al., 2014 demonstrated that significant changes in attachment anxiety did indeed occur by the end of therapy for a subset of partners (16 out of 32)—namely, those who were able to explicitly engage in a key change event in EFT, the *blamer-softening event*. The blamer-softening event occurs when a previously hostile/critical partner is able to openly ask for his or her attachment needs to be met from a position of soft vulnerability and a high level of emotional engagement (Johnson, 2004; Johnson & Best, 2002). A partner expressing needs in this manner pulls the previously withdrawn partner toward him or her, engages this partner in the process, and enables the partner to hear and respond to these needs. The blamer-softening event is a corrective emotional experience in which a new level of felt security is experienced with the partner. Since the withdrawer is helped to reengage before the blamer is asked to take a risk by openly asking for attachment needs to be met, both partners are responsive once the blamer-softening event occurs, and are able to risk, reach, and share attachment vulnerabilities and needs.

The task was now to reach a further understanding of how attachment orientations shift as a result of this key change event (Burgess Moser et al., 2014), which has been consistently linked to changes in relationship satisfaction and other positive outcomes at the end of EFT and at follow-up (Johnson & Greenberg, 1988; Dalgleish et al., 2014). A deeper understanding of this shift and its impact will enable therapists to guide partners confidently as they regulate difficult and unfamiliar affect, mine their emotional vulnerability, and take risks with their loved ones. Interestingly, we found that couples who were able to complete a softening (as coded from the audio-recorded interactions in session) also reported a significant increase in relationship satisfaction and a decrease in attachment avoidance at the end of the softening session. Although these couples reported an initial increase in relationship-specific attachment anxiety in the softening session, this was followed by a significant decrease in attachment anxiety in the sessions that followed. It seems that anxiously attached partners have pressing and urgent fears about whether they matter to their loved ones; they are preoccupied with the fear of abandonment and of being unloved (Collins & Read, 1990; Davila & Kashy, 2009). For these individuals, the anger/protest in the negative interactional cycle of relationship distress arises as a result of not being able to seek comfort or have their normal needs for contact and intimacy met by their partners (Johnson, 2004). The softening event appears to disconfirm their belief that their partners will abandon them, and provides them with an experience of soothing responsiveness that directly leads to decreased attachment anxiety. Therapy modalities that emphasize and elaborate the importance of close relationships with significant others and emotions may fit particularly well with highly anxious individuals (Daniels, 2006). EFT interventions are designed to be soothing and provide an alternative to these partners' usual hyperactivating relationship strategies. In EFT, partners are constantly exploring, accessing, and reprocessing emotions such as reactive anger, sadness, loss, shame, and fears of rejection and abandonment, and formulating their attachment longings with their partners. Throughout EFT, these partners develop more emotional balance. They find more positive, less angry, and less controlling ways of expressing their emotions and needs and of inviting their partners to engage with them. In a softening event, a previously withdrawn partner's new accessibility and responsiveness are carefully made explicit by the EFT therapist, and this actively challenges the more anxiously attached partner's cognitive belief that he or she will be abandoned and is essentially defective and therefore unlovable. This belief is a key element of the negative model of self in anxious attachment (Mikulincer & Shaver, 2007). The more anxious partner's awareness of vulnerability and the emotional risk associated with reaching for a partner in a softening event (Johnson, 2004) seems to explain the temporary increase in attachment anxiety reported by such a partner in this specific session.

The results of these two key studies from our lab support the notion that key events and interventions in the process of change in EFT are effective in facilitating changes in relationship-specific attachment security and relationship satisfaction. It is crucial for therapists to understand the process of change, so that they are able to select their interventions appropriately for the many couples dealing with significant issues of insecure attachment and chronic emotional disconnection, and to focus on the completion of successful softening events where both partners are open, engaged, and responsive. Understanding the probability that attachment anxiety will peak in a softening session should help therapists normalize, validate, and soothe this anxiety. In contrast to the effects on attachment anxiety, partners' attachment avoidance slowly decreases in every session over the entire course of EFT. This result emphasizes the importance of constantly supporting the more withdrawn member of a couple to slowly but surely become more actively engaged in the therapeutic process, and to gradually learn to express emotions to the partner. A therapist should also ensure that the avoidant, withdrawn partner is able to hear that his or her lack of emotional presence is a trigger for the other partner to experience panic and rejection, and that this other indeed truly values and desires the avoidant partner's love and care.

These findings support the idea that the softening event acts as a classic corrective emotional experience, as described in the general psychotherapy literature (Johnson & Best, 2002). This corrective experience demonstrates the powerful impact of sharing fears and vulnerabilities in an emotionally expressive and affiliative manner that elicits attuned caregiving rather than avoidance or rejection. The softening event is, then, a pivotal moment of intrapsychic and interpersonal change that therapists must actively shape in order to create changes in relationship-specific attachment orientations and relationship satisfaction. Preliminary follow-up analyses suggest that the changes discussed here, as found in other EFT follow-up studies, remain stable across time. Once partners have found the path to a deeply satisfying felt sense of security, they are likely to seek and find this path again and again. Thus attachment is amenable to change—to the integration of new experiences, and to revised internal working models of self and other—throughout EFT in general and through the blamer-softening event in particular.

Attachment, Caregiving, and Sex

This section addresses the impact that strengthening attachment can have on other key aspects of a bonding relationship. Attachment theory, as extended to include romantic attachments in adulthood (Mikulincer & Shaver, 2007; Shaver, Hazan, & Bradshaw, 1988), suggests that three independent, interconnected, innate behavioral systems are necessary in order to establish optimal functioning in romantic relationships: the attachment, caregiving, and sexual systems. Each of these three systems is influenced by the others, and together they encompass the behavioral responses that have generally promoted the survival, adaptation, and reproduction of humanity in the context of social relationships. The attachment system is focused on the provision of comfort and security in times of hardship. According to the theory, the caregiving system is considered complementary to the attachment system and is expressed by humans in order to ensure the safety and longevity of those they depend upon. In a romantic relationship, the activation of one partner's attachment system (by a threat to well-being or perceived security) triggers the activation of the other partner's caregiving system, and this partner attempts to alleviate the loved one's distress and restore a sense of safety (Collins, Guichard, Ford, & Feeney, 2006). Within a secure couple relationship, loved ones weave between expressing the need for security and comfort, and providing such care to their partners (Schachner, Shaver, & Mikulincer, 2003). The sexual system includes individuals' emotions, motives for engaging in sexual interactions, and sexual behaviors (Birnbaum, 2010; Mikulincer, 2006). A person's attachment and caregiving experiences have an impact on sexuality that is likely to develop in early adolescence. The sexual system is of substantial importance to both the development and maintenance of most couple relationships, as it promotes feelings of attraction and provides early bonding experiences; in addition to enhancing long-term relationship quality (Birnbaum, 2010, Davis, Shaver, & Vernon, 2004; Schachner & Shaver, 2004).

Empirical evidence of the links between the attachment and caregiving systems indicates that more anxious individuals report being less able to recognize and interpret their partners' needs, more willingness to provide needed care, and use of more controlling and compulsive caregiving strategies. Their responses tend to be less contingent and thus less effective. Avoidantly attached individuals report being less able to recognize and interpret their partners' needs, less willingness to answer to their partners' signals of need, and a greater tendency to be domineering when trying to help their partners. Individuals with such attachment patterns tend to become distant and dismissing of both their own and others' needs for care and security. These findings have been found across numerous populations, including dating couples (Feeney & Collins, 2001), couples in long-term relationships (Feeney, 1996; Millings & Walsh, 2009), and adults involved in same-sex couple relationships (Bouaziz, Lafontaine, Gabbay, & Caron, 2013). Similarly, research has revealed that subliminal priming procedures aimed at experimentally enhancing individuals' sense of security effectively elicit compassionate and supportive behavior (Mikulincer et al., 2001; Mikulincer, Shaver, Gillath, & Nitzberg, 2005).

The association between attachment and sexuality has also become better and better substantiated (for reviews, see Dewitte, 2012; Mikulincer & Shaver, 2007; Stefanou & McCabe, 2012). For example, security shapes the experience of positive emotions in sexual relationships, and it increases the capacity to let go and enjoy sex for itself (Birnbaum, Reis, Mikulincer, Gillath, & Orpaz, 2006; Shaver & Mikulincer, 2006). Casual, detached sex and low levels of intimacy; avoidance of sexual interactions; and engaging in fewer sexual fantasies about the partner are more predominant in avoidant people (Birnbaum et al., 2006; Brassard, Shaver, & Lussier, 2007). However, the importance of the partner's emotional involvement during sex, and sex motivated by the fear of losing a partner, is more associated with attachment anxiety (Tracy, Shaver, Albino, & Cooper, 2003). Anxious and avoidant individuals both report lower sexual satisfaction, and these attachment insecurities in women are related to lower sexual self-esteem and higher sexual anxiety (Birnbaum, 2007; Brassard, Péloquin, Dupuy, Wright, & Shaver, 2012; Brassard, Dupuy, Bergeron, & Shaver, 2014). All in all, a secure, connected relationship appears to be the best recipe for sexual fulfillment (Johnson & Zuccarini, 2010).

Only a few studies have directly examined the relations among attachment, caregiving, and sexual functioning (Péloquin, Brassard, Delisle, & Bédard, 2013; Péloquin, Brassard, Lafontaine, & Shaver, 2014). Results show that caregiving, mostly in the form of proximity and sensitivity, mediates the association between attachment insecurities and lower sexual satisfaction in both distressed and nondistressed romantic partners. In short, there is no doubt that there are theoretical and empirical links among the attachment, caregiving, and sexual systems. We also know that unhappy couples report to their couple therapists issues related to these three systems, thus indicating a real therapeutic need to promote attachment security and the integration of attachment, caregiving, and sexual responses by using an influential theory of adult love—namely, attachment theory. The integration of caregiving, sexuality, and attachment has to start with the attachment system and the creation of safe emotional connection, as privileged within EFT.

How does attachment affect caregiving? According to Bowlby (1969/1982), a primed attachment system is likely to inhibit effective caregiving. Under these conditions, a romantic partner will be focused on restoring his or her own sense of security, before attending to the other partner's need for comfort. In particular, partners with higher levels of attachment avoidance appear to express less empathy, reciprocate less supportive actions, and are less apt to consider others as deserving of their care, in comparison to individuals embodying other attachment patterns. Partners with higher levels of attachment anxiety may have difficulty responding to the needs of their loved ones, as their cognitive resources tend to be exhausted on their preoccupation with their own distress and attachment-related needs. In opposition, partners with secure attachment are not worried with regulating anxiety and doubts about self-worth, and they have more attention and resources to offer their partners. Securely attached individuals also perceive their partners to be available in times of need or distress, and in turn may be more likely to consider their partners as meriting compassion and help when needed (Mikulincer & Shaver, 2007). In this vein, it is only when a sense of security is established or restored within a romantic relationship that the caregiving system may be effectively activated in response to a partner's distress (Mikulincer & Shaver, 2005).

As mentioned earlier, results from clinical studies support the notion that EFT provokes changes toward attachment security in partners' views of themselves and others. These major changes will then be noticeable in terms of seeking connection and in terms of sensitive caregiving and contingent responsive behaviors in their relationships. In Stage 1 of EFT, where members of a couple are guided to reframe their problems in the terms of how they are stuck in cycles of distance that spark emotional starvation, separation distress, and deprivation around attachment needs, this meta-perspective "sets the table" for becoming more attuned and supportive of each other. For instance, Carol states in session, "I never realized that he was lonely too and felt rejected. I guess I have complained and blamed a lot. I feel more generous now, more caring toward him. He needs positive messages from me. We are not so different after all." In Stage 2 of EFT, the therapist helps the withdrawn partner to reengage in the relationship and to assertively state the conditions of this deeper engagement. The therapist will also encourage the critical partner to take a more vulnerable position that facilitates attempts to have the other partner respond to his or her attachment needs. By the end of Stage 2 of EFT, each partner is more able to trust and find comfort with the loved one, who is now more accessible, attentive, and supportive. For example, Ted, Carol's partner, is able to tell her, "I want some acceptance from you. I want you to support me when I am stressed and not assume I am going to let you down. I need caring too. Then I can let you in." Later, Carol can softly ask Ted, "When I get all lonely, I need you to be there. I don't need advice. I need you to take me in your arms and really comfort me." In Stage 3 of EFT, consolidation, partners can actively empathize with each other and develop new solutions to old problems that take each person's needs for closeness, security, and caring into account. These problems are no longer tainted with overwhelming negative emotions and active triggers for rejection and abandonment; they can be solved cooperatively.

In regard to sexuality, Heiman (2007) declared that unmet attachment needs will lead to undermined sexual arousal, because sexuality involves the exploration of the body and mind in both partners. Although Heiman (2007) specifically discussed arousal, this declaration is also relevant to the other dimensions of sexual functioning: desire, orgasm, and satisfaction. Therefore, secure attachment characterized by attunement and responsiveness to emotional and physiological cues provides a foundation for partners' experience of satisfying sex, which may in turn influence a sense of felt security. Sex can represent intimate play and a safe adventure in the context of a relationship where partners are emotionally accessible, responsive, and engaged (Johnson, 2008a, 2008b). This may be particularly true for women, due to the highly contextual nature of their desire (Basson, 2007). The view of optimal sexual satisfaction is often that of a relationship filled with passion, novelty, and a certain level of danger and thrill—a notion that is present in the dominant culture of romance. This is contradictory to the view of a secure, familiar, and predictable relationship in which security promotes exploration and attunement to one another's needs in the moment (Johnson & Zuccarini, 2010). The solution to seemingly inevitable sexual boredom and dissatisfaction in long-term attachments seems, then, to focus on sexual technique or to somehow inject distance or attempts at sexual novelty into a relationship. Unfortunately, this goal is often not achieved, as it does not promote attunement to a partner or the ability to be completely present. Focused attention and full engagement in the moment, however, tend to intensify eroticism and can overrule technique issues (Kleinplatz, 2001).

In many distressed couples, partners are trapped in cycles of critical demanding and defensive withdrawal. These cycles have a negative impact on overall couple functioning, but also on sexual interactions. The more demanding partner (typically the female partner) is usually more anxiously attached, looking for support and affection in and out of the bedroom, while the more withdrawn partner (typically the male partner) may start sexual contact but avoid closeness and remain emotionally distant and unavailable (Johnson & Zuccarini, 2010). In this negative cycle marked by attachment insecurity, the demanding partner's attention is on affection and reassurance, whereas the more withdrawn partner focuses on sensation and performance, which leads to more anxiety and disconnection from the demanding partner. In this circumstance, the EFT therapist deescalates the negative cycle and promotes secure bonding interactions between the partners. More positive and integrated sexual experiences begin to stem from new levels of emotional safety and connection. For example, a withdrawn husband is able to disclose how he longs to feel desired by his partner, and how he ejaculates fast to avoid any signals of disappointment or rejection from his partner. He shares that he only asks for sex because he does not know how to initiate closeness in any other way. This disclosure allows his wife to perceive him in a new way and fosters reciprocal sharing about their sexual and emotional relationship.

Improving attachment security and relationship satisfaction leads to new avenues in a couple's sexual interaction. Understanding love as attachment gives a picture of optimal, healthy relatedness and sexuality. In a secure relationship, positive emotional experiences of joy and excitement, tender touch, and erotic playfulness can all come together (Johnson & Zuccarini, 2010). The first step for the EFT therapist is to increase emotional safety and secure connection between partners, regardless of whether their sex life plays a role in their relationship distress (Johnson & Zuccarini, 2010). In Stage 1 of EFT, the therapist will first explore the quality of the couple's physical relationship and integrate this information into the context of the negative interaction cycle. Here it is important for the EFT therapist to give an attachment frame to partners' sexual responses—for instance, by connecting the lack of satisfaction and difficulty having an orgasm to the lack of safety and fears of abandonment. If partners do not report any sexual difficulty, but sex has deteriorated as a result of the negative cycle, their sex life begins to improve at the end of Stage 1, when both partners can work together against the negative impact of their cycle both inside and outside the bedroom. In Stage 2, the EFT therapist helps the partners initiate positive cycles of emotional responsiveness, as they are able to risk, confide attachment needs and fears (i.e., physical closeness and sexuality), and reach for and respond to each other. In a case where sexuality is experienced as dangerous, partners will be invited to preclude having intercourse and focus on safe, pleasurable touch. In order to normalize sexual experiences, the EFT therapist may need to offer the couple some information, with the goal of supporting the transfer of safe emotional engagement and exploration into the sexual area. For example, a husband may be reassured to find out that orgasms vary in intensity and character, and that it's perfectly natural for him to feel different from time to time. Mutual accessibility and responsiveness between partners helps them to engage in a new kind of satisfying and connected sexual experience. In Stage 3 of EFT, the therapist helps partners to create a joint story of the repair of their relationship that includes the enhancement of their sexual bond. The therapist may also help partners solve concrete problems, such as modifying a lifestyle that excludes time for enjoyable and pleasurable sexual play. Satisfying sexual encounters now strengthen the couple's bond, and a more secure bond continues to build more erotic and more satisfying sex.

In sum, by creating changes in attachment security, EFT helps romantic partners alter the explicit ways in which they seek support and provide support and care, as well as their sexual connection. Couple therapists will find in EFT a powerful guide that can help partners integrate attachment, caregiving, and sex, in a way that leads to a powerful, resilient, and satisfying bond.

Case Example: A Clinical Snapshot of a Moment of Change[1]

Prue is sent to couple therapy by her individual therapist, who is concerned about her recent but unremitting depression and her hopelessness about her marriage to Larry. After 25 years of marriage and the successful launching of four children, she has lapsed into extreme silent withdrawal, and his temper tantrums and lists of "concerned" directives for his wife have escalated. She admits that she feels "flawed" and unable to please her husband, who is, she believes, more verbal, more active, more fit, and more competent than she is. Larry lectures and reasons in the first therapy sessions, pointing out that she became depressed 2 years before when she went away to care for a dying aunt, and she should simply exercise more and try harder to combat her negative thoughts. When asked by the therapist, Prue states that her depression began on a day exactly a year ago, after a strenuous hiking holiday where she had fallen and hurt her leg, much to Larry's chagrin. "In fact," she states, "it began with the train—at that train station." Larry sighs, raising his eyes in exasperation.

Prue had gone to get coffee and was standing with a coffee cup in her hand, holding her pull-along luggage, when Larry realized that the train was moving. Alarmed, he sprinted along the platform and leapt onto the train while shouting at the conductor to stop the train. He then turned and screamed at his wife, "Run!" Prue froze, disoriented. Finally, she did indeed run, and with great difficulty she managed to clamber onto the moving train. Larry then screamed at her, "Why are you so damned slow?" At this moment, their relationship plummeted into unremitting distress and despair. Larry believes that his wife will soon leave him or harm herself.

There are many different ways to see this pivotal incident and this couple's problems. The EFT therapist, using an attachment perspective, builds an alliance as a secure base. The therapist then delineates the interactional dance that has taken over their relationship as a "criticize-and-complain, followed by defend-and-withdraw" cycle that leaves them both isolated, helpless, and dejected. As these partners are encouraged to explore and deepen their emotions, unspoken attachment sensitivities and fears emerge. Prue admits that she has "given up" on being accepted by her husband, since she will never be active and fit enough to meet his expectations. She feels overwhelmed by sadness and shame. Larry does not understand this response or the impact he has on his wife. In the therapy session, the therapist slowly replays and reviews the train station incident as a microcosm of the attachment reality of Larry and Prue's relationship.

As the station incident is slowly reviewed, the therapist asks evocative questions, orders and reflects emotional responses and statements,

---

[1] The case and the incident described in this section were first outlined in modified form in Johnson (2013).

and conjectures as to the attachment meanings associated with different moments. Prue becomes able to explicitly formulate and express her sense of condemnation and rejection, and her acceptance of herself as inadequate. The therapist validates that at the moment, this is the only sense she can make out of Larry's "desperate" exhortations and arguments that her perceptions are mistaken and her emotions inappropriate. Prue starts at the word "desperate" and looks at her husband intently.

The therapist slowly unfolds the elements of Larry's emotional experience and places it in an attachment framework. With help, Larry recalls the triggering image of Prue's standing still as the distance between them grew second by second. He is encouraged to tune into his body, and he now identifies "panic" and "breathlessness" in his chest. As the therapist asks him what he sees as he recalls this event, he says, "She isn't coming. She isn't running. She isn't trying to reach me—to be with me. She won't try." The therapist comments, "And so you are . . . ?" Larry calls out, "All alone," and collapses in tears. He then begins to recognize the compelling fears that arise when his wife is physically or emotionally absent or shows any sign of weakness or illness. He usually dismisses such feelings as "pathetic and foolish," but he is now able to shape his experience into a coherent whole and tell his wife that she is the only one he has ever turned to or felt safe with. As Larry owns and communicates his separation distress and links it to his controlling behaviors, Prue expresses amazement. She articulates that she is now seeing him differently, and as she recounts the times when her strength and responsiveness helped him through difficulties and earned his trust and respect, she straightens up and becomes more engaged and less subdued. In the next session, Prue is now able to firmly express her sense of rejection at his criticism, but now frames these in terms of his fears and how much he needs her, rather than any inadequacy on her part. Her depression, which Bowlby identified as an inherent part of separation distress, begins to lift. In the following sessions, Prue moves into asserting her need to be respected and accepted as "different" from Larry, but as a good and valued partner.

This husband and wife, who always had much genuine caring and respect for each other, have thus swiftly contained their pattern of negative interactions and, when directed by the therapist, have begun to tune into the channel of their attachment emotions and needs and to reach for each other. Both are then able to help each other stay calm, find their emotional balance, express attachment needs, and move into a place of mutual care and reassurance. In Session 9, the final session, Larry is able to articulate a view of himself as a lonely man who can now accept that he depends on his wife and needs to be able to turn to her, especially as he grows older and confronts his own vulnerability. The therapist helps him frame this ability to turn to his partner as strength.

At the end of therapy, both partners have expanded their model of self and other. Both are more trusting and able to deal with their emotions in a way that fosters open engagement and allows for empathic responsiveness to each other. Both now frame themselves as more confident and competent, and as able to offer more sensitive caregiving. Larry reports being less driven to exercise compulsively and less anxious in the relationship. Prue emerges from her clinical depression and becomes more assertive about her own needs with Larry and with others. In the final session, the partners also report that their new ways to communicate with each other seem to have improved their sexual relationship. In summary, the deepening of key attachment-oriented experiences in this case has resulted in new perspectives and new ways to send signals to each other that have pulled these partners closer and shaped a new dance of mutual accessibility and responsiveness—the elements of a secure bond.

Conclusion

Attachment theory and science are changing the way we view and treat adult love relationships. Attachment offers a systematic protocol for relationship repair that has already proven effective on many different levels and is more and more broadly adopted by couple therapists across the globe. It also expands the scope of couple therapy as a modality. If couple therapy can help partners not only repair their relationships, but shift from basically insecure working models and affect regulation strategies to secure connection, this therapy modality can begin a cascade of change and individual growth, evoking all the positive effects associated with more secure loving bonds. This not only offers a new direction for couple therapists and their clients; it also validates attachment theorists and researchers in their formulations of exactly how the most precious connections people have with others work, and how they may be honored and fostered in the future.

References

Acevedo, B., & Aron, A. (2009). Does a long-term relationship kill romantic love? *Review of General Psychology, 13,* 59–65.

Baldwin, M. W., Keelan, J. P. R., Fehr, B., Enns, V., & Koh-Rangarajoo, E. (1996). Social-cognitive conceptualization of attachment working models: Availability and accessibility effects. *Journal of Personality and Social Psychology, 71,* 94–109.

Basson, R. (2007). Sexual desire arousal disorders in women. In S. Leiblum (Ed.), *Principles and practice of sex therapy* (4th ed., pp. 25–53). New York: Guilford Press.

Benjamin, L. S. (1981). *Manual for coding social interaction in terms of Structural Analysis of Social Behavior (SASB).* Madison: University of Wisconsin Press.

Birnbaum, G. E. (2007). Attachment orientations, sexual functioning, and relationship satisfaction in a community sample of women. *Journal of Social and Personal Relationships, 24,* 21–35.

Birnbaum, G. E. (2010). Bound to interact: The divergent goals and complex interplay of attachment and sex within romantic relationships. *Journal of Social and Personal Relationships, 27,* 245–252.

Birnbaum, G. E., Reis, H. T., Mikulincer, M., Gillath, O., & Orpaz, A. (2006). When sex is more than just sex: Attachment orientations, sexual experience, and relationship quality. *Journal of Personality and Social Psychology, 91,* 929–943.

Bouaziz, A.-R., Lafontaine, M.-F., Gabbay, N., & Caron, A. (2013). Investigating the validity and reliability of the caregiving questionnaire with individuals in same-sex couple relationships. *Journal of Relationships Research, 4,* e2.

Bowlby, J. (1969/1982). *Attachment and loss: Vol. 1. Attachment.* New York. Basic Books.

Bowlby, J. (1973). *Attachment and loss: Vol. 2. Separation: Anxiety and anger.* New York: Basic Books.

Bowlby, J. (1988). *A secure base.* New York: Basic Books.

Brassard, A., Dupuy, E., Bergeron, S., & Shaver, P. R. (2014). Attachment insecurities and women's sexual function and satisfaction: The mediating roles of sexual self-esteem, sexual anxiety, and sexual assertiveness. *Journal of Sex Research,* 1–10. Epub ahead of print.

Brassard, A., Péloquin, K., Dupuy, E., Wright, J., & Shaver, P. R. (2012). Romantic attachment insecurity predicts sexual dissatisfaction in couples seeking marital therapy. *Journal of Sex and Marital Therapy, 38,* 245–262.

Brassard, A., Shaver, P. R., & Lussier, Y. (2007). Attachment, sexual experience, and sexual pressure in romantic relationships: A dyadic approach. *Personal Relationships, 14,* 475–493.

Brennan, K. A., Clark, C. L., & Shaver, P. R. (1998). Self-report measurement of adult romantic attachment: An integrative overview. In J. A. Simpson & W. S. Rholes (Eds.), *Attachment theory and close relationships* (pp. 46–76). New York: Guilford Press.

Burgess Moser, M., Johnson, S. M., Dalgleish, T. L., Tasca, G. A., Lafontaine, M. F., & Wiebe, S. A. (in press). Changes in relationship-specific romantic attachment in emotionally focused couple therapy. *Journal of Family Psychology.*

Burgess Moser, M., Johnson, S. M., Dalgleish, T. L., Tasca, G. A., & Wiebe, S. A. (2014). *The impact of blamer-softening on romantic attachment in emotionally focused couples therapy.* Manuscript in preparation.

Caron, A., Lafontaine, M.-F., Bureau, J. F., Levesque, C., & Johnson, S. M. (2012). Comparisons of attachment in close relationships: An evaluation of attachment to parents, peers, and romantic partners in young adults. *Canadian Journal of Behavioural Science, 44,* 245–256.

Cassidy, J., & Shaver, P. R. (Eds.). (2008). *Handbook of attachment: Theory, research, and clinical applications* (2nd ed.). New York: Guilford Press.

Cobb, R., & Bradbury, T. (2003). Implications of adult attachment for preventing adverse marital outcomes. In S. M. Johnson & V. Whiffen (Eds.), *Attachment processes in couple and family therapy* (pp. 258–280). New York: Guilford Press.

Collins, N. L., Guichard, A. C., Ford, M. B., & Feeney, B. C. (2006). Responding to need in intimate relationships: Normative processes and individual differences. In M. Mikulincer & G. S. Goodman (Eds.), *Dynamics of romantic love: Attachment, caregiving, and sex* (pp. 149–189). New York: Guilford Press.

Collins, N. L., & Read, S. J. (1990). Adult attachment models and relationship quality in dating couples. *Journal of Personality and Social Psychology, 58,* 644–663.

Crowell, J. A., Treboux, D., Gao, Y., Fyffe, C., Pan, H., & Waters, E. (2002). Assessing secure base behavior in adulthood: Development of a measure, links to adult attachment representations, and relations to couples' communication and reports of relationships. *Developmental Psychology, 38,* 679–693.

Crowell, J. A., Treboux, D., & Waters, E. (2002). Stability of attachment representations: The transition to marriage. *Developmental Psychology, 38,* 467–479.

Dalgleish, T. L., Johnson, S. M., Burgess Moser, M., Wiebe, S. A., & Tasca, G. A. (2014). Predicting key change events in emotionally focused couple therapy. *Journal of Marital and Family Therapy.* Advance online publication.

Dalton, J., Greenman, P., Classen, C., & Johnson, S. M. (2013). Nurturing connections in the aftermath of childhood trauma: A randomized control trial of emotionally focused couple therapy (EFT) for female survivors of childhood abuse. *Couple and Family Psychology: Research and Practice, 2*(3), 209–221.

Daniels, S. I. F. (2006). Adult attachment patterns and individual psychotherapy: A review. *Clinical Psychology Review, 26,* 968–984.

Davila, J., & Cobb, R. (2003). Predicting change in self-reported and interviewer-assessed attachment security: Tests of the individual and life-stress model. *Personality and Social Psychology Bulletin, 29,* 859–870.

Davila, J., & Cobb, R. (2004). Predictors of change in attachment security during adulthood. In W. S. Rholes & J. A. Simpson (Eds.), *Adult attachment: Theory, research, and clinical implications* (pp. 133–156). New York: Guilford Press.

Davila, J., Karney, B. R., & Bradbury, T. N. (1999). Attachment change processes in the early years of marriage. *Journal of Personality and Social Psychology, 76,* 783–802.

Davila, J., & Kashy, D. A. (2009). Secure base processes in couples: Daily associations between support experiences and attachment security. *Journal of Family Psychology, 23,* 76–88.

Davis, D., Shaver, P. R., & Vernon, M. L. (2004). Attachment style and subjective motivations for sex. *Personality and Social Psychology Bulletin, 30,* 1076–1090.

Denton, W., Wittenborn, A., & Golden, R. (2012). Augmenting antidepressant medication treatment of depressed women with emotionally focused therapy for couples: A randomized pilot study. *Journal of Marital and Family Therapy, 38,* 23–38.

Dewitte, M. (2012). Different perspectives on the sex–attachment link: Towards an emotion-motivational account. *Journal of Sex Research, 49,* 105–124.

Diamond, D., Stovall-McClough, C., Clarkin, J. F., & Levy, K. (2003). Patient–therapist attachment in the treatment of borderline personality disorder. *Bulletin of the Menninger Clinic, 67,* 227–260.

Eisenberger, N., Lieberman, M., Matthew, D., & Williams K. (2003). Does rejection hurt?: An fMRI study of social exclusion. *Science, 302*, 290–293.

Ekman. P. (2003). *Emotions revealed.* New York: Holt.

Feeney, B. C., & Collins, N. L. (2001). Predictors of caregiving in adult intimate relationships: An attachment theoretical perspective. *Journal of Personality and Social Psychology, 80*, 972–994.

Feeney, J. A. (1996). Attachment, caregiving, and marital satisfaction. *Personal Relationships, 3*, 401–416.

Fonagy, P., Steele, M., Steele, H., Leigh, T., Kennedy, R., Matton, G., et al. (1995). Attachment, the reflective self and borderline states: The predictive specificity of the Adult Attachment Interview and pathological emotional development. In S. Goldberg, R. Muir, & J. Kerr (Eds.), *Attachment theory: Social, developmental and clinical perspectives* (pp. 233–279). Hillsdale, NJ: Analytic Press.

Fosha, D. (2000). *The transforming power of affect: A model for accelerated change.* New York: Basic Books.

Fraley, R. C. (2002). Attachment stability from infancy to adulthood: Meta-analysis and dynamic modeling of developmental mechanisms. *Personality and Social Psychology Review, 6*, 123–151.

Fraley, R. C., Vicary, A. M., Brumbaugh, C. C., & Roisman, G. I. (2011). Patterns of stability in adult attachment: An empirical test of two models of continuity and change. *Journal of Personality and Social Psychology, 101*, 974–992.

Gottman, J., Coan, J., Carriere, S., & Swanson, C. (1998). Predicting marital happiness and stability from newlywed interactions. *Journal of Marriage and the Family, 60*, 5–22.

Greenman, P., & Johnson, S. M. (2013). Process research on emotionally focused therapy: Linking theory to practice. *Family Process, 52*, 46–61.

Gross, P. (2001). Emotional regulation in adulthood: Timing is everything. *Current Directions in Psychological Science, 10*, 214–219.

Hawkley, L., Masi, C., Berry, J., & Cacioppo, J. (2006). Loneliness is a unique predictor of age-related differences in systolic blood pressure. *Journal of Psychology and Aging, 21*, 152–164.

Heiman, J. (2007). Orgasmic disorders in women. In S. Leiblum (Ed.), *Principles and practice of sex therapy* (4th ed., pp. 84–123). New York: Guilford Press.

Horowitz, L. M., Rosenberg, S. E., & Bartholomew, K. (1993). Interpersonal problems, attachment styles, and outcome in brief dynamic psychotherapy. *Journal of Consulting and Clinical Psychology, 61*, 549–560.

Johnson, S. M. (2004). *The practice of emotionally focused couple therapy: Creating connection.* New York: Routledge.

Johnson, S. M. (2008a). *Hold me tight: Seven conversations for a lifetime of love.* New York. Little, Brown.

Johnson, S. M. (2008b). Couple and family therapy: An attachment perspective. In J. Cassidy & P. R. Shaver (Eds.), *Handbook of attachment: Theory, research and clinical applications* (2nd ed., pp. 811–829). New York: Guilford Press.

Johnson, S. M. (2009a). Extravagant emotion: Understanding and transforming love relationships in emotionally focused therapy. In D. Fosha, D. Siegel, & M. Solomon (Eds.), *The healing power of emotion: Affective neuroscience, development and clinical practice* (pp. 257–279). New York: Norton.

Johnson, S. M. (2009b). Attachment and emotionally focused therapy: Perfect partners. In J. Obegi & E. Berant (Eds.), *Attachment theory and research in clinical work with adults* (pp. 410–433). New York: Guilford Press.

Johnson, S. M. (2010). *Hold me tight: Conversations for connection—Facilitators guide for small groups* (2nd ed.). Ottawa, Ontario, Canada: International Centre for Excellence in Emotionally Focused Therapy.

Johnson, S. M. (2011). The attachment perspective on the bonds of love: A prototype for relationship change. In J. Furrow, S. M. Johnson, & B. Bradley (Eds.), *The emotionally focused casebook: New directions in treating couples* (pp. 31–58). New York: Routledge.

Johnson, S. M. (2013). *Love sense: The new revolutionary science of romantic relationships*. New York: Little, Brown.

Johnson, S. M., & Best, M. (2002). A systemic approach to restructuring adult attachment: The EFT model of couples therapy. In P. Erdman & T. Caffery (Eds.), *Attachment and family systems: Conceptual, empirical and therapeutic relatedness* (pp. 165–192). New York: Springer.

Johnson, S. M., Coan, J., Burgess Moser, M., Beckes, L., Smith, A., Dalgleish, T., et al. (2013). Soothing the threatened brain: Leveraging contact comfort with emotionally focused therapy. *PLoS ONE, 8*(11), e79314.

Johnson, S. M., & Greenberg, L. S. (1988). Relating process to outcome in marital therapy. *Journal of Marital and Family Therapy, 14*, 175–183.

Johnson, S. M., & Talitman, E. (1997). Predictors of success in emotionally focused marital therapy. *Journal of Marital and Family Therapy, 23*, 135–152.

Johnson, S. M., & Zuccarini, D. (2010). Integrating sex and attachment in emotionally focused couple therapy. *Journal of Marital and Family Therapy, 36*, 431–445.

Kirkpatrick, L. A., & Hazan, C. (1994). Attachment styles and close relationships: A four-year prospective study. *Personal Relationships, 1*, 123–142.

Kleinplatz, P. J. (2001). *New directions in sex therapy: Innovations and alternatives*. Philadelphia: Brunner-Routledge.

Lebow, J., Chambers, A. L., Christensen, A., & Johnson, S. M. (2012). Research on the treatment of marital couple distress. *Journal of Marital and Family Therapy, 38*, 145–168.

MacIntosh, H., & Johnson, S. M. (2008). Emotionally focused therapy for couples and childhood abuse survivors. *Journal of Marital and Family Therapy, 34*, 298–315.

Mackay, S. (1996). A neglected dimension in family therapy with adolescents. *Journal of Marital and Family Therapy, 22*, 489–508.

Main, M. (1991). Metacognitive knowledge, metacognitive monitoring, and singular (coherent) vs. multiple (incoherent) model of attachment: Findings and directions for future research. In C. M. Parkes, J. Stevenson-Hinde, & P. Marris (Eds.), *Attachment across the life cycle* (pp. 127–159). London: Tavistock/Routledge.

Makinen, J., & Johnson, S. M. (2006). Resolving attachment injuries in couples using emotionally focused therapy: Steps towards forgiveness and reconciliation. *Journal of Consulting and Clinical Psychology, 74*, 1005–1064.

Meyer, B., Pilkonis, P. A., Proietti, J. M., Heape, C. L., & Egan, M. (2001). Attachment styles and personality disorders as predictors of symptom course. *Journal of Personality Disorders, 15*, 371–389.

Mikulincer, M. (2006). Attachment, caregiving, and sex within romantic relationships: A behavioral systems perspective. In M. Mikulincer & G. S. Goodman (Eds.), *Dynamics of romantic love: Attachment, caregiving, and sex* (pp. 23–44). New York: Guilford Press.

Mikulincer, M., Gillath, O., Halevy, V., Avihou, N., Avidan, S., & Eshkoli, N. (2001). Attachment theory and reactions to others' needs: Evidence that activation of the sense of attachment security promotes empathic responses. *Journal of Personality and Social Psychology, 81,* 1205–1224.

Mikulincer, M., & Shaver, P. R. (2005). Attachment security, compassion, and altruism. *Current Directions in Psychological Science, 14,* 34–38.

Mikulincer, M., & Shaver, P. R. (2007). *Attachment in adulthood: Structure, dynamics, and change.* New York: Guilford Press.

Mikulincer, M., Shaver, P. R., Gillath, O., & Nitzberg, R. A. (2005). Attachment, caregiving, and altruism: Boosting attachment security increases compassion and helping. *Journal of Personality and Social Psychology, 89,* 817–839.

Millings, A., & Walsh, J. (2009). A dyadic exploration of attachment and caregiving in long-term couples. *Personal Relationships, 16,* 437–453.

Neumann, E., & Tress, W. (2007). [Close relationships in childhood and adulthood from the viewpoint of Structural Analysis of Social Behavior (SASB) and attachment theory]. *Psychotherapie, Psychosomatik, Medizinische Psychologie, 57,* 145–153.

Panksepp, J. (2003). Feeling the pain of social loss. *Science, 302,* 237–239.

Péloquin, K., Brassard, A., Delisle, G., & Bédard, M.-M. (2013). Integrating the attachment, caregiving and sexual systems into the understanding of sexual satisfaction. *Canadian Journal of Behavioural Science, 45,* 185–195.

Péloquin, K., Brassard, A., Lafontaine, M.-F., & Shaver, P. R. (2014). Sexuality examined through the lens of attachment theory: Attachment, caregiving, and sexual satisfaction. *Journal of Sex Research, 51*(5), 561–576.

Rogers, C. (1961). *On becoming a person.* Boston: Houghton Mifflin.

Schachner, D. A., & Shaver, P. R. (2004). Attachment dimensions and sexual motives. *Personal Relationships, 11,* 179–195.

Schachner, D. A., Shaver, P. R., & Mikulincer, M. (2003). Adult attachment theory, psychodynamics, and couple relationships: An overview. In S. M. Johnson & V. E. Whiffen (Eds.), *Attachment processes in couple and family therapy* (pp. 18–42). New York: Guilford Press.

Sexton, T., Gordon, K. C., Gurman, A., Lebow, J., Holtzworth-Munroe, A., & Johnson, S. (2011). Guidelines for classifying evidence-based treatments in couple and family therapy. *Family Process, 50,* 377–392.

Shaver, P. R., Hazan, C., & Bradshaw, D. (1988). Love as attachment: The integration of three behavioral systems. In R. J. Sternberg & M. Barnes (Eds.), *The anatomy of love* (pp. 68–98). New Haven, CT: Yale University Press.

Shaver, P. R., & Mikulincer, M. (2006). A behavioral systems approach to romantic love relationships: Attachment, caregiving, and sex. In R. J. Sternberg & K. Weis (Eds.), *The new psychology of love* (2nd ed., pp. 35–64). New Haven, CT: Yale University Press.

Simpson, J. A., Rholes, W. S., Campbell, L., & Wilson, C. L. (2003). Changes in attachment orientations across the transition to parenthood. *Journal of Experimental Social Psychology, 39,* 317–331.

Singer, J. D., & Willett, J. B. (2003). *Applied longitudinal data analysis: Methods for studying change and event occurrence.* New York: Oxford University Press.

Spanier, G. B. (1976). Measuring relational adjustment: New scales for assessing the quality of marriage and similar dyads. *Journal of Marriage and the Family, 38,* 15–28.

Stefanou, C., & McCabe, M. P. (2012). Adult attachment and sexual functioning: A review of past research. *Journal of Sexual Medicine, 9,* 2499–2507.

Tasca, G. A., Balfour, L., Ritchie, K., & Bissada, H. (2007). Change in attachment anxiety is associated with improved depression among women with binge eating disorder. *Psychotherapy, 44,* 423–433.

Tracy, J. L., Shaver, P. R., Albino, A. W., & Cooper, M. L. (2003). Attachment styles and adolescent sexuality. In P. Florsheim (Ed.), *Adolescent romantic relations and sexual behavior: Theory, research, and practical implications* (pp. 137–159). Mahwah, NJ: Erlbaum.

Travis, L. A., Binder, J. L., Bliwise, N. G., & Horne-Moyer, H. L. (2001). Changes in clients' attachment orientations over the course of time-limited dynamic psychotherapy. *Psychotherapy, 38,* 149–159.

Wallin, D. J. (2007) *Attachment in psychotherapy.* New York: Guilford Press.

Wei, M., Russell, D. W., Mallinckrodt, B., & Vogel, D. L. (2007). The Experiences in Close Relationships Scale (ECR)—Short Form: Reliability, validity, and factor structure. *Journal of Personality Assessment, 88,* 187–204.

Zuccarini, D., Johnson, S. M., Dalgleish, T. L., & Makinen, J. A. (2013). Forgiveness and reconciliation in emotionally focused therapy for couples: The client change process and therapist interventions. *Journal of Marital and Family Therapy, 39,* 148–162.

Author Index

Subject Index

The letter *f* following a page number indicates figure; the letter *t* indicates table.